Setting up
Community Health Programmes

A Practical Manual for Use in

Developing Countries

THIRD EDITION,
FULLY REVISED 2007

Ted Lankester MA, MB, BChir, MRCGP
Director of Health Care, InterHealth, International Health Centre, London
Director Community Health Global Network
Formerly, Founder-Director, SHARE Community Health Programme, North India

With
a chapter on AIDS by

Ian D. Campbell
International Health Programme Consultant

and

Alison Rader Campbell
Community Development Consultant (HIV/AIDS and Health), Salvation Army
International Headquarters, London

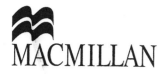

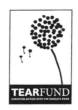

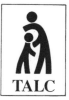

Macmillan Education
Between Towns Road, Oxford 0X4 3PP
A division of Macmillan Publishers Limited
Companies and representatives throughout the world

www.macmillan-africa.com

ISBN: 978-1-4050-8602-8

Text © T. E. Lankester 2000, 2007
Design and illustration © Macmillan Publishers
Limited and David Gifford 2000, 2007
Figure 20.5 © Marie-Thérèse Feuerstein 2000, 2007

First published 1992
Second edition published 2000
Reprinted with revisions 2002
This edition published 2007

Designed by Macmillan Education
Typeset by EXPO Holdings, Malaysia
Cover design by Charles Design Associates
Illustrated by David Gifford with additional
illustrations for the third edition by Tasha St John Reid
Cover photographs by Panos Pictures

Tearfund is an evangelical Christian relief and
development charity working through local partners to
bring help and hope to communities in need around
the world. It also publishes *Footsteps*, a regular
development newsletter, in English, French, Spanish
and Portuguese.

Further information is available from: Tearfund, 100
Church Road, Teddington, Middlesex, TW11 8QE, UK.

Community Health Global Network is an initiative of
InterHealth Worldwide. The mission of CHGN is to
maximise the impact of community based health care
worldwide through information sharing, training,
capacity building and advocacy.
Website: www.communityhealthglobal.net.

Printed and bound in Malaysia

2011 2010 2009 2008
10 9 8 7 6 5 4 3 2

DEDICATION

This book is dedicated to Community Health
Workers worldwide who work sacrificially in
service to their communities.

READERS, PLEASE HELP US

This book is designed to be a living resource in
a fast-changing field. Those of us involved in
community based health care are a community of those who learn from each other. We
are keen to hear from readers, whatever their
background or experience, with comments,
ideas, experiences and examples relevant to
any chapter of the book – or to any other
health topic with a community based focus.

The Community Health Global Network
website will act as an ongoing source for
sharing information. We would strongly
encourage individuals, and organisations, to
become CHGN members so that together we
can share information, ideas, guidelines and
good practice.

Website: www.communityhealthglobal.net
And please contact us at: team@chgn.org.

Contents

Acknowledgements

The writing and publication of this book has only been possible because of the support of many people.

I would first like to thank the members of SHARE, OPEN and TUSHAR projects for all that I learnt through them, along with the members of the Himalayan villages with whom they work in partnership. I am greatly indebted to Dr Alton Olson and Dr Pat Wakeham for their apprenticeship into community based health care.

Mr Lalchuangliana, formerly of the Emmanuel Hospital Association, has been a long-standing friend and steady inspiration as has Dr Kiran Martin of the ASHA programme.

I am indebted to Professor Andrew Tomkins for his encouragement to proceed with the book, and to Professor David Morley for his helpful comments and for writing the foreword to the first edition.

A number of people advised on the text of the first edition, including Dr Stephen Brown, Drs Richard and Judith Brown, Professor Duncan Vere, Dr Richard Franceys, Professor Malcolm Molyneux and Sir John Crofton.

I am grateful to Tearfund for its support in helping to bring the book to publication.

Dr Ian Campbell and Alison Rader Campbell deserve special thanks for sharing their radical approach to HIV/AIDS originally developed in their outstanding programme in Zambia.

A number of people have sent in helpful comments since the first edition was published: my thanks to all of them.

I would also like to thank most warmly both Shirley Hamber, my original editor at Macmillan, and Indira Benbow, formerly Director of TALC, for their affirming partnership in helping the first and second editions to see the light of day.

Chapters in this third and radically revised edition have been read through and commented on by a number of experts and colleagues, to all of whom I am extremely grateful. They include Professor Ann Ashworth of the London School of Hygiene and Tropical Medicine; Dr Nicholas Beeching, Consultant in Tropical and Infectious Diseases, Royal Liverpool University Hospital; Dr Colin Bullough, Senior Clinical Research Fellow, University of Aberdeen; Dr Isabel Carter, Editor of *Footsteps* magazine and Director of Resources at Tearfund; Dr Richard Franceys, Senior Lecturer in Water and Sanitation Management, Cranfield University; Dr Giuliano Gargioni of the TB Strategy and Operations Unit of Stop TB, World Health Organization; Dr John Guillebaud, Emeritus Professor of Family Planning and Reproductive Health, University College London; Dr Nick Henwood, public health specialist and co-director of Community Health Global Network; Dr Penelope Key OBE, formerly Chief Public Health Advisor to DFID; Revd Dr Pat Nickson OBE, founder of the Pan-African Institute of Community Health; Andrew Tomkins, Professor of International Child Health at the University of London; Dr Catriona Waddington of the HLSP Institute, London; David White, Management Consultant and Executive Director of InterHealth Worldwide and Dr Nick Wooding, recently director of Kiwoko Hospital in Uganda.

Finally a very big thank you to Liz Paren, my editor at Macmillan, and Lesley Butland, copy-editor.

Acknowledgements for illustrations

The author and publishers wish to acknowledge with thanks, the following sources:
Camera Press for Figure 2.13.
Richard Franceys/WEDC for Figures 16.10, 16.11 and 16.12 (from *Waterlines* 8(3): 18–19, 1990).
The Hesperian Foundation for Figures 1.7, 3.4, 3.5, 3.7, 3.8, 3.9, 5.3, 6.1, 7.5, 7.10, 7.18, 8.18, 9.15, 11.5, 11.8, 17.3 and 19.5 (from *Helping Health Workers Learn*).
John and Penny Hubley for Figures 7.4, 7.6, 7.12, 12.9, 13.11 and 20.10.

Oxford University Press for Figures 10.5 and 20.4 (from *Practising Health for All*) and for Figures 10.3, 10.6 and 14.11 (from *Immunization in Practice*).
PANOS Pictures for Figures 5.1 and 12.5.
PATH, Seattle, Washington, USA for Figure 16.7 (Path adaptation from *Peace Corps Times*).
TALC for Figures 8.7, 8.8, 9.6, 9.8, 9.9, 9.16, 9.18, 13.1, 13.2, 20.6, 20.8 and 20.9.
WHO for Figures 9.5, 9.10, 11.6, 11.12, 15.1, 15.6 and 20.12 (WHO photographs); Figures 16.2, 16.3 and 16.8 (from *The Community Health Worker*); and Figures 17.8, 19.1, 19.2, 19.7 and 19.9 (from *On Being in Charge*).
WHO Expanded Programme on Immunization for Figure 10.3.
Footsteps, Tearfund for 21.3.

Cover photographs courtesy of Panos Pictures

The publishers have made every effort to trace the copyright holders, but if they have inadvertently overlooked any, they will be pleased to make the necessary arrangements at the first opportunity.

Author to reader

This book is aimed at any group setting up or developing community health programmes. This includes government, Non-Governmental Organisations (NGOs), Faith-Based Organisations (FBOs), Community-Based Organsiations (CBOs) or Public-Private Partnerships (PPPs).

This is a radically revised third edition of a book I first wrote in 1992.

In the 1980s, I first became involved in working with colleagues to help start community based health programmes in remote areas where there was little effective health care. The first edition started as my scribbled field notes and gradually took shape as, together with colleagues and local community members, we developed the initial stages of a health programme. It finally saw the light of day as I was encouraged to broaden the scope of the book by including the accumulated experiences of many others.

It is now nearly 14 years since the first edition of this book was published. I am glad that despite its inadequacies the book has proved useful for many, seen several reprints and that a separate Indian edition and Hindi translation of the second edition have become available.

Many of us involved in global health feel exasperated that accessible health care is still beyond the reach of so many. But we are also encouraged that so many individuals, organisations and governments are determined to tackle poverty and ill health head-on.

It is also encouraging to see many worldwide initiatives taking shape that can make a real impact, the majority guided and empowered by the World Health Organization, UNICEF, and supported by generous funders. But as I study, lecture and travel, I see a gaping hole in global health – a giant jigsaw puzzle with the central pieces missing. This great omission is the community – the community as an empowered group of individuals able to help plan, manage and own health care in a way that works for its members – and which also connects into government programmes. This book is all about how communities, local health initiatives and appropriately trained health workers can help fill this hole, and become the missing pieces of the jigsaw; how community members must not be seen simply as beneficiaries to whom we deliver a product – health care – but how they can be intimately involved in the solutions, as they learn to use their skills, abilities and knowledge.

I have tried to combine guidelines, evidence, good practice and case histories so this book will be as useful as possible to as wide a range of people as possible. I have tried to incorporate the latest thinking on all the topics covered, ensure that guidelines follow those of WHO and other specialist agencies so that community health can be seen as something that works in harmony with programmes such as The Integrated Management of Childhood Illness, EPI, Stop TB and Roll Back Malaria.

Although aimed primarily at programme directors and field leaders in both NGOs and government programmes, this book is also designed to be of value on training courses, for managers and planners and for the increasing number of health care workers everywhere helping to achieve the Millennium Development Goals.

Those looking for omissions will certainly find some. The one that troubles me most is having no section on Community Mental Health Care. Some subjects have not been given the coverage they deserve, and some have been mentioned only in passing. Owing to its wide scope, certain sections may be less relevant to some than to others. And whereas some areas of the world have material and human resources to develop a stable primary health care system, others are disintegrating, as famine, civil strife, economic decline and HIV/AIDS frustrate attempts to provide even basic health care. For some such areas, even the simple procedures suggested in this book, may be beyond reach.

In the Bible we have an account of how Jesus used what was available – five loaves and two fish – to feed a crowd of 5000. My hope and prayer is this: that those of us who are committed to bringing accessible health care within reach of all will not be paralysed into inaction by the size of the task. Rather that we will realise that by working in partnership with local communities we can make an extremely significant difference. As the Chinese proverb states with brave simplicity: 'Many little things done in many little places by many little people will change the face of the world.'

Ted Lankester, 2006

Foreword to the First Edition

Over the last 50 years there has been a tremendous change in health care worldwide. On one side we see increasing sophistication with new technologies and new drugs being available. On the other side we see growing concern over the extent to which health services provide coverage to the communities they serve. In the countries of the South the very poor coverage provided by existing health services has led to much greater emphasis on community based health care. Here the communities are seen no longer as just consumers but as active partners in the planning, creation and supervision of health care.

Much of the early writing on this has been undertaken by those from outside the medical profession and among these David Werner has pride of place with his books *Where There Is No Doctor*, *Helping Health Workers Learn* and *Disabled Village Children*. The first of these has been translated into over 40 languages and more than a million copies have been distributed. This movement of health care away from dependence on doctors to a more family and community based health care is illustrated in one of David Werner's diagrams to which a further drawing has been added (Figure overleaf). In the last drawing emphasis is placed on the mother in the family who has always played such a major part in traditional as well as Western health care.

Although David Werner has played a leading role with his writings there are many others who, from a relatively lay background, have written on this subject. Dr Lankester, in this book, is one of the first doctors to write an extensive manual on community based health care. As you read this book you will see that much of it is quite unrelated to the traditional training of doctors. The author has shared his own experience and that of others for the benefit of all health workers who are concerned that the health care they provide should be community based and related to the desires and needs of the population they are serving. Such health care can only be successful when it is preceded by a dialogue between those being served and the health workers – a dialogue that has to be maintained as the health care programme develops. Dr Lankester gives ideas as to how such communication can be achieved.

The book is particularly aimed at non-governmental organisations as they are fortunate in having a greater ability to vary and develop services. Such non-governmental services are however having an increasing influence not only on how governments provide health care, but also in stimulating a more appropriate training of doctors and other health care workers. Perhaps those in developing countries who find the existing training they receive in medical schools irrelevant to the real needs of the country, will also find this a book they can usefully turn to for answers on how to create community based health care.

Thoughts on all forms of health care are in a stage of rapid change but few are developing so fast as in the area of community health. Moreover stages achieved by different communities, even within the same country will vary widely, meaning that no community health manual can ever be 'fully relevant to every stage of every project'. As you discuss and put into practice guidelines given in this book remember that the Author is eager to hear your own suggestions and ideas so that these in turn can be passed on to others.

Emeritus Professor David Morley
Institute of Child Health
London

Encourage independence

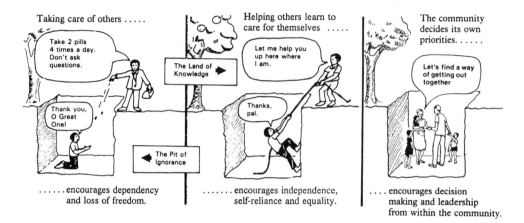

PART I
Basic Principles

1
Setting the Scene

This book is about Community Based Health Care (CBHC). It shows how CBHC, if well managed and based on good practice, can have a major impact on global health. This first chapter sets out to explain the unique features of CBHC, and how it links in with other health care models. It outlines the key role CBHC can play in helping to meet the health crisis now facing the world.

To help us understand what role CBHC can play, we need to be aware of the global and countrywide situations in which our programmes will be working.

This chapter tries to answer:

1. Where are we now?
2. Where have we come from?
3. What wider health challenges do we face?
4. How can CBHC help meet these challenges?
5. What are the special features of CBHC?
6. How does CBHC fit into other health care systems?
7. How can CBHC tackle poverty – the root cause of ill health?
8. What are the Millennium Development Goals?
9. Setting up new programmes or strengthening and scaling up existing ones?
10. Long-term commitment or quick wins?
11. What new challenges are now emerging?

Where are we now?

After a century of the most spectacular health advances in human history, some of the world's poorest countries face rising death rates, and falling life expectancy. Gains are being lost because of feeble health systems. On the front line we see over-worked and overstressed health workers too few in numbers, losing the fight, with many collapsing under the strain.
(*Lancet*, Vol. 364, 2004, p. 1984)

More than one billion people, one sixth of the world's population – live in extreme poverty, lacking the safe water, proper nutrition, basic health care and social services needed to survive. Almost 11 million children die each year, six million of them under 5, from preventable diseases, 500,000 women per year do not survive pregnancy or childbirth, and there are presently 40 million people living with HIV/AIDS.
(Press release, WHO, 2005)

This situation is completely unacceptable. We must be moved by the human suffering that underlies these figures and challenged to use our skills and knowledge to take effective action without delay.

This book attempts to show some ways of doing this, based on evidence, good practice and experience from around the world, and using the model of CBHC.

Where have we come from?

The answer is from a long way back in history. Health care based in communities dates back thousands of years. But in the second half of the

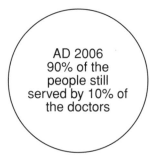

AD 2006
90% of the people still served by 10% of the doctors

Figure 1.1 Urgently needed: a new model of health care.

twentieth century many specific models of CBHC started to emerge, with India and China taking a lead.

However, we will take as our starting point 1978, famous in primary health care circles as the year of the Alma-Ata Declaration. Here, under the joint leadership of WHO and UNICEF, health planners from 134 member states of the United Nations met at Alma-Ata in the then Soviet Union (now Almaty, former capital of Kazakhstan). They drew up a charter with the aim of bringing basic health services within reach of every community and individual.

Target 5 of the declaration stated that a main social target should be:

> … the attainment by all the people of the world of a level of health that will permit them to lead a socially and economically productive life. Primary health care is the key to attaining this target. (See ref. 2, page 16.)

Out of this was coined the catchphrase 'Health for All by the Year 2000'.

Alma-Ata gave great encouragement to many health workers. A number of effective and far reaching programmes were started. Many of these continue today and have achieved spectacular results, a good example being the Comprehensive Rural Health Programme in Jamkhed, India.

However, as a worldwide movement, the 1978 Declaration did not bring about the largescale improvements that many people hoped for. Health for All (HFA) was based on developing strong community based partnerships but it lacked the aims, expertise and political will to be successful.

HFA followed what was known as a horizontal, comprehensive approach to health. In other words there was a strong emphasis on services at community level covering a very wide range of health-related topics. But because on its own this approach was not sufficient, many planners started to think of a different model. This caused them to concentrate on a single topic or illness, set up guidelines, train health workers from government down to community level and then deliver the intervention. This approach was, and still is, known as a vertical programme.

During the 1980s a famous example was UNICEF's Expanded Programme on Immunisation

(see Chapter 10), aiming to deliver immunisations against six key diseases to all the children of the world. It continues today.

During the 1990s many other vertical programmes were added, including Roll Back Malaria, The Safe Motherhood Initiative and what is now known as Stop TB.

Table 1.1 shows the pros and cons of these two approaches. In summary, vertical approaches work best for tackling single complex issues but they tend to undermine community action and initiative. They focus more on delivery than on empowerment. The result is that benefits last only as long as the programme is funded. However, some have also made spectacular gains – the virtual elimination of polio being an impressive example.

In the 1990s, WHO and UNICEF realised that the vertical and horizontal had to be combined to meet the health needs of children. This led on to a groundbreaking initiative known as The Integrated Management of Childhood Illness (IMCI). This programme starts vertically – in other words it is planned, managed and financed by donors, governments and health authorities. But at community level it becomes more comprehensive and horizontal as first-level workers are trained to provide a number of activities that increase child survival. IMCI is a model that, in its community based form (in distinction to its clinic-based form), combines many of the advantages of horizontal and vertical approaches.

The future direction of health care over the coming years is likely to combine the vertical and the horizontal. But we will need to make sure that community involvement remains central, and in particular that local people are involved in planning, management and monitoring.

What wider health challenges do we face?

Many of the big health challenges we face can be divided into specific topics such as childhood nutrition, HIV/AIDS and maternity care. These and other topics form the titles of many chapters in this book.

However, there are wider challenges that throw a shadow over all the topics that we try to address. It is helpful to understand what these are.

Table 1.1   Advantages and disadvantages of vertical and horizontal programmes

Vertical programmes	**Horizontal programmes**
Advantages Single topic or illness means programmes can more easily be expertly designed, managed, monitored and delivered Priority illnesses can be effectively targeted Effective in implementing programmes dependent on evidence based clinical guidelines, e.g. Stop TB Popular with donors	*Advantages* More opportunity for community partnership, design and management Based on empowerment and behavioural change alongside delivery If well managed more likely to be sustainable Less dependent on donors Emphasis given to strengthening health systems so that a wide range of problems can be addressed Easier to focus on prevention as well as cure Community and family members can be involved as formal or informal health workers Interventions often technically simple
Disadvantages Often undermine community involvement Often bypass traditional healers Can impose western models of health care Often driven by donors and planners rather than by local priorities May be inefficient at community level as health workers are trained exclusively in one programme Often unsustainable when funding stops, or another health priority is considered more important Many health workers working at community level leave to join better paid vertical programmes. The success of vertical programmes is in danger of being at the expense of horizontal approaches. (Put less politely, this means that the big vertical players sometimes steal staff, leaving basic health services almost destitute.)	*Disadvantages* Less focus. This is a problem where diseases are complex or a topic requires careful logistics and support Requires good quality local management and leadership Often require more time, training and patience to set up Funding is often harder to obtain

There are many, but from the CBHC viewpoint the most important include:

Lack of trained health workers

Experts estimate that there is a shortage of four million health workers worldwide, one million in sub-Saharan Africa alone.

There are many reasons for this shortage: countries do not have the resources either for training or for adequate payment. As a result, many health workers leave for better paid jobs as private practitioners, or join international organisations or vertical programmes that offer good salaries. Those more highly qualified, especially doctors and nurses, are recruited by developed countries who themselves need skilled workers. In many parts of Africa, large numbers of health workers die from HIV/AIDS or have to spend their time in caring for children or generating other sources of income.

That is the problem; here is part of a solution:

> Although hard evidence is difficult to obtain, many health workers estimate that about three out of four episodes of infectious illness in resource-poor communities can be prevented and treated by well trained community health workers supported by informed community members.

Poor planning and capacity at the national level

Planning health services is vastly complex and involves not only specific health related activities but also many other sectors such as agriculture, housing and the environment. Few countries have the capacity to draw up effective plans, let alone implement them successfully.

Weak or non-existent health systems

In most countries there may be agreed goals, and patchy implementation of vertical programmes. But in the neediest communities there are neither the systems nor the trained people for health care to happen at the local level. This paralysis at local level leads us back to the first point above, the desperate need for more health workers, especially at community level.

How can CBHC help meet these challenges?

Perhaps the answer has been emerging. CBHC is in a key position to make sure that health programmes actually work at local level, and that community members have access to effective care.

- CBHC goes a long way towards supplying the need for more health workers – most of whom will be community members who can be effectively and economically trained. *For example*: the Indian government announced a plan in 2005 to track and improve the health needs in rural communities. The national Rural Health Mission aims to raise a cadre of one quarter of a million women volunteers as accredited

social health activists over a three-year period.

- CBHC provides an answer to the setting up of health systems at local level so that IMCI, vertical programmes and other locally determined health needs can actually be tackled.

> One measure of the success of community based programmes is how effectively they can provide a local health system, into which vertical programmes can integrate and through which vertical programmes can function.

- CBHC involves communities in planning and management so that, even if programmes cease, donors withdraw their funds or corruption affects government planning, there will still be health systems in place at the community level.

> - CBHC will work most effectively if it is expertly set up and managed, and works in close cooperation with government health services, national plans and vertical programmes.

Beyond these obvious benefits, CBHC offers radical ways of meeting health needs, based on two powerful tools – *empowerment* and *transformation*. The meaning of these will emerge as we look at the distinctive features of a community based approach below.

What are the special features of CBHC?

A director in the World Health Organization recently wrote these words:

> Poverty is the reason why babies are not vaccinated, clean water and sanitation are not provided, curative treatment is not available and mothers die in childbirth.

CBHC tackles poverty head-on. Through empowerment it helps communities to overcome it. Through partnership it enables communities to share their skills and resources, to everyone's benefit.

CBHC emphasises – community

1. **CBHC encourages ownership by the community.**
   The community participates, the community becomes a partner, and the community eventually owns the programme.
   Conventional medical care is delivered by doctors and health workers *to* the people. CBHC is a genuine partnership of health workers and community members.

2. **CBHC responds to the needs of the people.**
   Conventional medical care starts with planners, projects and governments. CBHC starts with the people; it helps them identify their needs, and works with them in finding answers.

3. **CBHC leads to self-reliance.**
   Conventional medical care often introduces two unwanted side effects – a dependence on medicines and a dependence on doctors. CBHC aims to bring about healthy, self-reliant communities. People become armed with knowledge so they depend less on outsiders.

4. **CBHC helps to encourage community life.**
   CBHC encourages traditional practices unless they are actually harmful. New ideas are introduced with sensitivity. The aim of the health worker is always to build up confidence and dignity, never to cause offence or humiliation.

5. **CBHC moves outwards to where the people live.**
   Care, wherever possible, is based in the community, not the clinic or hospital. It is decided according to the needs of the community, rather than the convenience of the doctor or health worker.
   Sick people are treated in their homes or as near to their homes as possible.

6. **CBHC moves forwards to the next generation.**

   Children become a focal point of health activities. They are not simply targeted for improved health care but are involved in bringing it about.

   Healthy patterns of living absorbed by children today become the accepted practices of tomorrow.

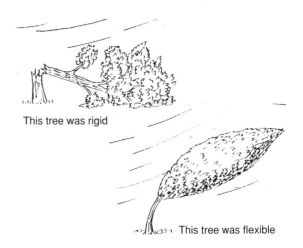

This tree was rigid

This tree was flexible

Figure 1.2   The flexibility of community based health programmes enables them to respond to changing needs and situations.

7. **CBHC helps to bring about behavioural change.**
   Through the excitement of discovering new ideas and different practices, real changes in lifestyle start to occur and health begins to improve.

8. **CBHC includes all community members.**
   The poorest, neediest and most at risk are given priority. Women are given equal status with men. The elderly and handicapped are cared for. Members of the least popular ethnic group, caste or religion are given full equality. The rich and powerful are included where possible, though never allowed to displace the poor or become too dominant.
   A person's need, rather than money or status, determines the type of health care received.

9. **CBHC depends on cooperation and integration.**
   Wherever possible, other doctors, practitioners and development workers are consulted and included. Other voluntary programmes are welcomed and ideas mutually shared.
   Without losing their unique strengths and values, CBHCs aim to integrate into the health services of the country.

10. **CBHC encourages a style of leadership that is committed to caring and sharing rather than being top-down and dominant.**

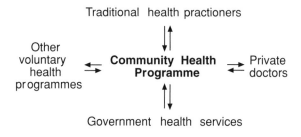

Figure 1.3 Community based health programmes work in partnership with others whenever possible.

11. **CBHC aims for a new community order.**
As the community takes initiatives, as health standards improve and as other forms of development emerge, a new order starts to take shape. This is based on:
- Justice, where the rich are no longer allowed to exploit the poor, nor the strong allowed to oppress the weak;
- Equity, where all have sufficient, and the differences between rich and poor are reduced; and
- Reconciliation, where individuals and community groups learn mutual respect. As communities work towards common goals conflict tends to lessen.

CBHC emphasises – health

1. **CBHC is involved more in health care than in medical care.**
CBHC opposes 'PPNN' – a Pill for every Problem, a Needle for every Need. Instead it emphasises that well-being is largely brought about through healthy living patterns and enlightened attitudes.

2. **CBHC emphasises appropriate cure.**
Most health workers use too many medicines and injections, many of them unnecessary and some of them harmful.
CBHC tries to ensure that a rational list of essential, life-saving drugs is always available, affordable and appropriately used.

3. **CBHC follows a comprehensive and integrated model of health care.**
It aims to include:

- Health education
- Mother and child health services

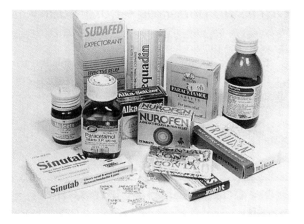

Figure 1.4 Most medicines are unnecessary, some are dangerous, a few are essential. CBHC promotes essential drugs and uses them effectively.

- Diagnostic and curative care
- Control of infectious diseases
- Adequate nutrition
- Immunisation
- Improvements in water supply and sanitation
- Referral systems
- Control of non-communicable illness
- The care of the disabled and the elderly
- Monitoring and evaluation
- Effective management.

CBHC links in to other forms of community development.

What CBHC is not

1. **CBHC is not opposed to doctors, hospitals and vertical programmes** – unless they disempower the community and impose inappropriate or short-lasting solutions.
CBHC releases hospital doctors and senior health professionals to fulfil their rightful function. By concentrating on effective primary care in the community, it releases doctors and other senior health workers to use their training more effectively, and enables hospitals to use their facilities more efficiently.

2. **CBHC is not simply adding new structures on to old foundations.**
CBHC is not an extension of a hospital into the four walls of a village clinic. It is a

complete restructuring of the health care system so that the people become partners with the providers.

3. **CBHC is not a second-rate health service for the poor** – as long as it is correctly set up and adequately supervised.

The charter of the People's Health Assembly expands and explains many of these principles (see Further reading and resources below).

How does CBHC fit into other health care systems?

It is helpful to look at this according to three stages:

Stage 1: The traditional health system

Health care takes place in the community, according to the wishes and convenience of people and patients.

Senior family members such as grandmothers are often the traditional source of wisdom. In serious situations other health workers are called in. These are usually community members using traditional skills or knowledge. Each community has its own traditional health practitioners. Examples include herbalists, shamans, priests, traditional midwives and ayurvedic practitioners.

Payment is made in cash or kind, usually, but not always, at a level the patient can afford.

This system has value when no better alternative exists, and when people's expectations are low. Many remedies bring comfort, and some are effective. Today many rural societies still function largely on this system. As health infrastructure collapses in some countries, many communities are turning back to this system.

Stage 2: The conventional 'western' medical system

Health care takes place in the hospital or clinic at the convenience of the doctor or private practitioner.

The health worker is an outsider with specialist and scientific knowledge, who tends to direct and dominate the treatment of the patient. Often he/she will demand high fees, which the poor cannot afford.

Although often effective, this approach may be frightening, inconvenient and expensive. The poor may never use it at all.

Stage 3: The integrated system

Health care returns to the community, with referral to clinic or hospital only when necessary.

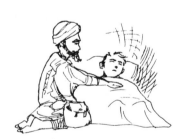 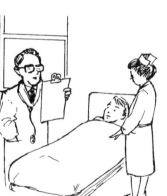 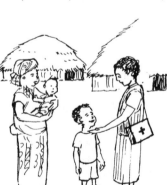

The traditional health system is	Convenient Affordable	The 'Western' medical system is	Inconvenient Expensive	Community based health care is	Convenient Affordable
but not very	Effective		Effective for the few who can afford it	and	Effective as part of an integrated health system

Figure 1.5   Three forms of health care.

The health worker, usually a Community Health Worker (CHW), is an insider who lives in the community, understands its traditions and provides effective health care at a fee that most can afford.

Stage 3 health care at its best combines the finest features of stages 1 and 2. Good quality care is available in the community, from a friendly provider at an affordable cost. A referral system ensures that those who need clinic or hospital care are able to receive it. Prevention of ill health becomes the dominant theme.

Although it may seem that Stage 3 is the most appropriate model for resource-poor communities, there are many who wish to anchor the process at Stage 2.

Whether Stage 3 health care actually becomes the new norm will depend on many factors, especially how sustainable and effective CBHC programmes prove to be. Each successful programme, however small, helps to tilt the balance in favour of Stage 3.

One vital way to strengthen CBHC is to form health care networks that will help us to share information, develop good practice, base our work on evidence, and share examples. Community Health Global Network is an example of this (see pages 406, 412 and ii).

CBHC comes about as all health workers realise that they have as much to learn from the community as they have to teach it.

Here is a comment from *The Lancet* medical journal about CBHC:

The focus of all strategies should be to ensure access by every family to a motivated, skilled and supported health worker system. The basis of this system consists of family members, relatives and friends, an invisible work force consisting mostly of women. They are backed by diverse informal and traditional healers and in many settings by formal community workers. Beyond these front line workers are doctors, nurses, midwives, professional associates, managers and non medical workers who support effective practice. All strategies should seek to promote community engagement.
('Human Resources for Health', *Lancet*, Vol. 364, 2004, page 1987)

How can CBHC tackle poverty – the root cause of ill health?

The problem (see Figure 1.6)

Health workers soon come to realise that the diseases they see are usually symptoms of a much greater 'illness' that affects their communities. Health planners call this The Social Determinants of Health and a great deal of research and action is focused on trying to understand these issues in more detail. *For example*: the reason why under-five mortality rates in children vary from 316 per 1000 live births in one country to 3 in another is in part a health care issue but largely depends on these 'social determinants'. Many are mentioned in Figure 1.6.

Most disease in developing countries is a direct result of poverty. Poor people have little money, little food, or little power; the rich consider them 'little people'. They become used and abused by those who own more land and more money. Such exploitation is always found in association with poverty and both causes it and results from it.

Poverty does not usually disappear when a country becomes prosperous. Most commonly the rich become richer still, and the poor stay the same or slide deeper into poverty and dependence.

As health workers we must be aware of the forces that act against the poor and lock them into lifestyles of poverty. We must come to see how other forms of development that reduce poverty and exploitation may be even more important than the health programmes we help to bring about.

We can look beyond the causes in Figure 1.6 and notice another thread weaving its way through all the problems listed – human corruptibility. This multiplies still further the problems facing the poor. Here are some examples:

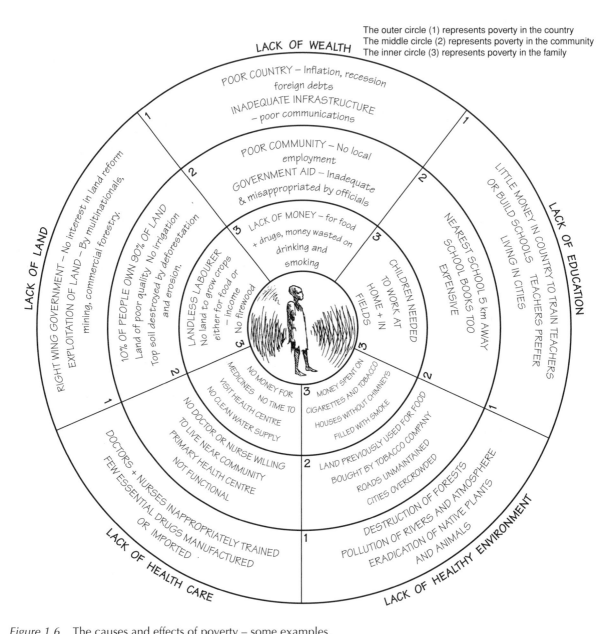

LACK OF WEALTH

The outer circle (1) represents poverty in the country
The middle circle (2) represents poverty in the community
The inner circle (3) represents poverty in the family

POOR COUNTRY – Inflation, recession foreign debts
INADEQUATE INFRASTRUCTURE – poor communications

POOR COMMUNITY – No local employment
GOVERNMENT AID – Inadequate & misappropriated by officials

LACK OF MONEY – for food + drugs, money wasted on drinking and smoking

LACK OF LAND

RIGHT WING GOVERNMENT – No interest in land reform
EXPLOITATION OF LAND – By multinationals, mining, commercial forestry.

10% OF PEOPLE OWN 90% OF LAND
Land of poor quality No irrigation
Top soil destroyed by deforestation and erosion.

LANDLESS LABOURER
No land to grow crops either for food or income – No firewood

LACK OF EDUCATION

LITTLE MONEY IN COUNTRY TO TRAIN TEACHERS
OR BUILD SCHOOLS   TEACHERS PREFER LIVING IN CITIES

NEAREST SCHOOL 5 km AWAY
SCHOOL BOOKS TOO EXPENSIVE

CHILDREN NEEDED TO WORK AT HOME + IN FIELDS

NO MONEY FOR MEDICINES   NO TIME TO VISIT HEALTH CENTRE
NO CLEAN WATER SUPPLY

NO DOCTOR OR NURSE WILLING TO LIVE NEAR COMMUNITY
PRIMARY HEALTH CENTRE NOT FUNCTIONAL

DOCTORS + NURSES INAPPROPRIATELY TRAINED
FEW ESSENTIAL DRUGS MANUFACTURED OR IMPORTED

LACK OF HEALTH CARE

MONEY SPENT ON CIGARETTES AND TOBACCO
HOUSES WITHOUT CHIMNEYS FILLED WITH SMOKE

LAND PREVIOUSLY USED FOR FOOD BOUGHT BY TOBACCO COMPANY
ROADS UNMAINTAINED   CITIES OVERCROWDED

DESTRUCTION OF FORESTS
POLLUTION OF RIVERS AND ATMOSPHERE
ERADICATION OF NATIVE PLANTS AND ANIMALS

LACK OF HEALTHY ENVIRONMENT

Figure 1.6   The causes and effects of poverty – some examples.

- **greed**, which brings about a wealthy minority at the expense of a poor majority;
- **dishonesty**, where broken promises and pledges are most keenly felt by the poor;
- **corruption**, where those unable to offer a bribe suffer the most; and
- **pride**, where the rich and clever tend to despise the weak and poor, so refusing to share their resources or help in time of need.

Our approach

In planning our attack on poverty and exploitation we must consciously resist becoming discouraged or intimidated. Anyone fighting poverty is liable to threats and opposition. We should simply see this as part of our job description.

Here are some approaches we can follow:
1. Understand the causes of poverty.

This will help us to be more compassionate towards the community and more realistic in our planning.

2. Realise that, although we can do little by ourselves, we can do a great deal as we work together with others, and form local, national and global networks.

3. See CBHC as a multiplication process, not an addition process.

   Stage 2 health care, where health workers merely treat patients, is an addition process. Someone has described it as trying to empty the ocean with a teaspoon.

   Stage 3 health care is a multiplication process. Health workers teach others, who teach others, who teach others. A stone is set in motion at the top of a hill, which moves faster and faster the further it travels.

4. Start with the skills that we do have.

   Each community is rich in ideas, skills and creative talent. These can be released as we empower and affirm community members.

5. Include community development in addition to health as soon as we are able.

   This may mean either expanding our own health programmes or linking the community with other agencies and experts. Agriculture, forestry, education, adult literacy, micro-enterprise, appropriate technology, improved housing, urban renewal and housing cooperatives will have a far greater effect on improving the health of our communities than health interventions alone.

6. Encourage people to claim their rights under the laws of the country.

   There may be many promises on paper designed to help the poor but little happening in practice. We can help community members to claim the services and supplies that are due to them.

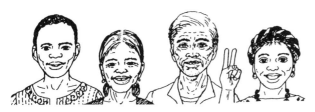

Figure 1.7

7. Alter traditional patterns of life as little as possible unless they are actually harmful.

   This becomes harder every year as 'globalisation' brings the promises of riches and glamour to those who will never afford them.

> Income generation schemes, sports clubs and other community initiatives can help to strengthen village communities and reduce migration to the cities.

8. Resist injustice, and show solidarity with the people where important principles are involved.

The Millennium Development Goals

Faced with so many health needs, we need a system to define clearly what these needs are and ways in which we can try to meet them.

The Millennium Development Goals (MDGs) are an example on a massive scale of what are known as SMART objectives (see Chapter 6): Specific, Measurable, Achievable, Results orientated and Time bound. We may not be able to achieve all these goals but, even if targets are missed, the MDGs focus our minds and help us to maximise our efforts.

The eight MDGs were formulated in United Nations conferences in the 1990s. In September 2000, 189 Heads of State adopted the UN Millennium Declaration translating this into a road map with goals to be reached by the year 2015. The Millennium Project is a three-year programme started in 2005 that established ten task forces to identify strategies likely to bring successful results.

There are eight goals, each covering one major area of development. Each goal has a number of specific targets that state clearly and concisely what we must aim for. In addition there are a number of indicators or measures (agreed by the United Nations system in 2001), which are a means of showing how successfully we are meeting those targets. (Ref. 1, page 16.)

Out of 8 goals, 3 (numbers 4, 5 and 6) relate *directly* to health, along with 8 out of 18 targets, and 18 out of 48 indicators. Table 1.2 lists the goals and targets as they relate to health, and these are taken up later in relevant chapters in this book.

Table 1.2   The 8 Millennium Development Goals with Targets and Indicators relating to Health*

	Health Targets	Health Indicators
	GOAL 1:	**ERADICATE EXTREME POVERTY AND HUNGER**	
	Target 1	Halve, between 1990 and 2015, the proportion of people whose income is less than one dollar a day.	

GOAL 1:	**ERADICATE EXTREME POVERTY AND HUNGER**	
Target 1	Halve, between 1990 and 2015, the proportion of people whose income is less than one dollar a day.	
Target 2	**Halve, between 1990 and 2015, the proportion of people who suffer from hunger**	4. **Prevalence of underweight children under five years of age** 5. **Proportion of population below minimum level of dietary energy consumption.**
GOAL 2:	**ACHIEVE UNIVERSAL PRIMARY EDUCATION**	
Target 3	Ensure that, by 2015, children everywhere, boys and girls alike, will be able to complete a full course of primary schooling.	
GOAL 3:	**PROMOTE GENDER EQUALITY AND EMPOWER WOMEN**	
Target 4	Eliminate gender disparity in primary and secondary education, preferably by 2005, and at all levels of education no later than 2015	
GOAL 4:	**REDUCE CHILD MORTALITY**	
Target 5	**Reduce by two-thirds, between 1990 and 2015, the under-five mortality rate**	13. **Under-five mortality rate** 14. **Infant mortality rate** 15. **Proportion of one-year-old children immunized against measles**
GOAL 5:	**IMPROVE MATERNAL HEALTH**	
Target 6	**Reduce by three-quarters, between 1990 and 2015, the maternal mortality ratio**	16. **Maternal mortality ratio** 17. **Proportion of births attended by skilled health personnel**
GOAL 6:	**COMBAT HIV/AIDS, MALARIA AND OTHER DISEASES**	
Target 7	**Have halted by 2015 and begun to reverse the spread of HIV/AIDS**	18. **HIV prevalence among pregnant women aged 15–24 years** 19. **Condom use rate of the contraceptive prevalence rate** 20. **Number of children orphaned by HIV/AIDS**
Target 8	**Have halted by 2015 and begun to reverse the incidence of malaria and other major diseases**	21. **Prevalence and death rates associated with malaria** 22. **Proportion of population in malaria-risk areas using effective malaria prevention and treatment measures** 23. **Prevalence and death rates associated with tuberculosis** 24. **Proportion of tuberculosis cases detected and cured under DOTS (Directly Observed Treatment Short-course)**
GOAL 7	**ENSURE ENVIRONMENTAL SUSTAINABILITY**	
Target 9	Integrate the principles of sustainable development into country policies and programmes and reverse the loss of environmental resources	29. **Proportion of population using solid fuels**

* Note 1. Targets related directly to health are in bold.

 Note 2. Only indicators for those targets are included and are numbered according to the official MDG system.

Target 10 Halve by 2015 the proportion of people without sustainable access to safe drinking-water and sanitation	30. Proportion of population with sustainable access to an improved water source, urban and rural
Target 11 By 2020 to have achieved a significant improvement in the lives of at least 100 million slum dwellers	31. Proportion of population with access to improved sanitation, urban and rural

GOAL 8:   DEVELOP A GLOBAL PARTNERSHIP FOR DEVELOPMENT

Target 12 Develop further an open, rule-based, predictable, non-discriminatory trading and financial system

Target 13 Address the special needs of the least developed countries

Target 14 Address the special needs of landlocked countries and small island developing states

Target 15 Deal comprehensively with the debt problems of developing countries through national and international measures in order to make debt sustainable in the long term

Target 16 In cooperation with developing countries, develop and implement strategies for decent and productive work for youth

Target 17 In cooperation with pharmaceutical companies, provide access to affordable essential drugs in developing countries	**46. Proportion of population with access to affordable essential drugs on a sustainable basis**

Target 18 In cooperation with the private sector, make available the benefits of new technologies, especially information and communications

Sources: 'Implementation of the United Nations Millennium Declaration', Report of the Secretary-General, A/57/270 (31 July 2002). First annual report based on the 'Road map towards the implementation of the United Nations Millennium Declaration', A/56/326 (6 September 2001). World Summit on Sustainable Development, plan of implementation, September 2002.

There are, however, some important aspects of health not covered in the MDGs that are essential in CBHC. Three of the most important are: the strengthening of health systems mentioned above, aspects of reproductive health, and the prevention and treatment of non-communicable diseases such as hypertension, diabetes and heart attacks. In addition, CBHC uses powerful social tools such as empowerment and transformation, which the MDGs do not specifically address.

Setting up new programmes or strengthening and scaling up existing ones?

These three activities are essential at both national and community levels. We will look at them from the specific viewpoint of CBHC:

Setting up refers to starting up new programmes where nothing effective exists. There are huge populations with no access to basic health care and in many areas there are no effective programmes working at community level. Examples include many urban slums, poor and remote communities (especially in mountainous and desert areas), or rural areas where infrastructure is poor. It includes poor and stigmatised communities, living amongst others who are relatively affluent. Equally important, it includes communities where conflict, disasters or the deadly progression of HIV/AIDS have undermined or overwhelmed health systems.

Strengthening refers to working with existing programmes, and building their capacity so that they have greater impact. This involves improving the knowledge and effectiveness of existing health workers, training new ones, improving systems, increasing quality, developing leadership skills, and enabling communities to use and trust their health services. It also involves bringing communities into planning and management so they start to see the programme as their own from an early stage.

Scaling up refers to making effective health programmes available on a wider scale to increasing numbers of people. Although governments will need to take a lead in this, we can make major contributions in CBHC. For example:

* Ideas can spread from one community to another nearby.
* Health planners and practitioners can visit and learn from existing programmes then start similar activities in their own areas.
* Governments can learn from effective CBHC approaches and implement them in other areas.

Scaling up needs to be higher on the priority list for community based programmes than it has been in the past.

Long-term commitment or quick wins?

CBHC is almost by definition a long-term commitment. However, as empowerment and behavioural change are tools we use, it does not mean that projects – or project leaders – need to 'last for ever'. Instead we should be looking at ways to enable communities set up, manage and sustain programmes with our help – considerable at the beginning, less as time goes on.

Within the context of CBHC there are some subjects that can bring about relatively quick and effective results. Apart from value in themselves, they can bring much needed encouragements both to project and community.

Figure 1.8 gives some examples.

What new challenges are now emerging?

Although there have been many advances in health care in the past 30 years, most of the poor have received little benefit. The WHO estimates that 1.2 billion people – one person in six – live in extreme poverty, and that half the world's population has no reliable access to health care.

In working with the poor we will need to develop creative solutions for some key challenges. Here are some examples:

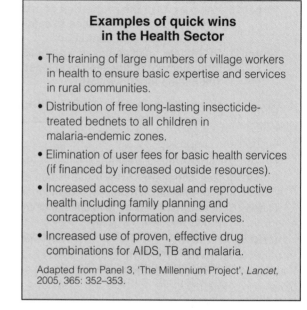

Examples of quick wins in the Health Sector

* The training of large numbers of village workers in health to ensure basic expertise and services in rural communities.
* Distribution of free long-lasting insecticide-treated bednets to all children in malaria-endemic zones.
* Elimination of user fees for basic health services (if financed by increased outside resources).
* Increased access to sexual and reproductive health including family planning and contraception information and services.
* Increased use of proven, effective drug combinations for AIDS, TB and malaria.

Adapted from Panel 3, 'The Millennium Project', *Lancet*, 2005, 365: 352–353.

Figure 1.8   Examples of quick wins in the health sector.

* **Emerging and re-emerging diseases.** Malaria, TB, HIV infection, dengue fever, schistosomiasis and antibiotic resistance are all getting worse and in some areas are out of control. Most of these problems need a strong community based element to be solved.

Table 1.3   Leading causes of death in low- and middle-income countries in 2000, for the two age groups most affected by injury

Age 5–14 years	Age 15–29 years
Childhood cluster diseases (200 131)	HIV/AIDS (852 793)
Road traffic injuries (114 087)	Road traffic injuries (317 654)
Drowning (112 512)	Tuberculosis (237 757)
Lower respiratory infections (112 307)	Self inflicted injuries (196 246)
Diarrhoeal diseases (88 411)	Interpersonal violence (178 651)

(Source: *Bulletin of the World Health Organization*, April 2005, 83(4), p. 295)

- **Non-communicable diseases**, which now account for 60 per cent of deaths worldwide, including heart attacks, strokes, cancer – and ageing itself. Most care will need to remain in the community but where family structures are breaking down we need to explore new models of care.
- **Mental health.** This is probably the most neglected area of health care worldwide and one that encompasses more human suffering than almost any other. The field is wide open for new and effective community based approaches to prevent, manage and cure a majority of mental illness in the community setting.
- **Increase in the use of drugs, alcohol and tobacco: growth in prostitution and sexual abuse of women and children.** These problems are now affecting communities almost world-wide – both urban and rural. Local community based solutions offer the best chance of control and of creating healthier lifestyles
- **Adolescent health.** WHO estimates there are 1.2 billion adolescents worldwide facing threats such as HIV/AIDS, tobacco and alcohol use, depression, suicide and violence. Community based programmes that tackle these issues will become increasingly important.
- **Obesity, lack of exercise and unhealthy lifestyles.** These are becoming more prevalent in developing countries as well as developed nations. They especially occur in urban areas and in situations where the cheapest food available is often the least healthy, especially if there is also a lack of affordable or home grown fruit and vegetables.
- **Road and industrial injuries** where so-called accidents, most largely preventable, are now one of the commonest causes of death world-wide (see Table 1.3).
- **Increase in war, civil strife, international terrorism and fear.** This can threaten years of development activity, in part because resources are used to support the war against terror rather than the war against poverty, which in part causes it.

War and conflict also generate vast refugee problems. But refugees themselves can be empowered and trained, whether they stay in

---

People living in crisis conditions

About 20 million people across the globe live in crisis conditions due to war, conflict or natural disaster while about two billion people are at risk of crisis conditions and face some threat to their health. Crisis can be caused by:

- catastrophic events: natural disasters like floods, earthquakes, hurricanes and tsunamis that often affect several countries or regions, and man-made disasters, for example, toxic spills.
- complex and continuing emergencies: violent conflicts and wars that often trigger displacement of communities.
- gradual breakdown of a country's social institutions due to economic decline; for example, the impact of high levels of a fatal disease, such as HIV/AIDS in sub-Saharan Africa; or widespread arsenic poisoning in the Ganges delta.

Source: WHO Bulletin, Feb. 2005, p. 89.

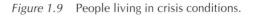

Figure 1.9 People living in crisis conditions.

semi-permanent camps or resettle elsewhere. Modified forms of CBHC are highly effective in refugee situations, and can help bridge the gap between disaster relief and long-term development.

- **Capacity to cope with disasters (see Figure 1.9).** Because natural disasters and human-generated conflicts affect an increasing number of communities, we need to build the capacity of all communities to cope with disasters and the effects of conflict. Such disaster preparedness will empower communities to cope with an increasing number of problems themselves and make them less dependent on outside aid and relief operations. This in turn will increase their dignity, respect and self-confidence.
- **International debt**, stripping the poorest countries of basic health services, and economic collapse, creating the 'new poor'. Here again low-cost CBHC, with an emphasis on prevention and treatment at an early stage, will reduce the numbers of those becoming seriously ill and needing unaffordable medical care.

• **Climate change** leading to global warming, rising sea levels and unpredictable weather patterns affecting the health of billions often through less reliable rainfall or through more frequently occurring climatic disasters such as flooding. The poor suffer disproportionately.

For all these challenges, action will need to be taken by government at national and regional levels. But as problems expand so do the opportunities for the voluntary, non-governmental sector, now increasingly known as 'Civil Society'. Our toolkit will remain the same – listening to the communities we serve, empowering them to devise and carry out their own solutions, and helping them to build their capacity so they can respond with sustainable solutions into the future.

The following chapters outline the tools we need, and some approaches we can use to prevent and cure some of the most important health problems in the community.

Further reading and resources

1. The UN Millennium Development Goals. Full and up-to-date details on the MDGs, the Millennium Task Force and a range of reports are available on several websites including www.un.org/ millenniumgoals, www.millenniumproject.org, www.undp.org.
2. 'Primary Health Care: Report of the International Conference on Primary Health Care', Alma-Ata, WHO, 1978.
   The report on the famous Alma-Ata Conference, which has guided the principles and practice of CBHC ever since.
   Available from: WHO. See Appendix E.
3. *Health for All in the Twenty-first Century*, WHO, 1998.
   Available from: WHO. See Appendix E.
4. *Poverty and Health: Reaping a Richer Harvest,* M.-T. Feuerstein, Macmillan, 1997.
   An excellent overview on poverty-related issues from both a global and a grassroots perspective.
   Available from: TALC. See Appendix E.
5. *Whose Reality Counts? Putting the First Last*, R. Chambers, IT Publications, 1997.
   A radical look at ways in which the needs and priorities of the poor can be understood, with the mapping of a future agenda.

Available from: IT Publications. See Appendix E.
6. *Community-based Health Care*, J. Rohde and J. Wyon (eds), Harvard School of Public Health, 2002.
   A wide ranging book suitable especially for primary care and public health practitioners.
7. *Community Health* (2nd edn), C. H. Wood, H. de Glanville and J. P. Vaughan, AMREF, 1997.
   An update of a popular and practical book first written in 1981 and widely applicable throughout East Africa.
   Available from: AMREF. See Appendix E.
8. *Refugee Health: An approach to emergency situations*, Médecins Sans Frontières, Macmillan, 1997.
   A guide for relief workers managing health care in refugee camps.
   Available from: TALC. See Appendix E.
9. 'Diagnosing Challenges: Health and the New Millennium', *Panos Briefing* No. 36, September, 1999.
   An excellent overview of the health of the world, with valuable statistics.
   Available from: Panos London, 9 White Lion Street, London, N1 9PD, UK.
   Email: panoslondon@gn.apc.org.
10. *Questioning the Solution*, D. Werner and D. Sanders, Healthwrights, 1997.
    This book explores primary health care and child survival in underprivileged communities.
    Available from: TALC. See Appendix E.
11. *Better Health for Poor People: Strategies for Achieving International Development Targets*, DFID, 2000.
    Has details of the G8 development targets relating to Health for All.
    Available from: DFID, 94 Victoria Street, London SW1 5JL or www.dfid.gov.uk.
12. The People's Health Movement.
    A radical coalition working towards people-centred health and development.
    Contact People's Health Assembly, Gonoshasthaya Kendra, PO Mirzanagar, Savar, Dhaka 1344, Bangladesh.
    Email: gksavar@citechco.net. Website: www. phmovement.org.
13. The Alternative World Health Report Global Health Watch, July 2005. Available from www.ghwatch.org.

See also Further references and guidelines, page 412.

2

Working as Partners with the Community

The key to Community Based Health Care (CBHC) is working as partners with the community. This includes, but goes beyond, the idea of people's participation.

In this chapter we shall consider:

1. **What we need to know**
   - How to make first contacts with the community
   - Why partnership is important
   - The effects of partnership
   - Partnership as the basis of all programme stages
   - Factors that obstruct partnership
2. **What we need to do**
   - Step 1 Prepare our own approach towards partnership
   - Step 2 Learn the skill of facilitating
   - Step 3 Learn how to set up community meetings
   - Step 4 Explain the importance of partnership
   - Step 5 Choose a subject
   - Step 6 Carry out the process
   - Avoid the pitfalls
   - Understand some models:
     - Village health committees
     - Women's' clubs

What we need to know

How to make first contacts with the community

The subject of this chapter, almost more than any other in the book, cannot be broken down into a formula that is bound to work or a series of steps that have to be followed. Rather the ideas and examples given in this chapter should be seen as guidelines and examples to stimulate the building of friendships and alliances on which the present and future impact of our work will largely depend.

We cannot just walk into a community and start asking questions. We need time to build trust and friendships before rushing in with questions and programmes. Quite apart from friendship for its own sake, we can never act as agents of change unless the community learns to trust both us and our motives. Poor people, after years of being cheated, are wary of outsiders bearing clever-sounding promises.

If we are making our first visits to a community, the people will be asking themselves:

- **'Who are these people anyway?'**
  Are they locals we haven't met before, outsiders, foreigners, government workers, family planning officers, spies?
- **'Why have they come?'**
  Just to do the job they claim, make money out of us, report on us, or because they can't get a better job elsewhere?
- **'What can we get from them?'**
  Free handouts, money, a hospital, a resident doctor, tonics for our children, cigarettes, foreign goods, guns?
  It is only by mixing with the people that they will learn to trust us and we will learn to appreciate them.

> As health and development workers our chief task is to enable communities to set up, manage and own their own health programmes.

We will learn from the community some of the secrets of living, relating, celebrating or enduring hardship, which 'health providers' have often forgotten. As we do this our own lives will be enriched, and the people will realise that we come as partners and fellow

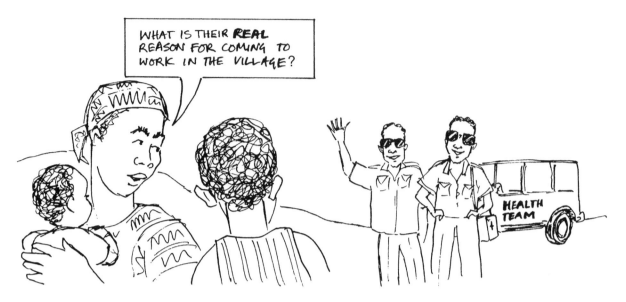

Figure 2.1

human beings, not just more outsiders with better ideas than others.

Twelve practical guidelines for when we enter a new community

1. Before going we find out first about any custom expected from us as a visitor.
2. On arrival we meet the leaders and explain who we are.
3. We are friendly and open, using the local greeting.
4. We dress appropriately and modestly wearing local-style clothes if possible.
5. We make the differences between ourselves and the people as small as possible, being careful not to show off expensive equipment.
6. We accept hospitality, eating and drinking with the people where possible.
7. We play and joke with the children, preferably within the family context.
8. We listen and learn, being slow to ask too many questions at the start.
9. We don't make plans or promises we may not be able to keep.
10. We praise and encourage good customs and practices, without being patronising.
11. We avoid argument or criticism both through our words and through our manner.
12. We don't take sides in any family or village dispute.

Why partnership is important

As we saw in Chapter 1, CBHC has come about because other models of health care have largely failed to bring basic health services to the poor. In developing countries medical care usually follows a top-down model, is mainly curative, often dominated by doctors and officials, and frequently subsidised by donations from governments and outside agencies. People come to expect things to be given to them and done for them. Although in the process they may gain a degree of improved health, they often lose something far more important – control over their own lives. An approach where people participate is the opposite of this.

> Our aim will be to promote health care with the people, not only provide medical care for the people. The community is the starting point, their leaders the chief partners.

Community involvement is the basis of almost every successful health programme. A recent worldwide study of programmes that really worked and really lasted showed that participation was the single most important reason for success.

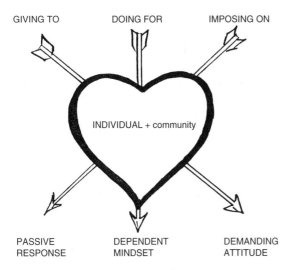

GIVING TO   DOING FOR   IMPOSING ON

INDIVIDUAL + community

PASSIVE   DEPENDENT   DEMANDING
RESPONSE   MINDSET   ATTITUDE

Figure 2.2   The effects of top-down development.

The effects of partnership

1. **Partnership helps make a project sustainable.**
   If people themselves learn to change unhelpful health patterns and adopt improved ones, then when the experts go and the funding stops their health will be permanently improved. As a famous book character once said: 'Why, Tom, us people must go on living, when all these people are gone.' (See Chapter 21.)
2. **Partnership helps to protect the people.**
   The poor are always exploited:
   • Doctors want them as patients – for a profit.
   • Drug companies sell them medicines – also for a profit.
   • The rich loan money – for high interest.
   • Politicians make false promises – for votes.
   Participation acts as armour against these forces.
   For example: In the treatment of diarrhoea in poor communities there is little value in only teaching mothers to buy packets of oral rehydration salts (ORS) from pharmacies. Supplies will often be exhausted or prices raised. Family members, in addition, should be taught how to make their own ORS from materials available in the home. In this way they will be self-sufficient and free from dependence on expensive, unreliable supplies. (See also Chapter 11.)
3. **Partnership gives dignity to the poor.**
   People soon realise that they no longer need others to do things for them or give things to them. They come to see they can bring about change and obtain things, for themselves.
   This new self-reliance gives a sense of value and worth to the poor. Instead of being passive receivers they become active participants.
   For example: In one project in western India it was found that newly selected Community Health Workers (CHWs) covered their faces, looked down to the ground and said: 'We are only useful for making bread and carrying water.' After a few months these same women, armed with practical health knowledge and new self-confidence, were teaching their communities, and caring for their health needs.

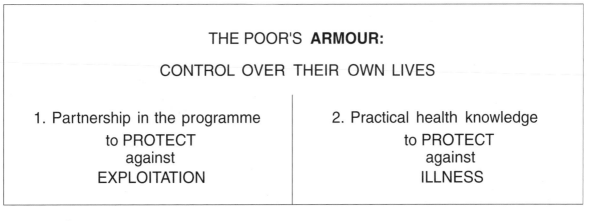

THE POOR'S **ARMOUR:**

CONrOL OVER THEIR OWN LIVES

| 1. Partnership in the programme to PROTECT against EXPLOITATION | 2. Practical health knowledge to PROTECT against ILLNESS |

Figure 2.3   The poor's armour.

4. **Local people become effective health workers.**

Members of a community already have a great store of wisdom and skills. With good training CHWs can often provide more appropriate primary care than health professionals: community members can understand local needs better than social workers.

An old Chinese proverb says: 'Outsiders can help, but insiders must do the job.'

5. **Partnership acts as a 'multiplier'.**

When local people become excited by what they have achieved, they will want to spread the news to others. They themselves will become agents of change, taking new health patterns and new ideas to other communities.

For example: a project in a large south Asian city recently bought a mobile clinic van to extend health care into city slums near to areas where they had previously been working. On the first day the mobile van went to the new area, community health volunteers from neighbouring areas had already arrived to encourage the local people to participate. As the clinic got under way, these volunteers took the lead in giving the health teaching.

Community partnership often seems a slow process at the start. Later this multiplier effect often causes a rapid increase in growth (see Figure 2.4).

6. **Equipment is better looked after.**

When people feel it is their clinic, their forestry plantation, their water pump, they will take pride in looking after it.

7. **Partnership helps to empower community members** and to build the capacity of local organisations.

8. **Partnership helps to give stability at the grass roots level.**

When civil war and instability cause changes in national and regional government, community programmes will often continue because of their strength and self-reliance.

Partnership as the basis of all programme stages

Partnership can be defined as:

a relationship based on mutual respect where responsibilities, benefits and costs are shared, leading to outcomes that benefit all partners.

All activities and all project stages involve the community – not just as beneficiaries but as partners (see Figure 2.5).

The community will form partnerships both with the facilitating agency – often a Non-Governmental Organisation – and with govern-

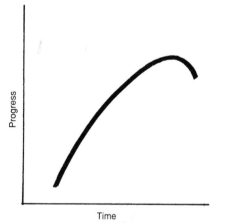

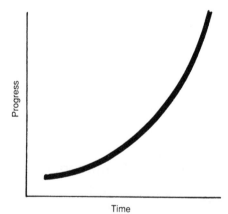

Project A: 'Community passive'. Project itself provides health care, gives to the poor, does things for people.
Result: apparent rapid progress at first – stagnation and decline later.

Project B: 'Community active'. Community participates at every stage. Project a facilitator, not a provider.
Result: slow progress at first – sustained and accelerating progress later.

Figure 2.4   Comparison between 'community passive' and 'community active' programmes.

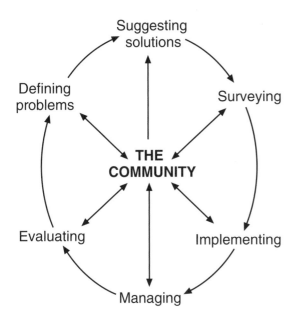

Figure 2.5   The community is central in all programme activities.

ment health services at local or district level. Other alliances may develop with groups such as private companies, civic societies, college departments and with agencies working in other forms of community development.

Factors that obstruct partnership

Helping a community to manage a health project is not easy. Being a 'facilitator' requires social skills every bit as challenging as a surgeon's technical skills. Some problems we are likely to face are:

1. **Blocks within the community.**
   Most communities will be used to the 'charity and donation' approach. They will expect us to do things for them and give things to them. If we don't, they may lose interest.
   This is especially the case where a project started with a welfare approach and moves towards an approach based on transformation and behavioural change.
   For example: an urban project in Nairobi had been providing services and handing out supplies to people in need for many years. It took this project several years to move from a donation approach to one in which local

people were trained how to be self-reliant and to do things for themselves. There was much opposition to this change until people saw the benefits in this new way of working together.

2. **Blocks from professionals.**
   Health professionals usually want to hold on to their knowledge, their skills and, above all, their power. They may dislike or even oppose any system in which patients and people start learning about health or running a programme.

3. **Blocks from government.**
   Although virtually all governments support the idea of primary health care in theory, many have other health priorities that in practice may hinder community involvement.

4. **Blocks within ourselves.**
   It is often much easier for project members to run programmes themselves rather than share management with the community.

> The biggest block to participation is not the unwillingness of the community. It is the possessive attitude of the health worker wanting to gain credit and keep control.

What we need to do

Step 1. Prepare our own approach towards partnership

We will never work in genuine partnership unless our own minds and attitudes are carefully prepared. We will need to be:

1. Really committed to the idea of participation.
2. Ready to share knowledge and skills at every opportunity.
3. Flexible, being prepared for mistakes, delays and experiments.
4. Ready to trust others.
5. Ready to give respect and credit to others. 'Our job is not to be heroes ourselves but to make heroes of other people.'
6. Prepared for a long-term commitment as facilitators.
7. Willing to give up control, and stop being the boss.

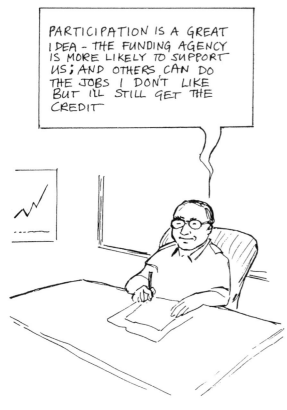

Figure 2.6

Step 2. Learn the skill of facilitating

1. **What is facilitation?** Most teaching follows the didactic model. One person teaches, the others listen, sometimes learn and often forget. Facilitation is a teaching process where everyone learns from each other under the skilled guidance of one person, the facilitator. It is based on respect for the gifts and knowledge of each group member. It is especially useful for those who have little formal education, status or confidence.

   Helping a group to identify problems and offer solutions is usually an important outcome.

   Learning to become a good facilitator is one of the most important skills we have to learn in CBHC. Some people do this naturally, most of us have to learn it.

2. **This is what a facilitator must be able to do:**
   * Enable each group member to feel welcomed, relaxed and able to share
   * Value each member's contribution
   * Help to steer the session in a useful direction
   * Remain friendly and patient at all times
   * Listen to others
   * Communicate clearly
   * Check everyone has understood what is being said
   * Summarise and draw together different ideas
   * Encourage humour and respect
   * Be well prepared but remain flexible
   * Keep to time but not be driven by it
   * Ensure the main findings and conclusions are recorded

   > A useful technique: the 'But Why' approach
   > 'The child has an infected foot.'
   > 'But why?'
   > 'She stepped on a thorn.'
   > 'But why?'
   > 'She has no shoes.'
   > 'But why?'
   > 'Her father is a landless worker and cannot afford them.'

3. **These are some important techniques a facilitator must learn:**
   * Helping everyone to agree to the ground rules at the beginning, for example: that everyone is free to share; each opinion is respected; minority views are not dismissed; no interruptions or harsh comments are allowed; no alcohol can be consumed.
   * Ensuring dominant people do not 'hijack' the conversation – instead facilitators can suggest specific tasks, such as making notes, or simple activities such as keeping the fire going on a cool evening.
   * Handling conflict and strong disagreement.
   * Coping with difficult questions.
   * Using 'energisers' – these are enjoyable activities that can be introduced at regular intervals to maintain interest and build relationships.

   Examples: (1) Playing 'mirrors': two people stand opposite each other – one does a certain action, the other mimics it: then they swap roles. (2) Singing: someone starts up a local song and everyone joins in. (3) Stretching, running and changing places: everyone gets up, stretches, runs or walks around the circle once or twice, then takes up a different position.

Skills checklist

Ask yourself these questions each time you lead a small group discussion. It will help you to assess the development of your skills in facilitation. Write down your answers and compare them over time.

- Did I use icebreakers or energisers to help people relax?
- Did I make sure everyone understood the questions and if necessary reword them?
- Was I comfortable with silence while people thought about the answers?
- How did I deal with someone who talked for a long time?
- Did I listen to everyone's responses?
- How did I encourage quiet people to join in the discussion?
- Did I make use of role play?
- How did I deal with someone who always answered the questions before anyone else had a chance to speak?
- How did I encourage useful points to be discussed further?
- How did I cope when I didn't understand the answers?
- How did I cope when I felt people's views were unhelpful?
- How did I handle differences of opinion?
- Did I bring the discussion to a satisfactory conclusion?
- How could I do this better?

Taken from *Footsteps*, No. 60, Tearfund, page 13.

Step 3. Learn how to set up community meetings

The elected or formal leaders should be present if possible. Informal leaders can also attend such as teachers, priests or others who have genuine influence or a sense of community welfare.

The real leaders may be different again. These are the community members who actually wield power. In practice these are often the rich, the 'bullies' or the upper class. We will need much

wisdom in knowing which if any of these should attend. Such people often try to dominate meetings, using them for their own personal ends or to strengthen their power base.

Usually it is better to let the community decide who should attend. We can try to encourage the whole community to come along, including women, and members of the poorest subgroup or caste. If this is not possible, each household can send a representative. In some societies women will need their own separate meeting.

Often meetings are quite easy to arrange but in remote or backward communities it may be hard to get people together. We must keep trying. There is no value in a health programme unless the community itself is involved and informed at every stage.

An example: Himalayan projects often have distant and scattered target villages. In one such project the health team was getting discouraged because, after many hours' driving, few villagers came to the meetings.

A solution was eventually found. A health film was shown at the beginning to draw people and create awareness; a humorous one was shown at the end to encourage them to stay. In the middle a useful dialogue was held with the whole village about the health problems they faced and how they might be solved.

In planning a meeting we need to make sure that:

1. The meeting is not too long. Farmers who have worked hard all day and drunk beer or homebrew with their supper will soon fall asleep. So will those living in urban slums, exhausted from trying to manage homes and earn income.
2. The meeting doesn't try to discuss too many things.
3. The meeting doesn't raise hopes that can't be met.
4. There is plenty of chance for people to talk.
5. Someone writes down what is decided. A member of both community and project can take notes.

Table 5.16 in Chapter 5 gives an example of how information can be presented to the community.

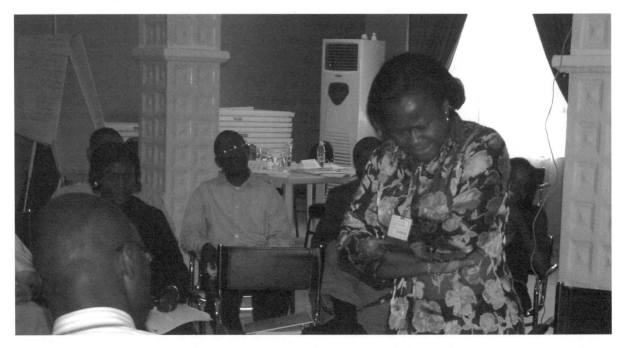

Figure 2.7   Collective decision-making and frequent use of energisers can help to make sessions interesting and enjoyable.

Step 4. Explain the importance of partnership

As we have mentioned, for many communities the idea of partnership still seems strange. Their past experience will often be with welfare-type projects that provided goods and services with little active participation from the community. There may also be mutual suspicion and even fear between project and community.

On the other hand, project members, unless well trained, may want to keep control and ensure successful results, often to satisfy their donors.

To overcome these suspicions we need to ensure that:

1. We prioritise plenty of contact time and dialogue between project and community.
2. We build trust through personal relationships and friendships.
3. When trust is growing, we work together on an activity, chosen by the community, which the project can help to facilitate.

Visiting a project in which participation is genuine can inspire others to aim for the same. Such a visit may act as an ideal stimulus for our own health team, CHWs or community leaders.

Step 5. Choose a subject

Partnership does not happen at once. Although our eventual aim is for people to manage the programme, this process has to come about in stages, and the technique of participation has to be taught.

The community should first learn how to take an active part in one main activity. As soon as possible this can be extended to others.

The community can suggest subjects – either through a discussion group, or in a meeting of leaders or community members (see pages 75–6). Suitable times may be after we have completed Participatory Appraisal (page 79) or planning with the results of a community survey (page 96).

The project will need to clarify that everyone understands and is prepared to work with locally

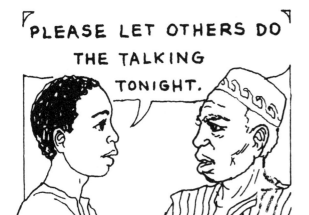

Figure 2.8

made decisions; also that the subject is workable and sustainable.

An appropriate subject for training communities in participation should be:

1. **A need strongly felt by the community.**
   There is no point in 'scratching where it's not itching', in choosing a subject in which the people have no interest.
2. **Within reach.**
   Any activity decided on must be easily within the abilities of the community. If it is too long or too difficult all will lose interest.
3. **Able to bring an early, obvious benefit.**
   For example: One project in central India was able to work with the community in sinking tubewells, so bringing drinking water and ridding the community of guinea worm. All were excited and wanted to work together on further activities.

> It is important to realise that many changes in community health are real but not obvious. The community may fail to notice any change unless they are helped to look back and see how much things have improved since they started.

Whatever activity is chosen, it must work and it must be enjoyable.

Some suggestions for 'starter subjects' include:

- Community survey (see pages 80–89).
- A community immunisation drive (see Chapter 10).

- Planning and building a community health post (see Chapter 8).
- Running a 'health fair' or baby show.
- Carrying out a CHW training programme (see Chapter 7).
- Improving a water supply (see Chapter 16).

Step 6. Carry out the process

1. **Generate enthusiasm.**
   Just as vehicles run on fuel, so projects run on enthusiasm.
   To increase enthusiasm:

   - do be friendly;
   - do create an atmosphere where people enjoy working together;
   - do give people the freedom to share their own ideas and do things their own way;
   - do give support when things are difficult;
   - do celebrate successes;
   - do give training and teaching so people feel they are making personal progress;
   - do be fair in making decisions and solving disputes;
   - don't blame people or become discouraged or angered.

2. **Involve others as early as possible.**

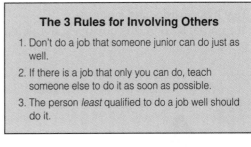

The 3 Rules for Involving Others

1. Don't do a job that someone junior can do just as well.
2. If there is a job that only you can do, teach someone else to do it as soon as possible.
3. The person *least* qualified to do a job well should do it.

Figure 2.9   The three rules for involving others.

In following these rules, we ensure that more and more of the skill pyramid is filled by community members (see Figure 2.11).

For example: In teaching CHWs:

- first, we teach CHWs;
- later, CHWs teach each other;
- eventually, senior CHWs start training new CHWs from new areas;

Enthusiasm ⟶ Unexpected ⟶ Learn from ⟶ Success ⟶ More
                    failure   mistakes   achieved   enthusiasm

Figure 2.10

For example: In running a clinic:

- from the very start, community members can learn to register patients and weigh babies, with project members acting as trainers;
- later, community members take over more skilled functions;
- eventually, the community takes over the management of the health post, but should share in this from the beginning so as to reduce dependence.

3. **Identify interest and abilities in community members.**
   Suggest names of people with special interest to the community and, if appropriate, train them and involve them.
4. **Lead from the middle, not from the front.**
5. **Keep outside money, resources and equipment to the minimum.**
6. **Be truthful and straightforward.**
   Never make promises that cannot be kept, or raise expectations that can't be met.
7. **Show respect to everyone**, even those it may seem difficult to trust.
8. **Teach generosity and kindness.**
9. **Stop an activity** if it is obviously not going to work.

Avoid the pitfalls

Common ones include:

Partnership in name, but not in practice

Participation may seem to be present but activities are only slanted towards the community, not based in the community. The community sees the branches, but the project keeps the roots.

Partnership is often surface rather than deep. Community members join in, but more as workers than as partners, more on the project's terms rather than on their own terms.

Partnership is often a pretence rather than genuine. This is usually in the hope that a good performance will be rewarded by a nice handout or new job opportunities.

Partnership fades away

We may originally aim for genuine community partnership. When the health committee chairperson runs off with the funds, we may quickly change our mind. We must keep encouraging participation even when problems arise and we are tempted to retake control.

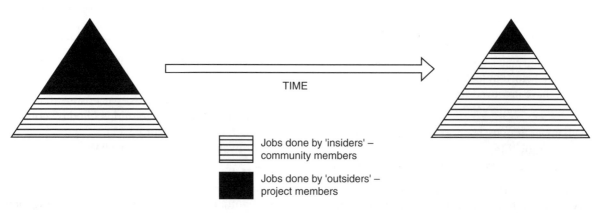

TIME

Jobs done by 'insiders' – community members

Jobs done by 'outsiders' – project members

Figure 2.11   Skills pyramids.

Partnership leads to division

Someone has written: 'Participation should release the energy to overcome the problems of poverty.' Although true, this process may start going in the wrong direction or get out of control.

- The poor may become so angered that they rise up against their exploiters.
- The rich may be so cunning that they use problems for their own gains.
- Issues raised may be so strong that they split and destroy communities.

> Participation is a powerful process. Carried forward correctly, it can help the poor, include the rich and benefit the community. Handled wrongly, it can leave a community wounded and unstable.

Understand some models

In order for partnership to succeed there need to be 'vehicles' to carry the process forwards.

There may already be community groups who meet from time to time. These might be formal groupings such as village elders, religious leaders, youth groups or social action committees. They may be informal gatherings such as women who meet regularly by the village well or borehole, and start sharing ideas about how to make their own lives easier.

If an appropriate group already exists, we may be able to build on this so that it forms the basis of a health or development committee. However, it must not represent vested interests, but genuinely speak for the whole community. Sometimes it will be easier to start from scratch.

The secrets of success for any community group include the following:

- Fair representation from within the community, not forgetting there is often a place for groups with special roles or functions, such as youth groups or women's groups;
- Regular training;
- Practical involvement of all members;
- Firm, but not dominating, leadership;
- Trustworthiness in handling money and resources;
- A task-orientated approach both in meetings and in carrying out what has been decided;

- Achievable aims and regular new challenges.

We will look in more detail at two common models for community action: Village Health Committees and Women's Clubs.

Village Health Committees (VHCs)

Although often known as Village Health Committees even in cities, these are equally relevant in both rural and urban areas. In fact, it is often better to call a VHC by a different name, such as Community Action Group. This helps the group to focus on goals rather than meetings or perks for members.

We will consider:

1. The functions of the VHC
2. How VHC members are chosen
3. The advantages and disadvantages of VHCs
4. The training of VHC members
5. How VHC members progress in their understanding
6. The need for new challenges

1. The functions of the VHC

There will be wide differences between projects. Usually a committee will start with one or two functions and learn to do these well. Later it can extend its activities. Here are some common examples of health committee functions:

CHW support

Members can encourage and support the CHW. They can help weigh children, keep records and accompany the CHW on night calls. They can stand with her in the face of any criticisms.

Health centre, post or dispensary: building and upkeep

The committee can help organise the construction of the health post. They can be responsible for its upkeep and repairs.

Health centre: clinic activities

Responsible VHC members can assist in the clinic. They can register patients, weigh children, help the health worker, and assist the dispenser. They can call patients and organise 'patient flow'.

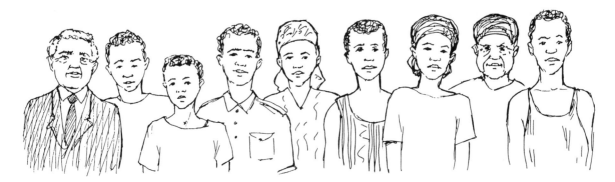

Figure 2.12   Village health committees must represent the whole community.

Within the community they can make sure that those needing to attend the clinic actually do so.

They can supervise TB 'DOTS' treatment in the community (see Chapter 14)

Where appropriate, members may supervise the regular taking of Antiretroviral Therapy (ART) for people living with HIV/AIDS (see Chapter 15).

They can accompany sick patients to hospital.

Immunisation campaigns

Committee members can arrange publicity and gather the children. They can assist the CHW and health team on community and national immunisation days by preparing the site and organising the campaign.

Community survey

Members can visit homes beforehand to explain why the survey is being done. They can work with project members in carrying out the survey. They can explain results to the community after the survey is finished. They can be involved in Participatory Appraisal (see Chapter 5).

Public health activities

Health committees can organise the digging of soakage pits, construction of latrines, and can take responsibility for community hygiene. They can help build and maintain water storage tanks, pumps and wells.

Contacts with government and outside agencies

They can claim grants and benefits on behalf of the people. They can make sure government plans and promises are actually carried out, and that the poor and underprivileged are treated fairly and receive any subsidies due. They can also participate in research with academic institutes to help prove the evidence-based value of community based activities.

For example: a rural health project in Makwanpur District, Nepal, worked alongside health researchers to see how the activities of VHCs and women's groups could reduce neonatal mortality rates through simple changes in practice. The research workers gained the information they needed over a five-year period and the communities learnt valuable skills to make their working practices even more effective. (See page 414, ref. Costello.)

Meetings

VHCs and projects should hold regular meetings for liaison, planning and training.

2. How VHC members are chosen

Who chooses them?

If possible, the whole community should be involved following the normal method of decision making used by the people. The process of selection is broadly similar to that used in choosing CHWs (see page 112).

The committee should not be chosen only by or from the rich, the powerful or those who speak the loudest.

What size should the committee be?

The committee should be large enough to represent the main social groups in the community and small enough to keep united and get things done.

Six to twelve members is ideal. Smaller 'social action groups' can be appointed in addition.

For example: at St John's Community Centre in Puwmani, Nairobi, specific groups have been formed for defined functions, each trained and encouraged by facilitators from the project. These groups include those responsible for collecting garbage, keeping the toilet complex clean, and washing cars. All these groups are youth led, and the community pays them small sums for their services.

In a Village Health Committee each main group in the community should be represented including women, the landless, the low-caste, and members of any minority tribe, subgroup or religion.

In very small communities each household can send one member.

> Every health committee, no matter how small, must include women, and at least one member of the poorest subgroup of the community.

What sized community should a committee represent?

This varies greatly. Usually each geographical community such as a village, a plantation or a city slum has its own committee.

This is not always possible. *For example (1)*: when villages are very small or scattered. In this case:

- either two or more villages can join together providing they are close enough for joint activities.
- or health committees can be set up for each health centre (often serving several villages), rather than for each village.

For example (2): in city slums or large towns. In such cases an appropriate area needs to be defined. This could be a street as in the People's Republic of China, or a cluster of dwellings. Some slums, especially illegal settlements, are often small enough for a single committee.

In mixed slum communities we must make sure that all communities and groups are represented.

Generally it is hard for a health committee to represent more than 1000 people and a much smaller number is preferable.

When should the committee be selected?

There are three possible times:

1. **At the start of the project.**
   Although this is a common practice, people are more likely at this stage to join for the wrong reasons.
2. **After a period of six months to a year.**
   By this time those with a genuine interest in health will be known both by the project and by the community.
3. **Before a special activity.**
   An example of this would be the building of a health post or the improving of a water supply. At such times members have a goal to aim for and are more likely to work effectively.

3. The advantages and disadvantages of VHCs

In some projects village health committees have proved successful, in others they have been disappointing.

Their advantages include:

1. They are a people's organisation. Their members are chosen by the community and live in the community.
2. They have authority to carry out health related activities.
3. They can liaise closely, or be integrated with, local or district health services. But they must still represent community interests.

VHCs can also have disadvantages:

1. Members join for the wrong reasons. They may be more interested in personal prestige than community welfare. They may join because of hoped-for perks and privileges, not because of any interest in health and development.
2. The committee may be slow and bureaucratic. Unless committees are small and their members enthusiastic 'a great deal of time can be spent doing a great deal of nothing'.
3. The committee may become politicised. Those with political ambitions, either local or national, may dominate the committee for their own personal campaign. Divisions in the community may be reflected in the committee. Meetings may turn into fights and power struggles. This is a particular risk in urban slums, or in the run-up to elections.

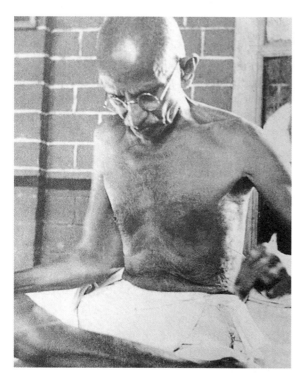

Figure 2.13   Mahatma Gandhi – a strong supporter of community involvement.

All these problems can be lessened by the careful choosing and training of VHC members.

In practice VHCs are often most successful when they take responsibility for community development as well as health. Health activities alone may not be sufficient to maintain their interest.

4. The training of VHC members

VHCs need thorough and regular training. This should include three components:

1. Ways of functioning together as a group, with an emphasis on team-building
2. Roles and responsibilities
3. Training for each specific task they undertake or supervise.

See also example on pages 317–320.

5. How VHC members progress in their understanding

An African health leader has described four stages through which VHCs usually pass:

Stage 1
Members are busy working out their own relationships and seeing which individual or which group will gain control.

Stage 2
Members test out the benefits to which they are entitled. Common ones include: lifts in project vehicles, free medicines, priority in clinics, and special access to the project doctor or director.

During this stage members may seem very interested in project activities, but only because of the privileges they are hoping to get.

Stage 3
Members start requesting special things for the community. Common examples are: a resident doctor, a well equipped hospital, a new vehicle or some special equipment. They may demand free food and handouts, supposedly for the poor.

If successful in these demands, members may hope to increase their own standing in the community.

If unsuccessful or if personal benefits fail to occur, members may lose interest.

Stage 4
Remaining members start working with the project and serving the community with genuine commitment.

Put another way, most teams go through these four stages: 'Forming, Storming, Norming, Performing'.

6. *The need for new challenges*
VHCs often lose interest and ultimately fail unless they regularly have new challenges and activities to maintain their interest.

Ideally suggestions should come from the group itself, so its members have ownership from the beginning. Once a new activity has been decided, we must ensure the VHC is given good quality training so it can carry out its new activity as effectively as possible

> Secrets of successful Village Health Committees are regular training and skills development, along with regular new activities to stimulate interest.

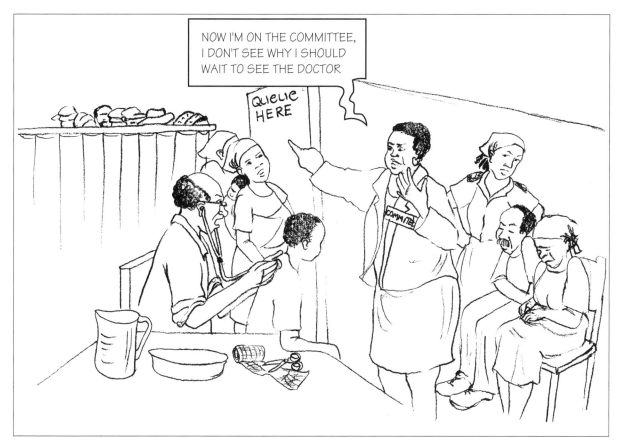

Figure 2.14

Women's clubs

We will consider:

1. The value of women's clubs
2. Club membership
3. How clubs are started
4. Activities that can be carried out
5. A simple constitution
6. Problems that have to be faced

The value of women's clubs

Clubs have one main advantage over committees: people usually join them out of genuine interest rather than to gain privileges.

Women's involvement in health care has one main advantage over men's: women are usually more interested in the welfare of their family than in personal gain.

> Women acting together can be highly effective. Not only can they claim justice for themselves but, if organised and united, they can help to overturn harmful community practices or resist exploitation from outside.

Club membership

Each project and community should set up its own guidelines. Some will encourage any woman who lives in the community to attend. Others will suggest that each household sends one female member, preferably a mother of small children.

Sometimes upper and lower age limits are set, or only married or partnered women are eligible.

How clubs are started

Here are some suggestions:

1. **A club should only be started if the people**

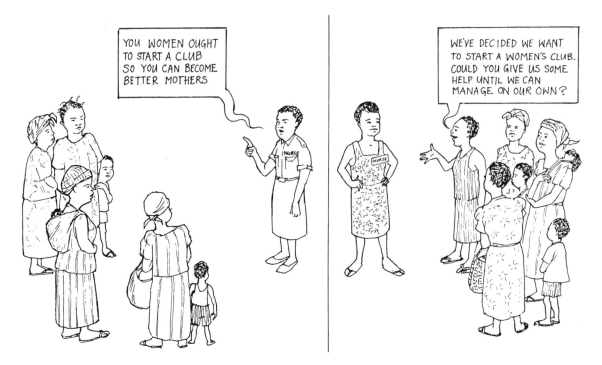

Figure 2.15   Clubs are more likely to succeed when the people themselves want to start them.

want it. However, if women lack interest, project staff could demonstrate the value to participants of starting a club.

2. **Appoint a facilitator from the project.** Community members may appreciate having one project member who can work with them, give them guidance and act as their teacher. Such a person will need to be sensitive, enthusiastic, and willing to let others lead. The facilitator's job might include:
   - encouraging interested women to call a first meeting;
   - helping women to come forward with their own ideas and suggestions;
   - enabling women to develop leadership skills;
   - giving advice and guidance when it is needed or when asked;
   - teaching club members about practical health matters;
   - assisting club members to seek loans, or pursue justice.
3. **Suggestions for a first meeting:**
   - Share a common religious observance. This is a good way to start a meeting, but we must make sure it is acceptable to all who are present.
   - Discuss a topic of current interest. *For example*: The CHW may have been beaten up the night before by her drunk husband, or a friend's child may have died from malaria. As causes and solutions are discussed, those present will see that such harmful events don't have to happen and that by working together they may be prevented.

   Other suitable topics might include:
   - How to prevent and treat common diseases of children, such as diarrhoea, measles or malnutrition.
   - Family planning.
   - How to raise more income for the use of the family.
   - How to start a kitchen garden.
   - How to prevent the spread of HIV/AIDS, by encouraging those who may be HIV positive to go for Voluntary Counselling and Testing (VCT).
   - Start a 'chit fund' or credit cooperative. Members contribute a small amount each month. Later, in turn or according to their needs, members receive a lump sum back.
   - Discuss future programmes and activities.

Activities that can be carried out

Worldwide, women's clubs carry out a huge variety of activities. Usually they will have started with just one or two activities that have proved to be successful or enjoyable. Here are some examples.

Health-related activities

> Women's clubs are ideal for giving practical support and encouragement to the CHW. This is especially needed when she first starts working and is finding the job difficult.

In addition, women's clubs will ·often take special interest in the following:

- the health needs and feeding of children;
- immunisation;
- health problems faced by women;
- family planning and child spacing;
- running a community health centre;
- problems in the home;
- home care of those with AIDS and of orphaned children;
- supervising TB 'DOTS' treatment, and the taking of ART;
- promoting personal hygiene.

For example: In rural Zimbabwe a new strategy to achieve safe hygiene practices has been developed using Community Health Clubs as 'vehicles for change'. A culture of health amongst 32 clubs totalling 2105 members prompted a 50 per cent hygiene behaviour change and huge demand for sanitation. (See www.wsp.org.)

Social activities

Examples might include:

- running a crèche for young children so mothers can work in the fields or earn a living;
- helping to organise festivals or cultural activities;
- starting a sewing circle, which could lead on to economic activities (below).

Educational activities

Women's clubs can arrange literacy classes or non-formal education for children or adults.

The club may have a member who is an effective teacher. Alternatively, a club member could be sent on a training course and then do the teaching herself.

Economic

These activities should not be started too soon. Club members should first establish trust among themselves and gain experience in club activities. Possibilities might include:

1. Starting a special savings fund into which each member pays a monthly amount. Funds could be used for:
   - Emergency grants to any member in special need, e.g. following the death of a husband.
   - An item of equipment that could be used by the club or hired out to others.
   For example: One club in Maharashtra, India, bought tents and musical instruments used for weddings. These were then available for the families of club members and hired out to others for a profit.
   - Giving repayable loans to members. These could be used for useful items that the family could not otherwise afford. Examples might include a sewing machine, farm animals, or improved seeds or fertilisers.
2. Income generation and community banking.
   For example: Project Hope, which works in many countries, encourages groups of about 25 women to take out loans from a village health bank to start small businesses. Health promotion is given priority whenever the bank meets. (See under Further Reading and Resources.)

Agricultural

Women's clubs can encourage and teach their members to start kitchen gardens. Nutritious vegetables can be grown on a plot near the house, kept damp by waste water from the kitchen and fertilised by kitchen compost.

Vegetables grown by women are more likely to be used as a food crop for the family, so benefiting the children.

Community action

Once a club is well established, women can stand together in joint action against social problems.

For example (1): Action against drunkenness. Women can make a united stand in the commu-

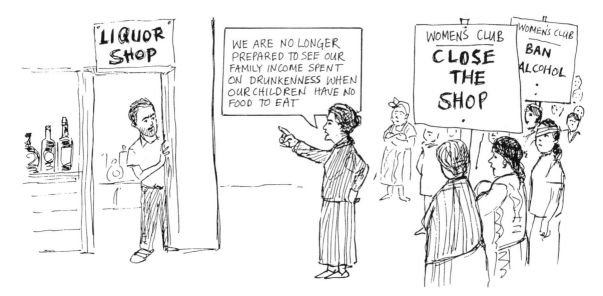

Figure 2.16   Women's clubs can act as effective pressure groups to overcome social evils.

nity to discourage husbands/partners and community members from abusing alcohol and drugs.

For example (2): Action to save the environment. A few years ago, women in the Himalayas banded together to prevent contractors cutting down trees and ruining the soil. When axemen appeared, they hugged the trees and when lorries arrived, they lay down in the road.

For example (3): Integrated action. The Murihi Project on the Kenyan coast was started in 2004 by a group of church members, mainly women, wishing to clean up the environment, reduce dependence on charcoal, which depletes the nearby forests, and generate some income. They do this through weaving baskets made of recycled plastic, selling briquettes for cooking made from renewable resources, and growing indigenous trees in a village nursery for each household to plant.

A simple constitution

At the start, members can simply meet together, the CHW acting as leader. No formal leadership is needed.

Later, the club may wish to appoint a secretary (often the CHW), a president and a treasurer.

Eventually, the club may wish to draw up a written constitution and become registered – usually in association with other clubs.

A small yearly membership fee can be paid by each member to cover costs.

Problems that have to be faced

Men oppose the clubs

The reasons for this are often jealousy and suspicion.

The remedies for this are to include and inform partners. Once they understand that activities are to benefit the whole family, the problem is often resolved.

Club members lose interest

One reason is because of wrong expectations. Club members expect great things to happen quickly. When they don't, interest drops and women stop coming.

The remedy is to start small with low expectations and for club members to know that it takes time (often about five years) to achieve useful results.

Members start to argue, factions develop, the club closes down

At the beginning, everyone must know and agree that learning to work together is the main purpose of the club and that, if this fails to happen, the club will achieve nothing.

The facilitator may be able to suggest a fair way of solving any serious dispute.

Other clubs

Clubs can be specially set up to give children a key role (see 5 under Further Reading and Resources).

For example: In Auguri, Nigeria, a group of 10–16-year-olds belonging to a child's rights club targeted the low rates of immunisation. In the area they covered, an average of 328 children was immunised each month over an eight-month period compared to only 8 per month before the children set to work.

These community groups can give valuable support to health and development activities in the community, sharing or replacing some of the functions of the health committees. They can act as vehicles for community participation in health care.

Summary

The ultimate aim of community based programmes is to hand over management of health and development activities to the community. Active participation of the community in all projects is the means of bringing this about.

Unless projects include the community in a genuine partnership, health patterns don't change and projects don't last. Participation protects people against exploitation, creating self-dependence and enabling communities to identify problems and devise solutions.

Partnership should be the basis of all project activities. Project members need to learn skills as facilitators so as to encourage ideas. Abilities present in the community should be used as widely as possible. One or two starter subjects should be chosen as a means of teaching the idea of participation to the community.

For participation to succeed, health team members must have clear aims and correct attitudes, making sure they give the community good quality training and preparation. Creating enthusiasm and showing trust are keys to bringing this about.

The process can be greatly helped by the setting up of health committees, women's clubs or similar community organisations.

Further reading and resources

1. *Jamkhed: A Comprehensive Rural Health Project*, M. and A. Arole, Macmillan, 1994.
   The story of Asia's most famous community health programme, compellingly told by the founders. This book is essential reading.
   Available from: TALC. See Appendix E.
2. *100 Ways to energize groups: games to use in workshops, meetings and the community. A Facilitator's Guide to Participatory Workshops with NGOs/CBOs responding to HIV/AIDS*, International HIV/AIDS Alliance, 2003.
   Available from 104–106 Queensbury House, Brighton, BN1 3XF UK; website: www.aidsalliance.org.
3. *Facilitation Skills Workbook*, Tearfund Resources Department, 2000, available from PO Box 200, Bridgnorth, Shropshire, UK; www.tearfund.org/tilz.
4. *Training for Transformation*, A. Hope and S. Timmel, Mambo Press, 1999.
   Incorporating four volumes to help field workers develop self-reliant communities. This is a radical and enlightening book, based on the work of Paulo Freire and widely applicable to a large range of programmes.
   Available from: IT Publications. See Appendix E.
5. *Children for Health: children as partners in health promotion*, Child-to-Child Trust and WHO, Macmillan, 2005.
   Recent examples of this inspiring approach.
   Available from TALC and Child to Child Trust. See also www.child-to-child.org.
6. *Partners in Planning*, S. Rifkin and P. Pridmore, Macmillan, 2001.
   A comprehensive guide with practical examples. Recommended for all community based health programmes.
   Available from: Macmillan. See Appendix E.
7. Project Hope. An international NGO carrying out a wide range of community based health and development. Project Hope, 255 Carter Hall Lane, Millwood, Virginia 22646, USA. Email: webmaster@projecthope.org; www.projecthope.org.
8. The following Pillars Guides: *Building the Capacity of Local Groups, Mobilizing the Community*. Available from Tearfund. See Appendix E.
9. *Child Participation: A Roots Guide*, Tearfund, 2004. See Appendix E.
10. *The Community is my University: a voice from the grass roots*, S. Maphogoro and E. Stutter, Kit Publishers, 2003.
    Available from: PO Box 95001, 1090 Amsterdam; www.kit.nl/publishers.

See Further references and guidelines, page 412.

3

Health Awareness and Motivation

In this chapter we shall consider:

1. The most important point of all: transformation of our own attitudes
2. The importance of raising health awareness
   - Health teaching
   - Awareness and motivation
3. Choosing an appropriate subject
4. Choosing an appropriate method
5. Making preparations
   - Teaching effectively
   - Materials needed
   - Equipment
   - The community
6. Methods of raising health awareness
   - Group discussions
   - Personal teaching at the point of need
   - Flashcards
   - Flipcharts
   - Flannelboards (flannelgraphs, cloth boards)
   - Stories and songs
   - Role play
   - Drama

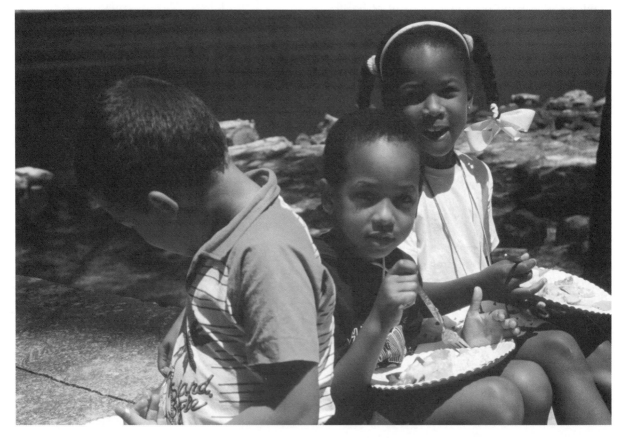

Figure 3.1   In health programmes, children become effective agents of change.

- Puppets
- Live examples
- Still images (slides and digital photographs)
- CD Roms and the internet
- Moving images (video, DVD and films)
- Radio and TV
- Other forms of health teaching
7. Evaluating progress

The most important point of all: transformation of our own attitudes

Most health workers can eventually learn how to give good health teaching. But in CBHC, teaching is not our primary aim. Rather it is to empower the community to become healthier, more united, and mutually supportive of the poorest and weakest members. In the period following war, famine or disaster this becomes even more important, and will also need to include reconciliation.

None of this will happen except through change or transformation in attitudes. And before this will occur in the community it has to take place in *us* – as project leaders and members.

Transformation means a radical and permament change from one set of attitudes to another. We have to change the negative ways in which we often look at ourselves and other people, to positive and affirmative ones. We must get rid of any cynical attitude we may have and adopt a can-do approach in order to deal with these issues.

For example: We may start with an attitude of feeling superior to the people we are working with because we are better educated, come from a city or belong to a different tribe or caste. We may blame community members for their ignorance and unhealthy habits. We may think less of others because they are poor, because we have never been poor ourselves, or because we have overcome poverty but have become arrogant of our success.

A health team that trusts, affirms and believes the best about the community it works with will automatically help to empower that community. Self-esteem and self-belief will grow.

It is easy to talk about the need for transformation, but much less easy to bring it about. How can we transform our attitudes?

- **Realise that it takes time**
  Changing attitudes is a long-term process, unlike learning a new skill or new piece of information. But in the early stages of a programme, when we are often more open to change, new attitudes will start to take root.

- **Engage in spiritual pilgrimage**
  From our own religious systems and values we may be able to draw strength and guidance, sometimes through prayer, self-awareness or the example of respected spiritual teachers.
  One famous religious teacher summed this up by saying:
  We should not become squeezed into the lifestyles and attitudes of those around us, but should continuously have our attitudes transformed by the renewing of our minds.

- **Live with those we are serving**
  For a period of time each project member, including those leading it, should live within the commmunity, experiencing the hardships – and joys – of community life. This will help us to understand why people live and act the way they do. When we grasp this, we are less likely to judge people and more likely to respect them.

We can ask ourselves two test questions: What would these community members have achieved if they had been given my opportunities? What would I have achieved if I had suffered their disadvantages?

- **Carry out an 'attitude brainstorm'**
  The team meets together and everyone shares ideas about unhelpful attitudes they have seen in themselves and appropriate attitudes they have seen in others (and themselves).
  Someone can list these in two columns on a flipchart. As people come to recognise helpful and unhelpful attitudes within the context of a supportive group, it helps the process of transformation.
  Later there can be a review session and members can share their experiences, and

ways in which their attitudes have changed. One golden rule must be understood: that no one is criticised or humiliated for anything personal they share.

- **Use the example of role models**
  People often say that attitudes are caught, not taught. Each person can be encouraged to think of one or two friends and community or national figures whose values they admire. Project leaders or members may themselves act as role models. For many of us, the dignified unselfishness of the villager or single mother in an urban slum who has successfully brought up a family brings its own inspiration.
- **Visit 'model' programmes**
  Sometimes there will be health programmes where we can observe the process of transformation or see the results of it in changed community attitudes. By living for a time in a new environment we will be more open than usual to new ideas, attitudes and practices.
- **Role play**
  This is an effective way of identifying the natural attitudes we possess, and learning how to change them. *For example*: We can role play the way we would naturally react to an uneducated village member who repeatedly fails to grasp our health teaching. Then, after group discussion, we could repeat the role play using a different and more affirmative approach in our conversation with the same villager.

The importance of raising health awareness

We must remember:

> In CBHC, teaching is always a two-way process. As we start teaching others about health, we ourselves must be ready to learn from the community. In doing this our understanding will grow, our attitudes will become more sensitive, and our own lives will be enriched.

Creating health awareness includes health teaching but goes beyond it. We will consider each in turn.

Health teaching

Many health programme staff spend most of their time running clinics and curing illnesses. They give health education only if there is time left over. Such an approach will never improve the health of a community.

Health teaching with the active involvement of the people is probably the most important of all community health activities. It must be top of our priority list, and should take place on all appropriate occasions, not only in clinics, but in schools, in meetings or whenever community members and health workers come together.

Awareness and motivation

The purpose of health teaching is not simply to increase people's knowledge about health. Even if people know more, it may not make any difference to what they actually do.

A community may have considerable health knowledge, but not be healthy; people may have heard endless health talks but not have changed incorrect practices.Our main aim, therefore, is not simply to teach or to share information but to create awareness and bring about behavioural change
For example:

> A mother may know she should wash her hands before preparing food but will not do so because no one has told her why it is necessary. She knows but she is not aware.

A person who has been made aware of a particular problem not only knows and understands it, but sees the importance of doing something about it. Such a person will be able to say: 'I know, I understand, I am motivated, I will take action.' *For example*: Consider a childhood immunisation programme:

- An unaware community may bring a few children because they have been told to.
- A partially aware community may bring several children because they begin to see its importance.
- A fully aware community will not only bring their children but may help to arrange the pro-

gramme and encourage defaulters. They may even have asked for the programme in the first place, because they realise it is essential.

Before starting to create awareness in the community we will need to start with ourselves and our team members. We may assume they are aware already, but this may not be the case, especially if they have worked only in hospitals or institutions.

Choosing an appropriate subject

Creating awareness is not a once and for all process. It starts with one or two concerns already important to the community, and grows from there.

Often such concerns will be known from discussions with the community or may become clear from the participatory appraisal (see page 72) or from the community diagnosis (see page 89).

Creating awareness about a felt need is usually quite easy. The people already understand the problem, now they must be encouraged to come up with solutions.

Creating awareness about a real, but often unfelt, need takes longer. Although the problem may be obvious to the health team, the community may have no understanding of how impor-

tant it is. *For example*: Consider the case of moderate malnutrition in children. Although the health team knows that children who are below the Road to Health on the Growth Chart are more likely to die from childhood illnesses, such children may look normal to members of the community, who will fail to understand the extra risk such children face.

Choosing an appropriate method

There are many ways of teaching and creating awareness, see pages 42–52. We should learn to use one or two effectively, rather than trying to master them all. Any method chosen should be:

1. **Appropriate to the local culture**
   For example: Storytelling or singing may be part of the local tradition. If so we can use these in our teaching.
   Equally we should avoid methods that are strange to the local people or which cause offence or give the wrong message.
   We must make sure that any teaching is in line with religious or social customs. Colours and symbols may have particular meanings in a community, and using a local language or dialect may help a community feel that this is THEIR programme.

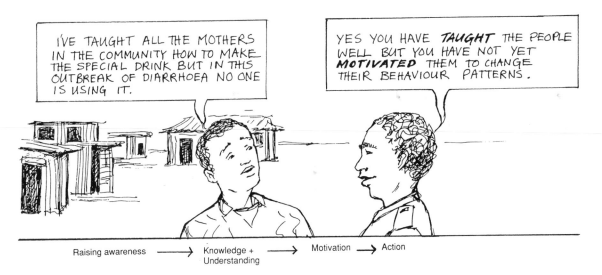

Figure 3.2

We should be prepared for unexpected results. *For example*: After watching a TV programme on how to prepare for a healthy delivery, instead of queuing up for the next antenatal clinic, community members may be consulting the local moneylenders about raising credit to buy their own TV set.

2. **Appropriate to the subject we are teaching**

   For example: 'How to overcome drunkenness' can be effectively shown through drama or puppets. Teaching is enjoyable, the audience feels involved and the message is clear. The drama can be paused at one or two key moments, and the audience asked to suggest what should happen next.

   For example: The use of oral rehydration solution is best shown by encouraging a mother to make it herself in the home or clinic, then feeding it to her child, and seeing its effect.

3. **Appropriate to the level of education**

   For example: Nurses and doctors may learn from lectures, but others become quickly bored and learn very little. Role play, health games or other action-based learning are more appropriate, especially for those with little education or who have difficulty in reading and writing.

4. **Appropriate to the gifts of the people**

   If there is a natural actor, teacher or storyteller, that person's gifts could be used, if they are willing to participate.

5. **Appropriate to the resources of the project and community**

   For example: Some projects consider that using films is an appropriate way of teaching. However, they should start doing this *only* if they have the money, resources, spare parts, fuel and expertise to make using and maintaining projectors successful.

> Try to use teaching methods that depend more on the gifts and active involvement of community members than on the resources of the project.

Making preparations

Teaching and creating awareness will only be successful if we are well organised beforehand. We will need to prepare: teachers, materials, equipment and the community itself.

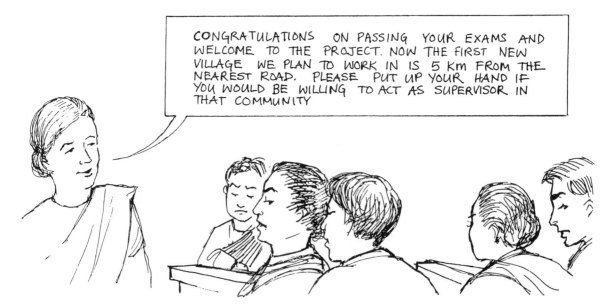

Figure 3.3   In CBHC, knowledge without enthusiasm has little value.

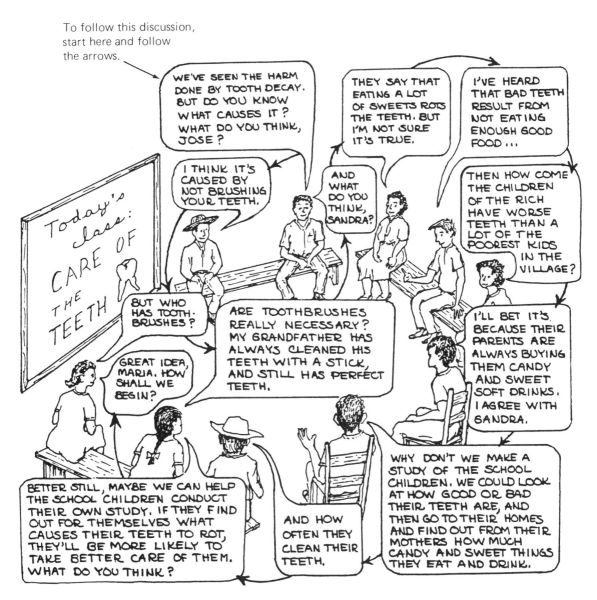

Figure 3.4   Creating awareness through group discussion.

Teaching effectively

This is obviously important if we are presenting a drama or puppet show, but it is equally necessary in leading a discussion or giving a talk with flashcards.

Team members should practise their skills in the classroom in front of each other before 'trying them out' on the community. Above all they must learn to teach in a way that involves the community (see Figure 3.4). Training of Trainers courses (TOTs) can help in this.

Materials needed

Teaching materials need to be both chosen and prepared with care. See if it is possible to adopt and adapt materials already being used in the community or in neighbouring projects.

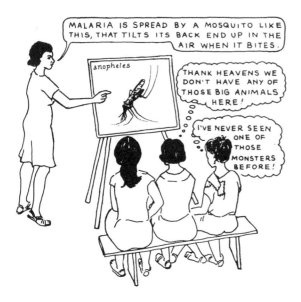

Figure 3.5   Make sure that people understand your pictures.

If choosing flashcards or pictures as visual aids, remember that many rural people are 'pictorially illiterate'. In other words they may not understand a picture's message even if it seems obvious to us.

Visual aids are best either prepared by local people, or field-tested with them.

For example: In one project in north India, local community members sketch out a series of flashcards on a specific topic in discussion with the health educator. These are then sent to a nearby large hospital to be produced in colour and on firm cardboard. This proves more effective than using standard flashcards from outside the project, which do not incorporate local images and scenes.

Equipment

Any special equipment such as projectors, generators or even props for a drama need to be well organised and checked carefully beforehand.

Make sure that everything works and that equipment is complete. Make a checklist of everything needed and read it through before setting out. Slide shows lose their message when the pictures are upside down and films don't impress the audience when the generator runs out of fuel halfway through the performance.

The community

We should aim to plan all health-teaching activities with the community, encouraging them to choose subjects, organise the programme and gather the people.

> Much energy, time and money has been wasted by the arrival of well prepared health teams to distant communities whose members were unaware of where, when and why the health team was coming.

It is important that we pre-test any form of health teaching we are planning to use. Without realising it, we may convey an unclear message or leave a community puzzled or offended. Although local people will usually be involved in preparing materials, we must still field-test our teaching method with a small group of community members.

We should encourage them to comment freely and then incorporate their suggestions into our final version. We can ask questions such as: What does this picture show? What do you like or dislike about the play or puppet show? What would you do to make the visual aid more easily understood? Does anything give an unclear message or cause offence?

Methods of raising health awareness

Group discussions

Team members can act as facilitators to enable community members both to share problems and suggest solutions (see Figure 3.4 and Chapter 2).

Practical guidelines:

1. Six to twelve people gather together in a circle.
2. A suitable subject is suggested – preferably a felt need of the people.
3. Guidance is given by the facilitator, who takes care never to dominate the discussion, and who makes sure that each person has a chance to speak, especially quieter members.

4. Good ideas are encouraged and useful suggestions discussed.
5. People are helped to think for themselves. This can be encouraged by asking Who? What? Where? Why? and How? questions.
6. The discussion is closed by selecting one or two important points for further discussion and possible action later.
7. Further meetings can be arranged for any community members with a special interest in health or development or who show leadership qualities. They themselves can be trained as facilitators who in turn help to extend health awareness in the community.

Discussion groups can also be adapted to a variety of special-need groups, such as heavy smokers, TB patients and support groups for people living with HIV/AIDS.

We must remember:

> Health team members need training in how to lead discussion groups. They must learn how to draw out ideas from others, rather than to share too many ideas of their own.

Personal teaching at the point of need

This takes place whenever a community member and health worker get together. The setting may be a clinic or a home, a village path, a city street, a local market, or during a community survey.

People listen best when they have a problem and want to find an answer.

For example: A mother comes to the clinic. She is worried about her child, now dehydrated from three days of diarrhoea. She listens and responds to a health worker who talks individually to her about the immediate problem.

Such teaching is often more effective than group talks at times when children are well and mothers less concerned.

Practical guidelines:

1. Make this type of teaching a priority.
2. Congratulate the patient or mother on any good health practice she has carried out, and build on that.

3. Talk in simple, non-medical language to the patient, making sure she understands.
4. Ask her to repeat back the main point that has been explained to her.
   In the case of a clinic:
5. Leave the door open, so other family members nearby can 'learn by overhearing'.
6. Teach by repetition. A good example of this is the use of 'Health drills' (see page 152).

Flashcards

Flashcards are cards with pictures, symbols or writing on them, used either singly or in sequence. They are a good way of unfolding a story that conveys a health message.

Practical guidelines:

Before using them make sure:
1. The message is relevant to the audience on the occasion it is being used. *For example*: In a Mother and Child Health clinic, show cards on conditions or problems being seen in the clinic on that day.
2. The pictures and script are easily understood.

> Use illustrations, ideas and words familiar to the people being taught, and not from another country, tribe or district.

3. The cards are in the right order. Check them through and practise holding them and telling the story beforehand.

While using them:

1. Know the subject and talk without reading.
2. Involve the audience.
   Ask questions, make jokes, and refer to recent events in the community, such as a death from diarrhoea, an injury from drunkenness or a measles epidemic.

After using them:

1. Develop a discussion.
2. Invite someone from the audience to retell the story or show the flashcards.
3. Stop before the people become bored, tired, too hot or too cold.

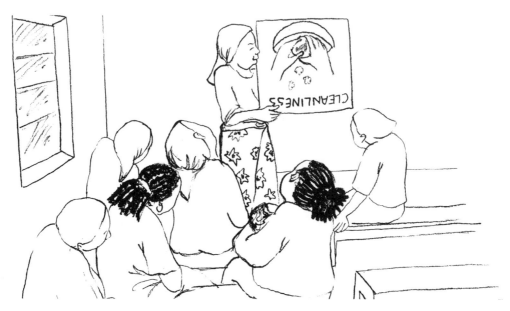

Figure 3.6   Flashcards can help give a health message, but practise using them first.

Flipcharts

These consist of several large sheets of good quality paper fastened together and bound with strong tape at the top of a board. After use the paper can be flipped over so that anything written down can be used later.

Flipcharts are very useful for recording ideas, to help brainstorming sessions and to help guide group discussions. They become even more useful if used by someone gifted at drawing cartoons.

Flannelboards (flannelgraphs, cloth boards)

A flannelboard consists of two parts:
1. A board covered in rough cloth or flannel and mounted in a frame.
2. Cutouts of people and objects with a rough backing such as sandpaper. Cutouts can be moved about to develop a health message.

Ready-made flannelboards with story ideas can be bought. Better still, the project and community can make their own.

Before using a flannelboard, good health stories must be prepared and practised, using the cutouts.

Otherwise follow guidelines for flashcards and flipcharts.

Stories and songs

These are excellent ways of teaching health, especially in communities where storytelling and singing are part of the culture.

One reason why stories are popular is because they use people, places and events that are familiar and often much loved by the people. Health teachings can be woven into traditional stories or folk epics or new stories made up using familiar characters and settings.

Practical guidelines:

1. Select or write a story that tells an important health message. Better still help a community member to write a story.
2. Tell the story to everyone gathered, for example to the CHW class.
3. Divide people into small groups of four to six and get members to retell the story to their group.
4. Encourage groups to act out the story as a drama, now or on another occasion.

5. Weave some true event into the story, which has happened in the community – either a bad event as a warning, a good event as an example, or an amusing one to help the people remember.
6. Discuss issues raised by the story.
7. Songs help to remind people of important health messages and can quickly be learnt by others. Set them to catchy or popular tunes. Encourage local people, such as CHWs, to make up their own words. Write a special song to mark an important event. Organise a competition between individuals or villages for the best health song, and arrange a cultural evening to hear and judge them.
For example: In the Prem Jyoti community health programme in Bihar, north India, singing is an important part of the culture. Few people can read or write. The village health workers and community, guided by the health team, have written nearly 30 songs (many set to popular tunes) to illustrate how to avoid and treat local illnesses and ways to lead a healthier life.

Role play

This is a simple form of drama where two people take on the roles of other people and act them out. *For example*: a health worker talks to a TB patient, a CHW talks to a pregnant woman, or a moneylender talks to a poor villager.

One of the main values of role play is to help those actually performing it to know how it feels to be the people they portray.

Practical guidelines:

1. Make sure the members of the group already know and trust each other.
2. Choose simple subjects and divide people into twos or threes. If groups of three are used, members take turns to observe the two doing the role play, make comments and then later feed back ideas to the class.
3. Give simple guidelines to each couple and a few minutes for them to plan.
4. Allow each pair five to ten minutes.

5. Discuss together at the end, drawing attention to the attitudes (both good and bad) acted out by the health worker.

Role play is often enjoyed most by the more outgoing members of a group, but they will often need a lot of encouragement to overcome their shyness and come to enjoy doing it. Don't force people to take part unless they wish to.

Drama

Drama is one of the best ways of all both to teach and to create awareness. It is fun, everyone feels involved and people can relate both to the characters and the things being said.

Drama or theatre is an especially good way of creating awareness and of motivating communities. Here are some reasons:

- Theatre does not require the audience to be literate or well informed.
- It appeals to all ages.
- It is fun and so holds people's attention.
- It appeals to our thoughts, ideas, emotions and wills.
- It challenges us to change our behaviours.

Short, simple dramas can be used in many situations, such as CHW teaching lessons, community meetings, marketplaces, school health lessons, or CHW box-giving ceremonies.

Longer dramas can be used during festivals or at special meetings.

For example: The Rampa Fund in Kyrgyzstan, Central Asia, produces an interactive street theatre programme that promotes local culture, healthy lifestyles and behaviour. We can find out if anything similar occurs in our country or region for use on special occasions such as a health fair.

Practical guidelines:

Please note before reading on: producing a drama takes a lot of time and energy. We should only do this if we really have the resources, including a team or community member with gifts and enthusiasm, able to take initiative. Using theatre on this scale is useful when there is a major issue

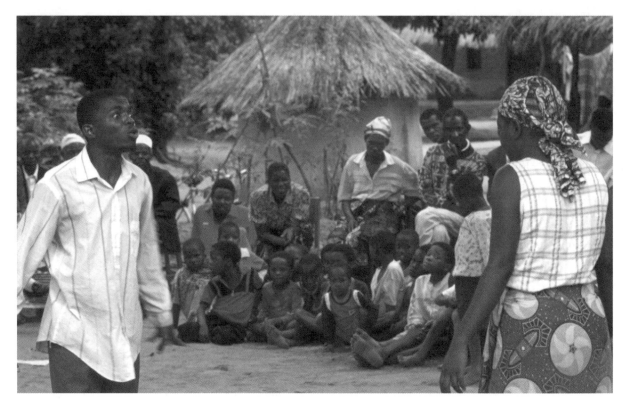

Figure 3.7   Theatre provides a creative way to engage with a local community and to learn from it.

the community needs to understand and when the drama can be used on a number of occasions.

1. Choose an appropriate theme.
2. Prepare and practise, using a script if necessary and leaving plenty of space for improvisation.
3. Start by using health team members as main characters. Later involve community members also.
4. Choose a site that has enough space both for actors and audience.
5. Make sure the audience can see properly. Hang lights blacked out towards the front, but shining on players.
6. Make sure the audience can hear properly. Actors must speak out and look forwards. Before starting, ask someone to sit at the back to make sure the play can easily be heard.
7. Use only simple props and costumes. *For example*: Dress a rich man in a T-shirt marked with a dollar sign, a poor man in rags, a crook can carry a toy gun, a health worker a stethoscope.
   Consider dressing up some of the characters as animals or making masks to represent some well known character, animal or emotion.
8. Write explanations and scene descriptions on a piece of cardboard. Hold this up between acts to explain what is going on and where the action is taking place.
9. Mix the serious with the funny. *For example*: After an important health or social statement, everyone can nod and look wise. After a wrong idea is given, other actors can boo or hiss.
10. Include songs and teach them to the audience, especially any with a useful health message.
11. Develop a discussion after the drama is over, or on another occasion to consider the issues raised or to plan community action.
12. Plan to repeat the play or perform it in another community if it proves popular.

13. Avoid causing offence to any community members either deliberately or in error. *For example*: A drama might very effectively compare a wise sister who cares well for her baby and a foolish one who makes many mistakes. This may teach a useful lesson to most mothers, but cause the minority who most need to understand the message to lose face and leave very discouraged.

Some important things to watch for

• Take care that nothing is being said or done in your organisation's name that could affect your reputation.
• Make time to train the actors and people who produce and direct the play so they do this as well as possible: poor performances can undermine the message.
• Make sure you get your facts right, especially important when the topic is HIV/AIDS.

• Ensure that the play highlights one or two simple messages, and that it is not too long or complicated.

Puppets

Puppets, like drama, are enjoyable and involve the audience. They can say almost anything, even strong, important and embarrassing things, without offending people. They are useful in sex education.

Practical guidelines:

1. Construct some puppets. These can be made out of papier mâché. Alternatively, stick or glove puppets can be made.
2. Arrange a puppet workshop. Call in someone with experience to lead a teaching session when team or community members can learn both how to make and to use puppets.

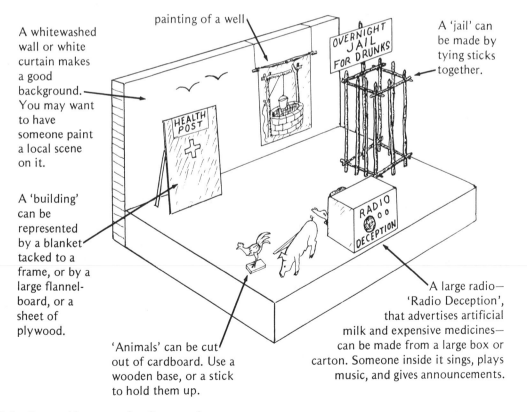

A whitewashed wall or white curtain makes a good background. You may want to have someone paint a local scene on it.

painting of a well

A 'jail' can be made by tying sticks together.

A 'building' can be represented by a blanket tacked to a frame, or by a large flannel-board, or a sheet of plywood.

'Animals' can be cut out of cardboard. Use a wooden base, or a stick to hold them up.

A large radio— 'Radio Deception', that advertises artificial milk and expensive medicines— can be made from a large box or carton. Someone inside it sings, plays music, and gives announcements.

Figure 3.8   Props add a sense of reality to a play.

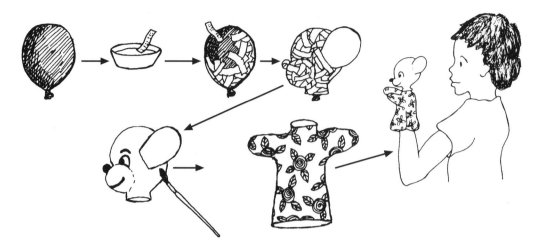

Figure 3.9   Making hand puppets out of papier mâché.

3. Prepare and practise a story outline leaving plenty of scope for adding in funny or topical extra lines.
4. Erect a screen at the right height. This can conveniently be a cloth stretched between two poles. The screen should completely hide the people holding the puppets.
5. Puppets should face the audience, opening their mouths, nodding their heads or making some movement when they speak.
6. A different voice should be used for each puppet.
7. Puppets should have exaggerated actions and characteristics, for example laughs should be loud, tempers should be bad, noses should be long.
8. Silences should be avoided.
9. Puppets can ask questions to the audience and encourage them to join in. They can lead a discussion afterwards.

Live examples

Actual people can make very effective visual aids.

For example: When giving a talk on malnutrition, present a child with obvious malnutrition (being sensitive to the feelings of the child and its parents). Such live models give a health message greater power.

For example: When giving an anatomy lesson, use a young man on which to draw the outlines of organs such as heart, lungs and liver. This will

be of greater interest than simply using a chalkboard.

For example: Cured TB patients can be trained to give brief health talks in the clinic. By explaining how they struggled but succeeded in taking medicine regularly, how they continued to support their family and how finally their illness was cured, their testimony can have great impact.

Still images (slides and digital photographs)

This is a good way to teach and create interest, if the equipment is available. People enjoy seeing photos, especially of people and places they recognise.

Practical guidelines:

1. Collect together good quality, relevant, slides or take a set of digital photographs. Many different sets of health slides and film strips can be bought. However, they may not be appropriate for the project area, and may not cover the exact subject we want to teach (see Appendix A).
   Some projects make their own sets of slides. This can be done as follows:
   • Choose a pair of health workers in the team with an interest in and gift at photography.
   • Decide together on the title(s) of the sequence to be made. Suitable subjects

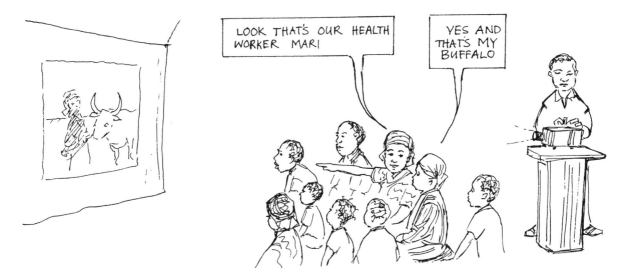

Figure 3.10   Teaching slides taken 'on location' always arouse great interest.

might be 'Immunise your child'; 'What happens in an MCH clinic'; 'A day in the life of a community health worker.'
- List the subjects and situations for which photographs are needed.
- Encourage the photographers to take action and close-up shots in the project area. Each photo should be of a specific subject or make a particular point: they also need to be good quality.

2. Link photos into a teaching sequence. Aim to put about 30 together. In the case of slides, each should be clearly numbered, labelled and marked the correct way for loading into the projector.
3. Practise giving the slide show to develop a good technique.
4. Photos can either be scanned or, if digital, downloaded and shown using a data projector.
5. Show the sequence to the audience, using each slide as a discussion starter.
   For example, we could ask:
   - What does this picture show?
   - What is the picture trying to teach us?
   - How could we do this in our community?

Before the presentation we should:
1. Practise showing the sequence, in the case of slides making sure they are in the right order and prepared the right way up.

2. Check the equipment is working and that nothing is left behind. Include a spare bulb for a slide projector.
3. Visit the meeting place beforehand, working out how the equipment will be set up and planning a power supply.

Finally, be aware that using photos of people limits how far away from the project area they can be shown. People like to see photos that represent their own cultural tradition.

> If used wrongly, photosequences become sleepy entertainment. If used correctly, they can arouse much interest and motivate the audience. Their success depends on the skill and enthusiasm of the teacher, and how much the people are involved in dialogue and discussion.

CD Roms and the internet

The use of CD Roms is increasingly valuable. Many relevant ones are now obtainable and they can be used individually or in small groups. They are a permanent, accessible and low-cost way of storing a considerable amount of information.

Where equipment is available and connections reliable, training individuals and groups to use the internet is an effective and popular way to increase knowledge.

Mobile phones can receive text messages on health or be used to download information from the internet. 'Wind up' low cost computers are becoming available.

Moving images (video, DVD and films)

More and more people are watching and making videos for health education. Find out what is available locally or within the country.

Practical guidelines:

1. Choose short, appropriate videos, DVDs or films with a clear health message.
2. View the showing to a selected audience to make sure the message is important, relevant, easy to understand and unlikely to cause offence.
3. Videos and DVDs on small screens can only be seen effectively by a limited number of people: make sure everyone can see and hear clearly.
4. Ensure that the video or DVD is the correct format for your equipment, with good quality image and sound.
5. Check all the equipment is in working order before starting.
6. Introduce the showing, indicating key things to look for, and explaining ideas that may be difficult for people to grasp.
7. Summarise key points afterwards and open up discussion on the issues raised.
8. Use videos and films where people naturally gather together, such as the village meeting hall, a bar, or room attached to a place of worship.
9. If no suitable video or DVD is available, consider making one with the community, using a camcorder. Call in outsiders with the necessary skills to help.

Radio and TV

Many TV and radio programmes reflect unhealthy values and consumerist lifestyles but with care and pre-planning we can still use the media for useful health education.

In some countries, Health Soap Operas are proving very popular and effective

For example: Urunana has been a popular radio programme broadcast in Rwanda, which also reaches neighbouring countries. One estimate suggested over half Rwanda's population originally tuned in. *Urunana* has a well written and entertaining storyline but includes valuable health lessons such as education about HIV/AIDS.

Similar programmes have also been produced in Somalia, Afghanistan and Cambodia.

> Health education by radio is more effective when combined with entertainment than if made in a standard teaching style.

Practical guidelines:

1. Publicise the times of any regular and relevant health-related TV or radio programmes.
2. Encourage people to watch in groups.
3. Arrange discussions on issues raised either immediately afterwards or within a few days.
4. Participate by:
   - writing to the producer with ideas, questions and suggestions;
   - sending in a health story or health song;
   - entering any publicised health competitions;
   - submitting a health script for radio or TV.

Other forms of health teaching

Posters

Buy or encourage the community to design posters with a clear message, a simple bold text and colourful pictures. Film stars or folk heroes, preferably making an appropriate health quote, are ideal subjects. Place in public places where people wait or stand around, such as clinic waiting areas, bus stops or in the community shop or meeting place. Do not leave the same poster up for too long. Pre-test any poster before printing large numbers.

Calendars

The community can design or buy these, writing in appropriate health texts and making illustrations. They can be placed on the walls of houses where family members will see them every day, and gradually absorb their message. Children can compete in a poster-drawing or calendar-making competition and the best ones can be displayed.

Printed leaflets and handbills

These should be short, well laid out, easy to read, with catchy illustrations. Comic strips can be used for teaching children (and adults). Leaflets are to remind people of something they have been taught about previously, such as how to make home-made oral rehydration solution (ORS).

Lecturing

Useful for more educated audiences. Maximum time one hour. Divide time into thirds – 20 minutes for teaching, 20 minutes for group discussion, 20 minutes for feedback. Alternatively, split into two – 30 minutes for teaching, 30 minutes for questions.

Use of chalkboards, whiteboards and overhead projectors

Good for giving a summary of what is being taught. Also helpful in developing a theme where the audience takes part, such as in the use of spider charts (see page 171).

Health quizzes and health games

Divide the health team, CHWs or other group into two or more teams. Set carefully worded questions and have a good question master. Give a prize at the end. This can be enjoyable and is a good way of revising a subject or of testing knowledge. A variety of games can be used or devised by the team or community.

Brains trusts

Those with expert knowledge answer questions. Questions are written out before but can also be asked 'from the floor'.

Books and journals

These are helpful for private study and useful for teachers in preparing lessons. Consider setting up a simple project library and show people suitable books and articles to read. The person in charge can mark helpful articles with different symbols or colour codes for levels of difficulty and subject matter and useful books can be listed out on a noticeboard. Many can be accessed online on the internet.

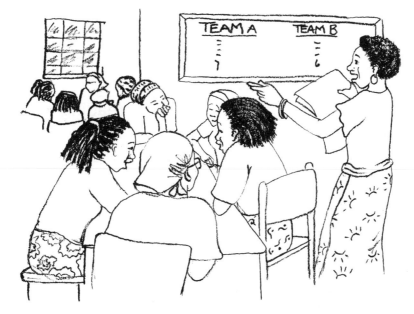

Figure 3.11   Learning together can be enjoyable.

Visits to seminars, conferences and other projects

Arrange for project members, CHWs or community leaders to attend seminars appropriate to their level and interest. Arrange visits to appropriate projects to stimulate interest and generate new ideas.

Finally, we can devise our own methods of teaching. Some of the best ways may be yet to be discovered.

Evaluating progress

It is helpful to know if our health teaching is effective. Here are some simple ways of finding out:

1. Talk with the community.
   We will soon get ideas and suggestions about ways in which we can improve our methods.
2. Make a questionnaire.
   This is good for evaluating CHW teaching or at the end of special courses for health workers. Ask which sessions or subjects were found to be the most interesting and most important. Discover which forms of teaching were the most enjoyable or helpful. Ask participants to grade their answers from 1 to 5 – 1 being the worst, 5 the best.
   Request written suggestions about how teaching could be improved.
   If questionnaires are kept unnamed, more reliable answers may be given.
3. Set an examination.
   This will test how much people have understood, and how much they remember. It tells little about how much knowledge is being put into practice.
4. Assess progress in the community.

The best way of evaluating our teaching will be the participation, enthusiasm and progress of both the health team and the community. Good teaching eventually leads to good statistics.

Summary

Our aim is to create awareness and teach effectively so that individuals develop healthier lifestyles, and communities become united, confident and inclusive of the poor and marginalised. Before doing this our own attitudes must undergo transformation. This process can be speeded up as we spend time living in the community, reflect on our attitudes, draw strength from spirituality, brainstorm ways of improving our attitudes, and learn from role models and through role play.

Creating health awareness includes teaching but extends beyond it. It is a two-way process in which the community learns about better health practices and the health team comes to appreciate the richness and value of community life.

Before carrying out health activities, both team and community members need to be well prepared. They must receive basic health teaching to increase their knowledge, and have their awareness raised to improve motivation.

Communities should be helped to understand about one major issue at a time, using a method that is appropriate both to their culture and to the subject being taught. Many methods are used but the best ones actively involve the community. These include group discussions, the use of storytelling, song, drama and puppets. CD Roms, films, radio and TV have a growing part to play.

Feedback on the success of health education programmes can be obtained through discussions with the community and by questionnaire. The real mark of success is a healthier, happier and more united community.

Further reading and resources

1. *Jamkhed: A Comprehensive Rural Health Project*, M. and R. Arole, Macmillan, 1994.
   This beautiful book describes the famous project where transformation has become central to all project activities.
   Available from: TALC. See Appendix E.
2. *Training for Transformation*, A. Hope and S. Timmel, Mambo Press, 1999.
   See description at end of Chapter 2.
3. *Helping Health Workers Learn*, D. Werner and B. Bower, Hesperian Foundation, 1982. Numerous reprints, the latest 1995.
   One of the great CBHC classics that every programme should own and use.
   Available from: TALC. See Appendix E.

4. *Teaching Health-care Workers* (2nd edn), F. Abbatt and R. McMahon, Macmillan, 1993. Available from: TALC. See Appendix E.

5. *How to Make and Use Visual Aids*, N. Harford and N. Baird, VSO Book, Heinemann, 1997. A clear and accurate how-to-do-it manual. Available from: TALC. See Appendix E.

6. *Pictures, People and Power: People-centred visual aids for development*, B. Linney, Macmillan, 1995. Available from: Macmillan. See Appendix E.

7. *Where There is no Artist: Development Drawings and How to Use Them*, P. Rohr-Rouendaal, IT Publications, 1997. More than 400 drawings are given, along with guidelines on using, adapting and enlarging them. Available from: IT Publications. See Appendix E.

8. *Appropriate Media for Training and Development*, J. Zeitlyn, Tool, 1995. A handbook to help teachers communicate using puppetry, TV, etc. Available from: IT Publications. See Appendix E.

9. *Health on Air*, G. Adam and N. Harford, Health Unlimited, 1998. A step-by-step guide on how to develop local radio programmes. Available from: TALC. See Appendix E.

10. *Footsteps*, Issue 58 (Tearfund) is available on www.tearfund.org/tilz.

11. *Healthlink Worldwide Resource Centre Manual*, 2nd Edition, 2004. Valuable information including use of electronic forms of communication. Can be downloaded from www.healthlink.org.uk/pubs.html or obtained from publications@healthlink.org.uk.

12. *Participatory Video: A Practical Approach to using Video Creatively in Group Development Work*, J. Shaw and C. Robertson, Routledge, 1997. Available from: IT Publications. See Appendix E.

13. Mobile development and the use of information is the theme of *Developments* magazine, issue 31, 2005, DFID, UK; www.developments.org.uk.

14. *Facilitation Skills Workbook*, S. Clarke, R. Blackman and I. Carter, Tearfund, 2004. Available from: Tearfund. See Appendix E.

See also Further references and guidelines, page 412.

Useful website

Creative Exchange
www.creativexchange.org.

Slides

A full list of slides, all useful for teaching health workers, is available from TALC.

PART II
Starting a Programme

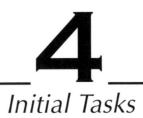

4

Initial Tasks

In Community Based Health Care (CBHC), we are helping communities identify and solve their own health problems. In some cases this means setting up health services where nothing appropriate exists. In others it involves developing health services from an existing hospital or health centre at the request of the community. It will often involve partnering with the government in helping to develop CBHC.

In order to be effective facilitators we need to be efficient and well organised. This chapter explains the first steps we need to take in responding to the needs of a community. The next chapter describes practical ways in which we can meet community members and start working with them.

There are six 'starter topics' we now need to consider:

1. Choosing a community to work with
2. Choosing a team
3. Understanding the project cycle
4. Obtaining funds
5. Setting up base
6. Ordering supplies

Choosing a community to work with

We should answer these questions:

1. **Has the community requested our help?**
   If the answer is no we should either choose another community or spend time building relationships with community members, in order to raise awareness of ways in which we can assist them.
2. **Is the community willing to work with us as partners?**
   Probably few community members will understand this idea at the beginning. As we mix with people and raise awareness they will move from trying to get things from us to a willingness to work in partnership with us.
3. **Do the leaders show genuine interest?**
   Signs of an effective community leader may include:
   • concern for the people's welfare, especially that of the poor;
   • willingness to plan and work together;
   • a reputation for honesty;
   • respect in the community.
4. **Do the people seem united?**
   Almost all communities have splits and divisions. If these are serious, follow racial or tribal lines or are very long-standing, it is hard to establish a useful partnership. However, working towards common health goals can sometimes bring reconciliation and encourage a united spirit.
5. **Is there serious ill health present?**
   Ask such questions as:
   • Do the people in general seem healthy or sick?
   • Do many of the children die young?
   • Is there year-round clean water?
   • Is there much disability or blindness?
   One effective way of doing this is through Participatory Appraisal (PA). See Chapter 5.
6. **Are existing health services adequate?**
   We may find that government services exist but are little used; that private doctors are present but not serving the poor; that other health programmes or hospitals are at work but offering only curative care.
7. **Have we sufficient resources**, especially in terms of personnel and expertise, to help the community set up its own health programme?
   • Can we help them to meet their felt needs? These are the illnesses people want cured, and the problems the people want answered.

- Can we help the community identify and solve actual causes of ill health, such as contaminated water, wrong feeding practices, lack of food, alcohol abuse, poverty and exploitation?
- Is there an existing referral system, such as with a health centre or hospital, for problems we cannot handle ourselves? If not, can we help set one up?

8. **Is the target area a suitable size?**
If it is too small, rapid health improvements may occur, but the project will not be cost-effective.

> If the communities we serve are too large we may get swamped with urgent problems and be unable to help the people bring about lasting health improvements.

At the start of a project we should usually confine our work to an area within a single Health District.

Figure 4.1

9. **Does the government approve the project plans?** If our project is not already working closely with the government, we will need to contact the District Medical Officer (DMO) to find out:

- if the government is already doing primary care in the area;
- if the DMO approves of our plans, feels able to work in partnership or is willing to draw up a written agreement.

Governments are often unable to provide adequate primary health care at community level. Providing we approach them in a cooperative spirit and outline an appropriate plan, they will usually welcome our assistance. If we gain a good reputation they may even 'contract out' aspects of primary health care for us to carry out, or ask us to help scale up existing programmes by working with them.

For example (1): A health programme in Sichuan, western China, where an NGO has been partnering with government health services since 1996, was so effective in training village doctors and other community based projects based in a few townships that the NGO was asked by the state government to work with them to cover the entire prefecture (district).

For example (2): It is estimated that, at the present time, between 30 and 40 per cent of health services in sub-Saharan Africa are provided by voluntary (non-governmental) agencies, many of them church related. With churches and other religious organisations often being the dominant civil society organisation, there is huge potential for more partnerships between such groups and government health services, which are often overwhelmed.

Having decided on a community to work alongside, we then need to decide whether to serve all the people in the target area or just the neediest groups within it.

It is generally better to work with the entire population but to give special attention to the poor and those with the greatest health needs. There are a few exceptions:

1. Where there is an obvious group that is deprived or different, such as refugees, nomads or the landless.

2. With certain health problems such as TB, HIV/AIDS, substance abuse or addiction, there may be value in specific targeting.

Although HIV/AIDS is the dominant problem in many areas, there is still much value in mainstreaming its prevention, care and cure into an integrated Community Based Health Programme (see Chapter 15).

Choosing a team

In the start-up phase, CBHC teams will usually develop three levels of worker: the community health worker, usually a member of the village or poor urban commmunity we are working in; middle level workers making up the main part of the project team; the senior staff members making up the project leadership, which will usually include a doctor, nurse and administrator.

Who should be selected?

Answer: those best able to respond to the help the community has asked for.

In choosing a staff team this will include:

Those with appropriate qualities

1. **A real interest in the community** – not just financial gain. Field workers will often work long and hard hours. They are more likely to continue in the project if they possess vision and enthusiasm.
2. **A willingness to learn.**
   It is better to have people who know little but want to know more, than those who believe they know everything. This is especially true of people who have been working in health institutions. They will need careful retraining and reorientation into the very different world of community health.
3. **A readiness to take on any job.**
   Health team members must be ready to take on any activity, ranging from the use of clinical skills to menial tasks. They must also be ready to take initiatives.
4. **A respect for and appreciation of the poor.**
   Many religious teachers have taught special love for the poor. Many of the best health

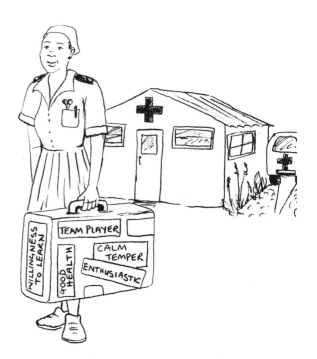

Figure 4.2   All CHWs, even those who have worked in institutions, need to bring the same qualities to the job.

workers are happy to be known as friends of the poor.

5. **An ability to work as part of a team.**
   This includes appreciating colleagues from different districts of the country, religions and tribes. It means being slow to become angry and being quick to forgive. Angry words in the community can destroy weeks of work. Hidden anger against a colleague can ruin team relationships.
6. **Good health.**
   Strong physical and mental health is important for many jobs. However, people with less good health may be given appropriate tasks. This includes those with disability, and people living with HIV/AIDS. The key question we need to ask from an occupational health viewpoint is whether the applicant is fit enough to do the job required.
7. **A balanced team.**
   Health teams will need a balance of those who have gifts in vision, ideas and networking (the ideas people), those able to find common ground and solve disputes (the smoothers), and those who are methodical and able to

complete tasks efficiently (the finishers). Each will need to recognise and respect the other's gifts and different approaches (see also pages 348–357 on Managing Personnel).

Those with appropriate qualifications

> Generally in community based health care character is more important than qualifications. Most community health skills can best be learnt on the job.

For middle level workers, basic education up to grade 10 or 12 combined with common sense and enthusiasm is a good profile to look for. Learning on the job and via appropriate training courses is often more appropriate than formal professional training.

Whatever the type of training given, health workers increasingly need documentation of their training, qualifications and continuing professional development.

Programmes will also need professionally trained staff:

- A doctor or medical advisor who can act as facilitator, trainer and part-time clinician. Only doctors gifted and trained in management should be overall project directors. Doctors must have sympathy and understanding of CBHC, otherwise they may 'hijack' the project, changing it into a curative programme for their own advantage (see pages 372–4).
- A nurse (medical assistant or equivalent) often makes the best team leader or director of a smaller programme.
- A manager or administrator is essential to coordinate tasks and manage finance for all but the smallest programmes.

> The ultimate success of projects is largely determined by how well the programme is managed.

> Managers will need personal gifts and training appropriate for the project. They will be managing people as well as supplies, so their style must be democratic and inclusive (see pages 348–9).

Where can suitable team members be recruited?

Here are some possible sources:
1. The local community.
   In genuine CBHC, most team members are drawn from the local community. As we mix with the people, we can look out for appropriate people to nurture and to train.
2. Networks.
   Through networks of friends and contacts suitable workers may be found from a wider area.
3. Training schools and institutions.
4. Voluntary health associations or religious bodies.
5. Transfers from hospitals, sister projects or government programmes, but only after careful assessment.
6. Through advertisements in papers and journals. This often attracts inappropriate people merely interested in having employment.

An emerging problem: in many least developed countries there is a serious shortage of health workers. There are several reasons for this: recruitment to work in higher paid jobs, either abroad, in city hospitals or with well funded aid agencies or 'vertical' programmes (see page 4), also from illness, especially untreated HIV/AIDS.

This is making it harder to find appropriate qualified staff, which in turn means we need to seek and train community members who show aptitude and interest. We also need to consider incorporating traditional and private practitioners providing they are willing to learn and are in agreement with the aims and values of the project.

How should team members be selected?

By personal recommendation or references

These should be from reliable sources. Relatives' comments should be treated with caution.

By interview

Many people appear attractive and talk well at interviews. It is therefore sensible in addition to spend time with applicants individually and informally.

By a trial period

This is very useful for non-professional staff. Invite applicants to spend a few days in the project where they can join in all activities. Assess how they get on with others and relate to the community.

Situations that require caution

Employing relatives

Existing team members may ask if their relatives can be employed in the project. This is usually not a good idea. Sometimes such relatives may have failed to find other jobs. Often two or more members of one family in a project may exert too much influence and cause division in the team.

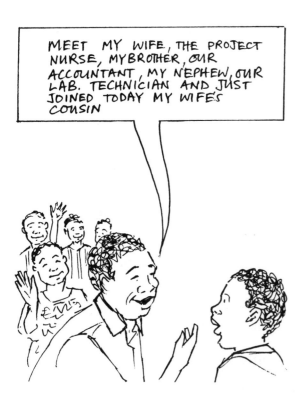

Figure 4.3

Overloading with members of one tribe or district

This can destroy a team's unity and cause suspicion among the community, especially if most team members are from outside the project area.

Unmarried women

Any young unpartnered women in the team will need safe working and living conditions. In some countries it is not appropriate to employ them and in others they will need to work in a group or in the company of older married women.

Employment laws

We must ensure that our personnel policy, including recruitment, is in line with the laws of the country we are working in.

Understanding the project cycle

At an early stage in setting up a programme it is helpful for us to understand the concept of the project cycle. First, this enables us to be methodical in our thinking and second, many outside donors tend to follow this pattern and will expect us to be aware of it and to follow it where possible.

Look at Figure 4.4 and start at the top.

We first *identify* both the problems and the solutions on which the health team and the community wish to work together. This is done largely by a needs assessment such as the Participatory Appraisal or the Community Survey described in Chapter 5.

We then need to *plan the project*, which is described in chapter 6, and which leads to a design best set out in a logical framework.

Next we need to *implement the project*, and various chapters in this book show us ways we can do this.

At regular intervals we will need to *evaluate the project*, see Chapter 18, and reflect on any changes we need to make in the next 'project cycle'. As the programme develops, and at least once yearly, we review and monitor our progress.

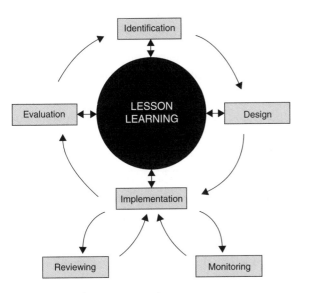

Figure 4.4   The Project Cycle.

Obtaining funds

> Setting up a project is difficult and expensive. It takes many years. It is better not to start at all than to start, then run out of funds and have to stop. The developing world is full of projects that have been abandoned, and people whose hopes have been disappointed.

Before making promises and raising hopes we must plan well ahead and work out how much funding will be needed. This can only be approximate. Our plans will be likely to change as we respond to the needs of the people.

We must make sure that programmes we help to set up can be sustained for a number of years ahead.

Chapter 21 looks at this in more detail. The following section in this chapter looks mainly at how we can get sufficient 'seed funding' so our project can make a start.

In obtaining funds we will first choose the source and, second, make an application.

Choosing the source (see also Chapter 21)

> Before writing off to foreign donors, identify sources of funds within the community and within the country.

For example: a project on the east coast of Africa, hoping to improve the health of communities through local income generation and improvements to the environment needed seed funding to get started. Before writing to sources outside the country they approached local tourist hotels in the area, explained the project and secured sufficient donations to enable the project to begin.

It may at least be possible to raise sufficient money from local sources or within the country to start the project or to cover a proportion of the costs. Although projects often look for foreign funds, these will not last for ever, and from the very beginning our project must aim to become self-sustaining, even though this is often hard to achieve in practice.

Main sources of funding include:

Sources within the project itself

Patient fees

One useful source is the fees patients pay for curative services, though this will only amount to a small proportion of the total project budget. Experience shows that charging nothing often causes community members to undervalue the services and medicines supplied to them. On the other hand, even relatively small charges can reduce the numbers attending clinics and usually the poorest and most needy are the first to stay away. For this reason some countries have abolished user fees and we need to be aware both of the laws and the practices in the region where we are working.

Here are some practical suggestions:

- Charge fees for medical services or supplies that the majority of the patients are willing and able to pay (estimate this by verbal comments and take-up of services rather than questionnaire).

- Ensure that those genuinely unable to pay some of or all the fee are not turned away.
- Consider charging higher fees to those outside the project area, or those who have bypassed their Village Health Worker or self-referred.
- Consider the use of a revolving drug fund. More details are on page 391.

Insurance schemes and income generation
These are relatively difficult to set up but may be possible later (see pages 391–4).

The base hospital

If the project is run by a hospital, some funds may be available. If the hospital has a high reputation, funds can flow in from private patients. In practice most hospitals are seriously short of funds and have little to give towards community health care (see pages 378–81).

Local organisations

Try any appropriate sources – churches, temples, mosques, cooperatives, Rotary and Lions clubs, charities, local business associations, the 'generous rich'.

The government – district, state or national

Funds are often available in theory, especially if working in cooperation with the government or on a specific project. However, such sources may be unreliable or may have 'strings' attached. In addition to funding, certain supplies may be available, usually immunisations, sometimes TB drugs, and increasingly antiretroviral therapy to treat HIV/AIDS. In many of the poorest countries, government health services have no funds available.

However, we must remember that one of our aims will be to set up strong community based health systems that can work alongside and receive support and funds from specific government health programmes. Many such programmes will themselves be part of worldwide health initiatives set up by the World Health

Organisation and UNICEF (see sections in the chapters of Part III of this book).

Sources outside the country

Before trying to obtain foreign funds, we must understand the laws concerning foreign contributions. Special registration is usually necessary. Sources may include:

Voluntary funding agencies
There are a large number of agencies holding funds to support projects in developing countries. These include aid agencies and other groups, both religious and secular. Most are based in developed countries, especially Europe, North America, Japan and Australasia. Such groups are often willing to support smaller-scale health and development projects. Lists can be obtained from national or voluntary health associations, and from embassies.

International aid agencies (multilateral aid)
These include the United Nations agencies such as WHO, UNICEF, UNDP, but these only rarely support voluntary health programmes. The European Community (EC) has funds available for certain types of project, through the European Community Humanitarian Office (ECHO). Increasingly, funds for larger programmes are becoming available from donor foundations such as the Bill and Melinda Gates Foundation and the Global Fund (see Further reading and resources).

Foreign government aid programmes and embassies (bilateral aid)
Large sums may be available but normally a national of that country needs to be connected with the project. Many voluntary funding agencies receive one-to-one matching grants (called co-funding) from their own governments so making more money available.

Before applying for foreign funds we must be aware of possible disadvantages:

Dependence
If foreign funds are available, community members may expect handouts. They may be less ready to contribute their own time, money and

Wise Funding Inc.
Bigtown
Anystate, USA
30 March 2006

Dear Project Leader

Thank you for the funding application which you sent on behalf of your organisation, "Cure all People" (CAP).

Although we do have funding available it is our policy only to release this if we have an assurance that all local and national sources have been tried first. We also require outline plans of how your project plans to become sustainable when outside funding stops ...

Figure 4.5

resources if they see foreign jeeps or receive foreign medicines.

Suspicion

In some countries rumours may spread that foreigners attached to projects may be involved in illegal activities or as undercover agents.

Applying for funds

Remember that funding takes time. We must start applying just as soon as our plans begin to take shape. In the case of government or foreign funds it may take six to twelve months or more before

funds are actually received (see Figure 4.7, The reply gap).

Follow this procedure:

1. **Write to the funding source as soon as possible.** Include a brief personal introduction and ask for an application form. This is best done through a mutual contact or by asking someone with influence to write in support of the application. Make three copies of the letter. Keep one and send the others to the agency, posted on different dates and from different places because postal services are often unreliable. Use email if you have it.

2. **Prepare the material the agency will require.** We can do this while waiting for its

Dependency, suspicion, separation from people as foreign funding increases

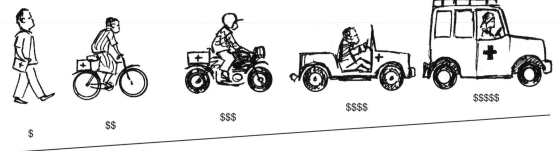

$

$$

$$$

$$$$

$$$$$

Figure 4.6   The effect of increasing foreign funding.

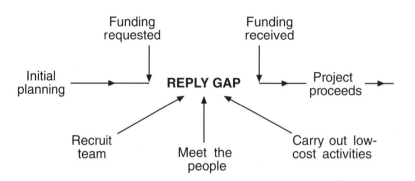

Figure 4.7   The reply gap.

reply. Although different agencies request different information and each has its own form, most will expect brief details of the following:

a) The name of the organisation and any larger group to which it belongs, the director's name, the project address.

b) The names and brief qualifications of senior team members.

c) Details of the project area – its location, terrain and climate.

d) Details of the target population:
   • Number (approx.) of people and villages or slum colonies to be served.
   • Social structure of the communities, including details of local employment, relative wealth, poor or neglected sub-groups, etc.
   • Religious make-up of the population.

e) Details of the people's health:
   • Present services available – both government and private.
   • Serious illnesses and health problems present.

f) Details of the programme:
   • Aims and objectives.
   • How these will be achieved.

Try to give an approximate framework (see programme planning using the logframe, pages 101–107). Details will be worked out later with the community. Mention any surveys planned, and any clinics, teaching or other programmes likely to be carried out.

g) Relationship with government:
   • Details of planned cooperation.
   • Whether written permission has been obtained.

h) Budget:
   Give details of planned income and expenditure. Include detailed budget for one year, and an approximate budget for two further years. For income, estimate total from other sources. For expenditure, divide into capital (non-recurring) and annual (recurring).

   Under recurring include: salaries, services, rent and buildings, supplies including medicines, travel and transport, training and administration.

   Include in the budget items that are essential, but do not ask for expensive or unnecessary equipment. There are more details on preparing budgets in Chapter 19, (pages 360–62).

   Figure 4.8 lists the questions used by one agency that supports a number of small-scale health programmes.

   Other information may be requested, such as the latest report and accounts of the parent organisation, photographs of the area and people, results of a sample population survey, etc.

3. **Maintain contact with the agency.**
   Having received funds, we must maintain close, friendly links with the sponsoring organisation:

   a) Write a letter of acknowledgement and thanks.

   b) Send in, on time, any regular reports, budgets or other information requested.

   c) Welcome any visitors from the funding agency.

   d) Participate in any training seminars or capacity building which they arrange.

HEALTH PROJECT APPLICATION FORM

Project title ....

Contact person ....

Job title ....

Background to the project
1. How did this project begin and why is it needed?
2. Who have you discussed the project with?
3. Are any other organisations working on the same problems?
4. How does your project fit into government health plans etc?

Aims and objectives
1. Write your project aim in one sentence.
2. Write your project objectives, which should be SMART (see page 98).
3. Include a logical framework if you have used one.

Does the project address priority health issues?
List what you think are the main health problems in your community.
What does the local community consider to be their main health problems?
(Attach sample survey or statistics if you have them.)

Who will benefit from the project?
1. Who are the main beneficiaries?
2. Have they been involved in the planning? How?

How has the local church been involved in the project?
1. How will the project support the local church's ministry?
2. How has the church been involved in developing the project proposal? How has the church shown its commitment to this project?

Project plan/activities/risks
Anticipated start and completion dates of project.
For how long will you be seeking funds?
Which other funders have you approached?
What plans do you have to make the project self-sustaining?

Who will manage the project?
1. Who will be the main project leader?
2. Do you have a management team/committee?

Sustainability
1. Once funding has finished, what are your specific aims to enable the project to be self-supporting?
2. Has the project been discussed with local government? How does it fit in with their objectives and funding?

Monitoring
How do you plan to monitor the work of your project? What systems will you use?

Evaluation
How do you plan to evaluate the work of your project?
How frequently?
Will you use internal or external people to evaluate your work?

Budget and financial management
1. Detail *all* the items in your budget.
2. Do you have a financial manager?
3. Do you have someone to audit/certify your accounts?
4. Have you approached other funders, and do you have any funding secured already?

Additional Information

Figure 4.8   Health questions asked by one funding agency.

Setting up base

No project will succeed unless it has a well organised project base. Before starting a field programme, we will need to carry out the following:

Ensure team members have adequate accommodation

Many team members will live locally with their families. Any team accommodation should be adequately equipped, within the project area, appropriate to the worker's level, and available until the member leaves the project.

Draw up an agreement with each worker that includes length of tenure, list of items supplied with the accommodation, details of rent and other charges such as fuel, water and electricity. These should be discussed, agreed, written down and signed by both parties.

In practice team members often live together on a campus, compound or hospital. This may be convenient but, where team members share work, leisure, worship and accommodation, relationships can easily become strained.

Set up office and stores

The project base may be located in a primary health centre or health post. Usually it will be in a separate building serving a wider area, but within the project area. Generally the base should be separate from any hospital to help retain some independence. Nothing big or expensive is needed; the simpler this is kept the better. Often three or four rooms will be enough to start with, for example, one for the office, one for meeting and training and one for storing and sterilising equipment.

The storeroom can be used for keeping both drugs and equipment. Make sure that this is:

- secure so that people cannot break in,
- dry even during the rainy season;
- large enough and well enough lit for convenience;
- accessible by vehicle for easy loading and
- rat-proof and bat-proof, and screened against mosquitoes.

Ordering supplies

Details on receiving, storing and issuing supplies are found on pages 156–7. At this stage we will

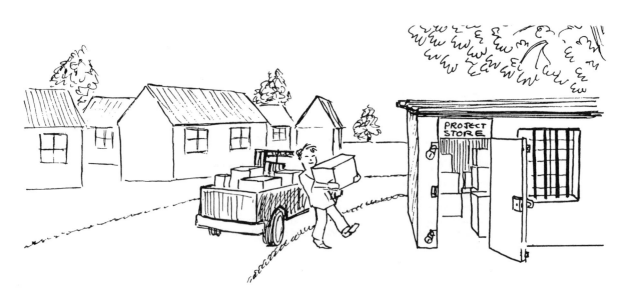

Figure 4.9   The project storerooms should be well sited and well protected.

simply consider what equipment and medicines need to be ordered.

Order equipment

1. **List out what supplies are required (see Appendix B):**
   a) Include all items that are really necessary.
   b) Decide on what type and what number of items are needed.
   c) Discuss this list with the leaders of other projects or anyone with suitable experience.
2. **Identify sources where supplies can be obtained.**
   a) Buy locally wherever possible.
   b) For each type of equipment compare prices and quality of different suppliers.
   c) Build a relationship with the main suppliers. Try to arrange discount prices.
   d) Find an alternative supplier for important items in case the main supplier runs out of stock.
   e) Order supplies in plenty of time. There is often a long delay between ordering and receiving.
   f) Avoid poor quality products even if alternatives are more expensive.

> Only obtain equipment from abroad if good quality supplies are not available or manufactured within the country.

3. **Carefully check all supplies on arrival**, making sure they are complete and intact. See Appendix A for a list of foreign suppliers. See Appendix B for a list of essential supplies.
4. **Two special pieces of equipment:**
   a) A Refrigerator. Solar powered fridges are increasingly used. They are most useful if solar power is also used for other community activities, so the cost can be shared and technicians are available to install and maintain them. Otherwise it is better to buy fridges that run on kerosene or electricity (via mains and/or generator). All fridges need regular maintenance, temperature monitoring and defrosting.

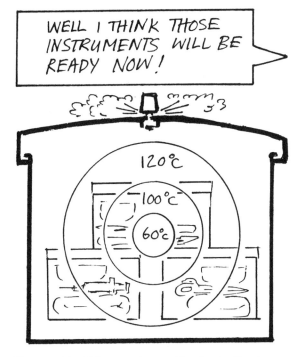

Figure 4.10   Take care that sterilisation is effective.

   b) A Steriliser. Unless we can arrange to use a nearby hospital's sterile supplies, a steam steriliser, autoclave or pressure cooker will be needed for sterilising any non-disposable instruments used in the clinic or community. Needles and syringes should only be reused if it is impossible to obtain disposable items. Take great care that health workers who use sterilisers fully understand how they work and the length of time supplies need to be heated.

Order medicines (see also Chapter 17)

1. Decide which medicines are needed. Together with the project medical adviser, draw up a suggested list and then compare it with:
   • the list used by the nearest hospital,
   • the national essential drugs list,
   • the WHO essential drugs list and
   • the suggested list in Appendix C.

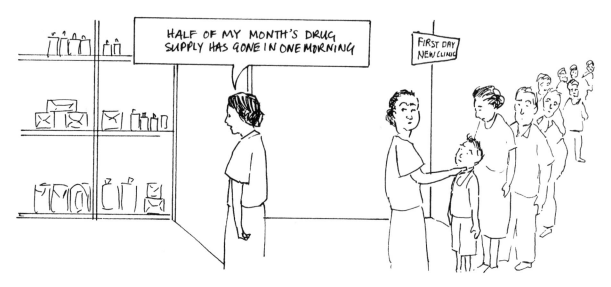

Figure 4.11

The drugs chosen should be:
a) appropriate for the health needs of the area;
b) appropriate for the level of health worker who will be using them;
c) single component, meaning that in most cases they should contain only a single drug. TB drugs, treatment for malaria and antiretroviral therapy to treat HIV/AIDS are important exceptions.
d) generic, meaning they should be ordered using the scientific, chemical name, and not the trade name (this saves money and confusion);
e) good quality. Many poor quality or fake drugs are being made. Make sure that any drugs used are made by good companies licensed by the government. This can include multinationals. Only use foreign supplies if good quality, essential medicines are not made within the country.

2. Calculate how much medicine will be needed. This can be done by working out both the likely number of patients to be seen and by knowing the likely drugs to be prescribed for each.
a) Estimate the likely number of patients that may be seen within a one-year period. One way we can do this is by discovering numbers attending clinics in neighbouring projects.

The proportion of a population attending a clinic is extremely variable. An approximate guide for communities with few existing health facilities might be an attendance of between a quarter and a half of the population within the first year for curative care (see also Chapter 8).

b) Estimate the numbers of each drug likely to be used per 100 patients seen. To do this look through the records of patients seen in similar clinics or outpatient departments, and list out the essential drugs used for each. Total up the numbers of each drug used per 100 patients. Remember that most clinics overprescribe and that patients will only rarely require more than two or three medicines. If there are no such clinics, we can work out from our knowledge of local illnesses the medicines likely to be needed. Drugs are otherwise ordered and received as with equipment. Expiry dates must be checked.

3. Keep a stock card.
We can keep a separate card for each recurrent item. One design is shown in Figure 4.12. It is divided into two sections: a supply section and a balance section. Cards (or sheets) can be filed alphabetically, and by subject, e.g. drugs in one card holder, medical supplies in another, laboratory supplies in a third.

Item .Amoxycillin. Code number ....AB5........ Monthly consumption ......2000.......

Re-order level .....3000........

| Supply section | | Suppliers | 1 .Best Generics Ltd............ | 2 .Deltamedicines Inc...... |
| | | | 3 .International Drug Co | 4 .... |

Date ordered	Rate per 1/10/(100)	Quantity	Total value		Supplier	Notes
5/11/05	USD 5	4000	USD 200		1	Slow supply last time.

Balance section

Date issued/ (received)	Where received from/issued to supplier	Amt issued	Amt received	Prev. balance	Present balance
6/12/05		0	4000	3000	7000

Figure 4.12 Example of a stock card.

Alternatively, computerised systems can be used. Once every six or twelve months we will need to stocktake. This means checking that the balance of each item on the stock card is the same as the amount on the shelf. In the case of medicines, we should also check expiry dates, making sure the oldest supplies are issued first.

Order a vehicle

A project vehicle may not be needed at the beginning, and may not be wise, as it suggests a project is wealthy or foreign. For as long as possible we should use local or public transport, a motorbike, bicycle or foot.

Only order a vehicle if there is no alternative system of transport that can be used by project members.

When deciding whether to buy a vehicle, ask these questions:

1. Are funds available to buy it?
2. Are funds available to maintain it?
3. Are spare parts available to mend it?
4. Is a skilled mechanic available to repair it?
5. Is fuel available to run it?

When choosing a vehicle, ask these questions:

1. Is it tough enough for the worst roads during the worst weather?
2. Is it large enough to carry project members, community health workers, patients, visitors and equipment?
3. Is it suitable for carrying seriously ill patients?
4. Is it cheap to run? In many countries diesel is cheaper than petrol. Some vehicles do many more kilometres per litre than others.
5. Is it reasonably dust-proof? Does it start well in cold weather?
6. Is it made in the country and can it be bought locally? Where countries manufacture vehicles, those made within the country are usually more appropriate than foreign models because:
   • They are cheaper to buy.
   • They are cheaper and easier to look after and spare parts may be obtained more easily.
   • They make the project look less foreign.
   • They may be available at a discount for registered charities.
   • There is no need for foreign exchange.
   However, locally made vehicles may be less strong or durable than foreign models. Second-hand vehicles should be carefully

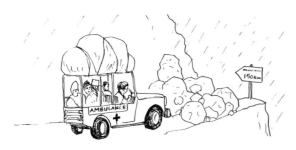

Figure 4.13   When choosing a project vehicle, consider the worst conditions it may have to encounter.

checked by a skilled mechanic before being bought.

7. Have seat belts been fitted? This is essential even if it is not the custom in the project area. Ensure the vehicle is regularly and expertly serviced. More development workers die in road accidents (many because of faulty vehicles, non-use of seat belts and drunken driving) than from any other cause.

Summary

When a project first receives requests to give help, several activities must be carried out and coordinated before fieldwork is actually begun.

This includes selecting an appropriate community, and selecting a suitable team on which so much of the project's future depends.

Funding needs to be obtained wherever possible from local and national sources before foreign agencies are approached. The goal of becoming financially self-sufficient should always be remembered.

A base needs to be established for storing supplies and setting up a project office. Accommodation for staff sometimes needs to be considered. The base should be within the target area or as near to it as possible so that the community can be involved in management at an early stage.

A list of essential equipment and drugs needs to be drawn up and supplies ordered in the correct amount from reliable sources. A refrigerator and steriliser will be needed and at some stage a four-wheel-drive vehicle will probably become necessary.

Further reading and resources

1. *Project Cycle Management*, Roots Book No. 5, Tearfund UK, 2003. Available in English, French, Spanish and Portuguese. Available from Tearfund. See Appendix E.
   An immensely useful book written from a practical viewpoint on many aspects of starting health and development programmes
2. *Fundraising*, Roots Book No. 6, Tearfund UK, 2004. Also available in above languages. Practical strategies on all aspects of fundraising.
3. *How to Look after a Refrigerator*, J. Elford, AHRTAG, 1992.
   Applies to kerosene, gas, electric, solar refrigerators. Available from: TALC. See Appendix E.
4. *How to Manage a Health Centre Store*, A. Battersby, AHRTAG, 1994, revised.
   Available from: TALC. See Appendix E.
5. *Care and Safe Use of Hospital Equipment*, M. Skeet and D. Fear, VSO, 1995.
   Available from: TALC. See Appendix E.
6. *Management Support for Primary Health Care*, P. Johnstone and J. Ranken, FSG Communications/ODA, 1994.
   This book has useful sections covering many aspects of this chapter. Limited supplies. Available from: TALC. See Appendix E.
7. *Good Driving, Safe Driving*, P. Stuart, Campion Press, 1998.
   Teaches good driving and maintenance, both of which can save the lives of workers and others. Available from: TALC. See Appendix E.
8. *Medical Supplies and Equipment for Primary Health Care*, M. Kaur and S. Hall, ECHO, 2001.
   All programmes should obtain a copy of this. Also produced on CD Rom. Available from: ECHO. See Appendix A.

The following two organisations publish lists of funding agencies:

- The Charities Aid Foundation,
  Kingshill, West Malling, Kent ME19 4TA, UK.
  Tel: + 44 (0) 1732 520000
  Fax: + 44 (0) 1732 520001
  Email: information@cafonline.org
  Website: www.cafonline.org
  CAF produces a wide range of information about fundraising, relevant for many countries of the world.
- The Directory of Social Change,
  24 Stephenson Way, London NW1 2DP, UK.
  Tel: + 44 (0) 207 209 5151
  Fax: + 44 (0) 207 209 5049
  Email: info@dsc.org.uk
  Website: www.dsc.org.uk.
  The DSC produces a huge range of information on fundraising as well as comprehensive publications giving details of grant-making trusts, companies and other sources of financial support.

CD Rom

Proposals that Make a Difference: How to write effective grant proposals – a manual for NGOs, Oxford Learning Space, 1998.
Expensive but very useful.
Available from: IT Publications. See Appendix E.

5

Learning about the Community

In this chapter we will be looking at the various ways we can get to know the community with which we will be partnering. Just how we do this will be different for each project. It will depend on factors such as how much trust we have already established, and how much information we need to gather. This chapter looks at two broad ways of learning about the community. The first is Participatory Appraisal, which collects a wide range of qualitative (descriptive) information. The second is a Community Survey and

Diagnosis, which provides more detailed quantitative information.

PARTICIPATORY APPRAISAL

In this section we will consider:
- What is Participatory Appraisal (PA)?
- Some basic principles

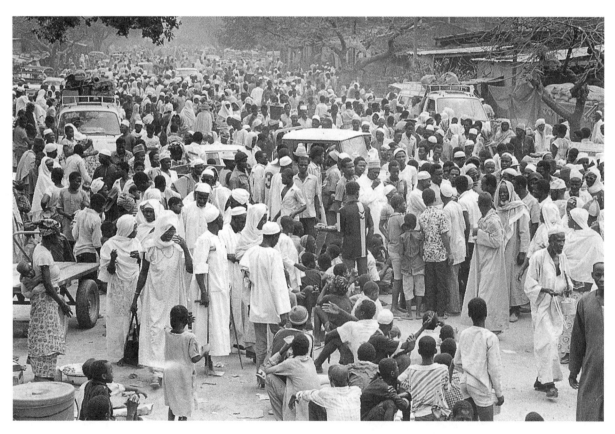

Figure 5.1 By the year 2000, half the population of developing countries was living in city communities. The photograph shows Ouagadougou, Burkina Faso, on a Friday.

- Deciding what information we need to find out
- Planning for PA
- Techniques used in PA
- How to analyse our information
- How to use our findings.

What is Participatory Appraisal (PA)?

PA is a method of gaining as much information as possible about a community in a limited period of time. PA is also sometimes known as Rural or Rapid Appraisal (RA) or Participatory Research and Action, or Participatory Rural Learning.

PA is often used early in a project to gain the general information needed to guide the way forward, help to write proposals and make preliminary plans. A survey often follows later when we need more detailed information so that we can discover the type and extent of the problems we wish to tackle. PA and surveys also give us a baseline for measuring our achievements when we come to resurvey at a later date. Each programme will need to select from the menu in this chapter the most appropriate way of gathering information and decide on the most appropriate sequence and timing.

Some basic principles

1. Explain to the community why we are wanting to gather information. Members may suspect our motives, or be surprised that yet another group is coming to ask questions. We need to ensure that both the community leaders and groups with whom we work understand why we have come.
2. Take care not to raise expectations. In poor communities, especially those who in the past have had donations, gifts and handouts, expectations can easily be raised by the mere mention of words such as health centres, medicines and doctors. People may jump to wrong conclusions and then be bitterly disappointed when the hoped-for benefit fails to occur.

Before meeting any individual or group we need to explain that nothing has yet been decided on; that we are gathering information so that with the community we can make future plans together.

3. Collect only as much information as is really essential. For every piece of information we gather we should answer these questions: What is the reason I need this data? Will knowing this data make any difference to the successful planning and implementation of the programme?
4. Carry out all activities with the full participation of the community. They should be involved at every stage: planning, training, carrying out the appraisal, presenting the results and drawing up plans.

PA must therefore be a joint effort that includes team members, the community and sometimes outside facilitators or experts. In countries with strong central control, as in the People's Republic of China, PA needs to be done in full partnership with government health workers and party cadres. PA works equally well in urban settings.

The purpose of gathering this information is to help the project choose the best ways of tackling health and development problems. It is not primarily to gain information for interest alone.

With the community involved at every stage, PA can generate interest and excitement as community members begin to understand the real nature of their problems, and even more important, realise that they can be part of the answer.

PA can take anything from a few days to several weeks, depending on the depth and scope of the analysis we need to make. One to two weeks would be a typical period of time for a new, small-scale programme.

Deciding what information we need to find out

PA needs to be planned carefully. Unless it answers the questions we want to know and builds relationships with the community, it will achieve little.

The information we are seeking may be a general understanding of how the community

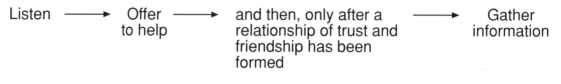

Listen ⟶ Offer to help ⟶ and then, only after a relationship of trust and friendship has been formed ⟶ Gather information

Figure 5.2

functions, its needs and wishes or it may be looking more specifically at one particular aspect, such as reasons for chronic malnutrition in children.

Here is a list of information it is useful to collect as a basis of understanding how a community functions. It should be adapted to the specific needs of each project:

1. **Family structure.** Marriage customs, including age at marriage, whether multiple partners, dowry customs. Authority figures in the family. Attitudes to the elderly, to in-laws and to children. Connection with tribe and extended family.
2. **Social patterns.** Power structures in the community. Leadership – formal and informal. Political, religious and economic groupings in the community. Caste, tribal grouping and its practical results. Ways by which disputes are sorted out. How the community makes a joint decision. Status and what determines it – wealth, land, education or tradition.
3. **Religion.** Beliefs and how they affect lifestyles, attitudes to others, to the environment and to health and nutrition. Local and national festivals: how and when they are celebrated.
4. **Daily routines.** Ways in which different members of the family spend their day. How work is divided among family members. School attendance among the children and attitudes towards it. Employment patterns of men, women and children.
5. **Yearly pattern of climate and farming.** When the rainy season starts and finishes. Months for ploughing, sowing and harvesting. Types of crop grown. Ways of coping with harvest failure. Use of labour – both outsiders coming in at busy times and insiders seeking outside work at less busy times of the year.
6. **Relation to nearest city or large town.** Whether used for employment, leisure or crime. Whether young people are leaving or wishing to leave their village or community.
7. **Health-related beliefs and practices.** Traditional beliefs about what (or who) causes and cures illness. Attitudes to traditional healers and remedies, and towards modern medicines and health workers. Whether health needs are considered a priority.
8. **Details of other programmes.** Past and present government programmes in health, agriculture and related development. How these are viewed. Details of other NGOs currently or recently working in the community. Achievements they have made and the community's perceptions. Location and effectiveness of nearest health posts, primary health centres or hospital.
9. **Causes of poverty.** Overall degree of poverty. Difference in earning power, lifestyle, ownership of land and animals between richest and poorest. Outside constraints that lock the community into poverty. Community problems that block solutions (see also Figure 1.6 on page 10).
10. **With urban programmes:** in addition, we need to discover how people are employed, the state of the environment including details on water, sanitation and garbage collection; specific hazards including threats to women and children; levels of crime, violence and prostitution; local power structures.

Planning for PA

For PA to be successful we need to think carefully about the best way of carrying it out in our own situations. For a detailed PA we can follow these phases (small-scale PA can be kept simpler and shorter: move to the next section – Techniques used in PA):

1. **Defining the objective.**

   Why are we doing the PA? This will inform what information we need to collect and what we do with it. PA is an active tool designed for later community action, so we want to gather only the information that is useful and relevant.

2. **Choosing the most appropriate techniques for the information we require.**

   This will include deciding the best methods for collecting each type of information we need. Identifying sources of information and listing topics for questions or interviews will always be part of this.

3. **Training the team.**

   The team will need training, ideally from someone with previous field experience of PA. Training should include how we can relate to the community, the best ways of asking questions, and how to use the various forms of PA described later. Training in how to conduct interviews and focus groups is especially useful.

   Because the community should be fully involved with PA, encourage them to send one or two intelligent members (e.g. high school students) to join in the training. A combined project/community team of three to six is a good number, ideally from different backgrounds and with differing areas of interest.

4. **Collating information by category.**

   PA generates large amounts of information. It is helpful if broad categories can be decided beforehand so that information can be written down under those categories. This helps systematic thinking and makes the analysis of information easier when PA is completed.

   We should choose categories that fit in with the particular information we wish to collect. Examples of categories might be: common causes of illness; reasons for low uptake of existing health services; causes of economic hardship (external and internal) affecting community members.

   We can also use the broad headings 1 to 10 from the previous section.

5. **Practicals.**

   This will include details such as: dates to begin, for mid-term reviews, for completion. Coordinating with community events and deciding on convenient times of day and seasons of year. Liaison with community about locations, facilities, and availability of participating members.

Techniques used in PA

Whichever technique we use, participants will need to remember, record in a notebook and reflect on information gathered each day.

1. **Simple, direct observation.**

   As we visit, drink tea, walk the paths and play with the children we are constantly observing and raising questions. We should record significant things we have heard, incidents we have seen and perceptions we have gathered. Later these will be compared with other observers.

2. **Semi-structured interviews.**

   These are informal interviews with various community members based on a checklist of questions we write down beforehand. By interviewing people of different backgrounds, wealth and age we can obtain a variety of information from different viewpoints.

   a) With key informants.

   We select several key members of the community.

   For example: When recently carrying out PA in a remote area of western China, we arranged for a Chinese government health official and project member jointly to interview a village doctor, a traditional birth attendant, the village chief and the local teacher.

   Secrets of success: The interviewer must be fluent in the local language or have a skilled interpreter. Choose a quiet location; introduce yourself and explain the purpose of the interview; have a checklist of questions to be answered but allow the answers to emerge through free-flowing conversation and appropriate prompting; allow 45–60 minutes; thank the informant; record answers during the interview or immediately afterwards.

   Key informant interviews tend to give an overall impression of the way things are –

or of the way the informants wish they should be. Information needs to be checked through other approaches.

'Useful' community members

Most communities contain 4 groups of people:
Gatekeepers – who decide what new people and new ideas are acceptable to the community.
Caretakers – to whom people turn when they have problems.
Newscatchers – who always know what is going on.
Brokers – who know key people and can get things done.
Together these people can be the change-makers in a community.

---

b) With community members.
   Information from key informants can be checked by similar interviews with other community members.
   The techniques are similar. It is valuable to include a cross-section of the community. *For example*: A teenage student, a middle aged woman and man, a member of the poorest subgroup, and one elderly person who can also give a historical perspective.
   We must be careful not to threaten or intimidate those we question. Sometimes one-to-one interviews are most appropriate, sometimes two-to-two, allowing a livelier discussion and helping to draw out different viewpoints.

c) With patients who have chronic illness.
   Most communities will have members who have had years of poor health and tried numerous remedies.
   For example: An in-depth discussion with a person living with HIV/AIDS or TB can reveal the full effects this disease has had on the patient's life, work, family and relationship with the community.

3. **Focus groups.**
   Focus groups are gatherings of between six to twelve people from similar backgrounds, discussing a particular topic under the guidance of a trained facilitator.
   They are a valuable tool in Community Based Health Care (CBHC) at various stages in project planning and evaluation. They are especially useful in PA. Two useful questions for focus groups are:
   • What are the main problems affecting your community?
   • How do you think those problems can be solved?
   These questions could both be asked in one meeting. As each problem is raised, members of the focus group suggest answers. Alternatively, two meetings could be held, one for problems, the other for solutions, with summarised notes from the first available to guide discussion in the second.
   Secrets of success: members should have similar backgrounds or interest, e.g. village women from a similar income group, landless labourers, nomadic herdsmen; the location should be quiet, comfortable and convenient; refreshments should be arranged; the facilitator explains the topic, ensures it is adhered to, encourages all to participate, prompts relevant questions and steers the discussion into productive approaches; detailed notes are recorded. See also page 22.

4. **Village or slum mapping.**
   This is a way of making community health enjoyable for all. Many members can get involved, leading to a lively discussion and fresh insights into community life. Mapping provides a surprising amount of information and is an excellent tool for involving a wide range of community members.
   Maps are best made on a flat piece of ground or, in the case of smaller groups, on a large piece of paper. Ideally, men, women and children should join in together. That is not always possible. *For example*: at a recent mapping in Ethiopia a crowd of up to 60 gathered spontaneously. Men did the mapping and the map size grew to 15 metres by 10. Meanwhile, the children who had been chased away by the men started making their own map. The two maps when added together gave valuable insights, the men tending to see the village from an economic viewpoint, the children more from a human and educational viewpoint.
   A special form of mapping known as Risk Mapping can be very valuable in areas prone

to floods, hurricanes, earthquakes or ethnic conflict. Buildings, water supplies, or vulnerable people and escape routes can be identified so that a community plan can be drawn up to help give special protection if a crisis occurs.

Secrets of success: choose an appropriate flat location, preferably out of the sun, wind and rain; gather materials (e.g. chalk or charcoal); explain either spontaneously or ahead of time the purpose of making a map; encourage the community to select two or three intelligent members who can draw the map and respond to instructions from the onlookers; agree symbols for different village facilities, e.g. for water sources, latrines, school; stones, coloured powders, leaves, twigs would be appropriate symbols in poor rural communities; allow at least one hour for the mapping, and up to two to three further hours if discussion follows; have someone copy the map onto paper or into a notebook, or, in addition, have it photographed, ideally with a digital camera as the process takes place.

Mapping will raise many interesting issues, which can be further discussed in focus groups, village meetings and can contribute to future action plans.

5. **Seasonal Health Calendars.**
   Community members can construct these. An example is shown in Figure 5.3. They are most useful when space for different variables such as rainfall, food availability and levels of sickness can be seen side by side.

   The calendar constructed in Sierra Leone (see Figure 5.3) showed that people often fell sick at three particular times: when there is most work to be done, least food to eat, and least money available for treatment.

   This information helps us to plan health programmes so they are as effective as possible.

6. **Daily activity charts.**
   Women and men can be asked to list out their normal daily activities. This alone gives a powerful picture of village life and raises numerous ideas for discussion and action. Table 5.1 shows a report by the Swedish International Development Agency from such an exercise carried out in sub-Saharan Africa.

7. **Review of existing records.**
   We can gain very useful information about disease patterns, etc. by reading through hospital and clinic records and other information kept in the community.

How to analyse our information

It is never easy to analyse a mass of information collected by several people from a variety of sources. Here are some suggestions:

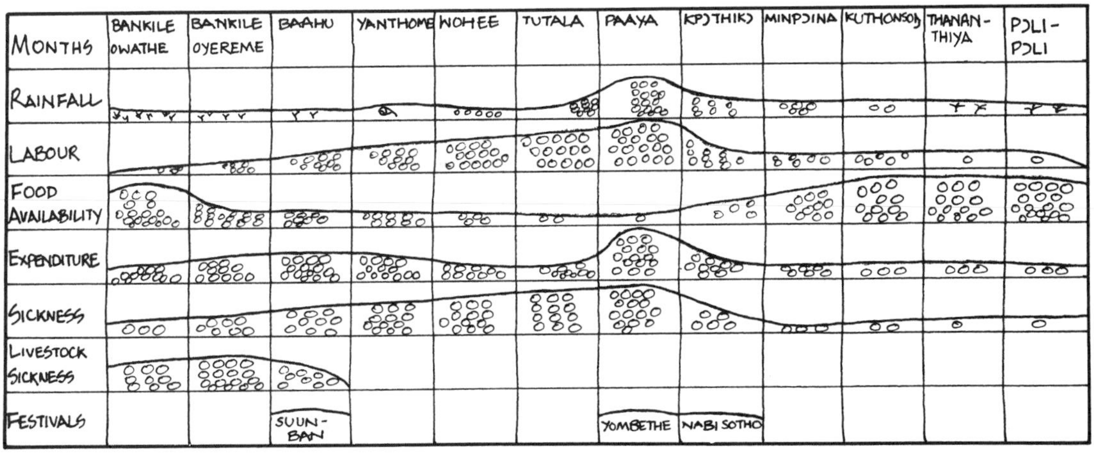

Figure 5.3   A seasonal health calendar made by young men in the village of Bubuya, Sierra Leone, through an Action Aid project.

Table 5.1   A woman's day or a man's day?

Woman's day	Man's day
Rises first	Rises when breakfast is ready
Kindles the fire	Eats
Breast-feeds baby	Walks 1 km to cotton field
Fixes breakfast/eats	Works in the field
Washes and dresses the children	Eats when wife arrives with food
Walks 1 km to fetch water	Works in the field
Walks 1 km home	Walks 1 km home
Gives the livestock feed and water	Eats
Washes cooking utensils, etc	Rests
Walks 1 km to fetch water	Walks to village to visit other men
Walks 1 km home	Walks home
Washes clothing	Goes to bed
Breast-feeds baby	
Pounds rice	
Sweeps the house and compound	
Kindles the fire	
Prepares meal/eats	
Breast-feeds baby	
Walks 1 km to cotton field with food for husband	
Walks 1 km back home	
Walks 1 km to her field	
Weeds field	
Breast-feeds baby	
Gathers firewood on the way home	
Walks 1 km home	
Pounds maize	
Walks 1 km to fetch water	
Walks 1 km home	
Kindles the fire	
Prepares meal/eats	
Breast-feeds baby	
Puts house in order	
Goes to bed last	

Source: *Safe Motherhood*, Issue 14 March–June 1994, originally from the Swedish International Development Agency.

- **Triangulation.** Ideally, important information collected from one source is validated or rejected by checking data from two other sources.
- **Daily recording.** Each observer records information at the time of the activity or immediately afterwards. Where possible they use the categories discussed at the PA training (see earlier).
- **Daily ranking.** Within 24 hours, observers rank or prioritise information under categories or using clear headings.

- **Numerical information.** This could include, for example: the number of patients attending the nearest health post per month, the number of children under five who have died in the past twelve months.
- **Workshop for all participants.** This is the forum where each individual presents findings as far as possible by category and rank. It is helpful if each person brings a legible summary of the main findings. During the workshop, information can be headlined and compared on flipcharts.

- **Summary report.** One or two members can document the information in report form using participants' written information and flipchart papers.
- **Report finalised.** Ideally the draft should be shared with all main participants to make sure nothing important has been left out or mistakes been made before the final document is produced.

How to use our findings

PA is a time-consuming exercise and the information we gain needs to be shared and used as widely as possible. The following groups can benefit:

1. **The PA observers**

   We can arrange a further workshop to present and discuss the findings. Other community members (if already appointed), such as CHWs, Village Health Committee members or teachers can be included, as well as health team members. Key points can then be fed into the programme's management process.

2. **The community**

   We should share results with the whole community. This is an important occasion when new information, new ideas and threatening implications may emerge, especially in urban settings. It may be helpful to meet with community leaders first, then a short time afterwards to meet with the community as a whole. *A word of warning: One project in Nepal recently carried out a detailed PA in many villages over several months. In the community feedback a village woman asked: 'Why have you brought an empty "doko" to our village?' (A doko is a traditional Nepali basket slung on the back.)*

   This incident highlights two dangers: The first is raising expectations through the whole process of PA. Ideas discussed are often taken as promises made; disappointment can be bitter when little seems to change. The second is the danger of much talk and little action. Many communities are crying out for basic necessities.

3. **The donor agencies**

   Agencies are usually pleased when we send them PA summaries. Information gained can also be used to complete the detailed application forms necessary to obtain funding (pages 63–65).

4. **Evaluation and research**

   Although ideally PA is done before programmes start, in modified form and with altered objectives PA can be repeated as a part of project evaluation (see Chapter 18).

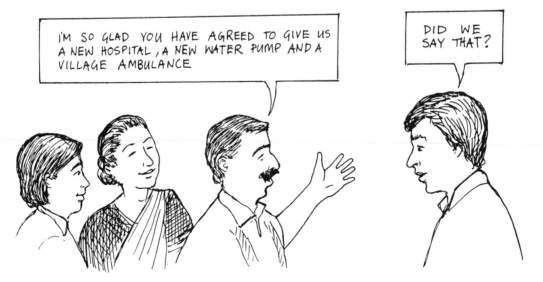

Figure 5.4   Ideas discussed in meetings are often taken as promises by the community.

Larger programmes may be able to use the information for research. *For example*: by linking with a student or faculty at a college or university, or by a student or researcher visiting from a different country or region.

5. **Government health services**
   The results of the PA can be shared with the District Medical Officer, District Management Team, or more local equivalents. Other government departments such as Agriculture, Education and Natural Resources can also be informed. The information gathered from PA will cross all developmental boundaries and help to stimulate a combined approach to problems of poverty. This helps to bring about one of CBHC's key aims – 'intersectoral collaboration'.

COMMUNITY SURVEY AND DIAGNOSIS

We may already have carried out PA and agreed together with the community about areas for joint action. Even if we have done this, a community survey gives more accurate, numerical, information and forms a valuable base for a longer-term programme.

A word of warning: Many communities have developed 'survey fatigue', especially if located in main cities or near main road or rail connections. Numerous outsiders may have arrived, notebooks in hand, asked questions, made vague promises, then disappeared.

THE COMMUNITY SURVEY

In this section we shall consider:
1. What we need to know
   • Why a survey is necessary
   • Types of survey that can be done
   • Who should do the survey?
   • When should the survey be done?
2. What we need to do
   • Prepare materials
   • Train the survey team

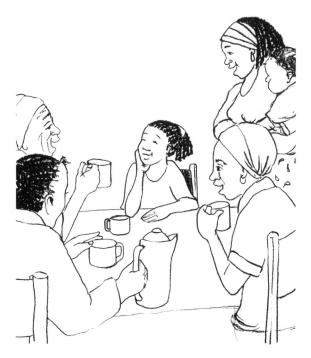

Figure 5.5   At the start of a project, it is important to get to know community members.

   • Carry out the survey
   • Use the results

What we need to know

Why a survey is necessary

There are several reasons for doing surveys:
1. **To discover the main health needs of the community.**
   Accurate baseline information on the community's health and population structure is best obtained before we help to bring solutions. Then by resurveying after a period of time, say three or five years later, we can estimate how much progress has been made.
2. **To discover those individuals and families with the greatest health needs.**

> This means that, at the start of a project, health workers may spend much of their time getting to know community members, playing with their children or challenging young people at the local sport. This is not time wasted.

They will usually include:

- children under five, especially those shown to be malnourished on the Growth Chart;
- pregnant and breastfeeding women;
- those with serious, chronic illnesses such as TB, leprosy and HIV/AIDS;
- the physically and mentally disabled; the elderly;
- any group, family or individual who is socially outcast, very poor, or abusing drugs.

3. **To build relationships.**

A survey done in a relaxed and friendly manner will help to build friendships and create trust. It will prove a good 'starter subject' for community participation (see Chapter 2).

4. **To teach and create awareness.**

We will have a chance to discuss health problems with individual families and create awareness about how they can be solved. We can encourage people to come forward for Voluntary Counselling and Testing (VCT), in areas where HIV/AIDS is common or on the increase.

Types of survey that can be done

There are several types of survey that can be carried out in CBHC, for example, surveys designed for evaluation (see Chapter 18). This chapter describes common types of community survey.

1. **Comprehensive surveys.**

Every home is visited and questions are asked concerning all family members.

The main advantages are that all individuals at risk can be discovered and comprehensive care can be started without delay. Information obtained is also more complete.

The main disadvantage is the length of time it takes.

2. **Sample surveys.**

Some, but not all, households are visited. Every fifth or tenth house can be chosen or houses selected at random, using a random number chart.

Sample surveys are used either if numbers in the project are very large or if a quick, initial survey at the time of fundraising is needed (see Chapter 4, page 63).

3. **Mixed surveys.**

Here we may visit each house to record certain important information such as the weight or mid-upper arm circumference of the children, but only some houses to record other details such as socioeconomic data (see pages 63–65).

4. **Pilot surveys.**

These are small-scale surveys carried out at the start of a project, either to estimate the needs of the people, obtain an approximate census or to pretest a surveying technique. All comprehensive surveys should be piloted first.

Who should do the survey?

Project and community members should work together. *For example*: A project member can record answers, a community member find out information.

The project member will need to be:

- open and friendly in manner;
- exact and neat in recording.

The community member could be one of the following:

- a community health worker, or Village Health Committee member;
- a high school student;
- any community member with a genuine interest and wanting to help for the right reasons.

Usually the community should select the surveyor.

When should the survey be done?

This will need to be:

1. **When the community is ready for it.**

We should make sure the community understands the reason for the survey and is ready to participate. A suspicious or unwilling community may give inaccurate answers.

If we have not done Participatory Appraisal (PA), the survey can be done at an early stage, and combined with some PA techniques. If, however, PA has been carried out and led to successful action, the survey can be done later and for a clearly defined purpose.

2. **When the project has enough resources.**
   At the very least we will need:
   • team member(s) who have been trained in surveying;
   • survey materials including forms or family folders;
   • time to do the job properly;
   • the ability to work with the community in response to the needs discovered;
   • sufficient funding.
3. **At a time of day and a time of year** when most people are at home, and not too busy with other activities, such as harvesting or seasonal employment.

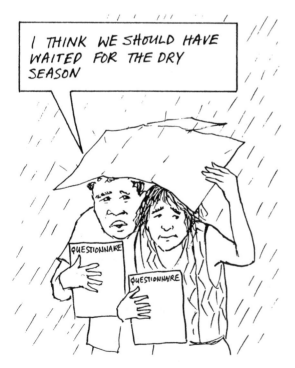

Figure 5.6

What we need to do

Prepare materials

Follow these guidelines:
1. **Decide what information needs to be gathered.**
   Such information should be:
   • Useful.
     Will it help in making plans?
     Can it be used to bring about improvements?

Great care must be taken that when doing surveys we do not falsely raise the people's expectations nor create hopes that cannot be met. Surveying a community carries with it an obligation to work with that community on the problems that are discovered (see Chapter 6).

   • Easily gathered.
     Questions should be simple to ask and easy to record. Where possible, answers should be yes, no, a number or a single word. This makes it much easier to analyse the data (see page 90 and Chapter 6).
2. **Study and adapt existing survey forms.**
   Find out if the government or any voluntary health association or nearby projects have materials available. Study the sample form given in Appendix F, and see if that or any other forms can be adapted and used. This can save a lot of time.
   If we are planning to do research or a detailed evaluation later, it is worth designing the form with the help of someone who understands statistics. If we plan to use a computer for analysis, the form must be compatible with (or the same as) the data input screen.
3. **Collect the materials needed.**
   Each surveyor must have:
   • A list of questions.
     These will need to be carefully worded so that the answers obtained are valid.
     For example:
     If we are enquiring about cough in a suspected TB patient, there are many ways we could ask a question:
     • Do you have a cough?

- Do you cough often?
- Have you been coughing for a long time?
- Have you been coughing for more than three weeks?

The last of these will give the most valid or useful answer in trying to discover which people have TB.

In order for all answers to be consistent, the same question must be asked to each community member with the same wording. If different team members use different questions (like those about coughing) answers cannot be compared and the results will not be accurate.

- A family folder.

This is made of stout paper and details about family members are filled in on the front. Other details such as those on socio-economic conditions can be recorded on the back or the inside. Each family has its own folder (see Appendix F for an example). This has proved to be useful in a number of projects but can be very time-taking when population numbers are high or when other documentation is needed for specific programmes.

- Insert cards.

If we use the family folder system, these will be needed for comprehensive surveys. Whenever a family member is found whose health is at risk, details are recorded on an insert card, which is then placed in the family folder (see pages 158–9).

In order to keep forms tidy it is better to record answers in pencil first and ink them in later when the survey is complete and folders have been checked.

4. **Obtain or make a community map, if possible.**

Train the survey team

Surveyors should be trained in two basic skills:

1. Relating to the community.
   Surveyors must be:
   - friendly so that they will be able to build lasting relationships with the community members they visit;
   - tactful so that they can ask questions without causing offence;
   - persistent so that they obtain the answers they need;
   - discreet so that they do not gossip about the health problems of those they visit.

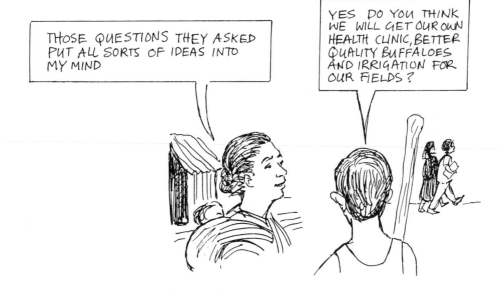

Figure 5.7   Surveys can easily raise false hopes in the community.

Before asking questions the surveyors will need to explain who they are, where they are from and why they are doing the survey. This will be easier when a community member is part of the survey team and has been involved in planning and design.

Survey skills are effectively taught by role play in the classroom (see page 45).

2. Obtaining the information.
   Surveyors will need to learn:
   • Questioning, both what to ask and how to ask it. They should carry a list until they have reliably memorised the correct wording for each question.
   • Recording, making sure that each answer is written down correctly (see page 88).
   • Measuring, e.g. the mid-upper arm circumference (MUAC) of children aged one to five, or the child's weight or anything else required.
   Skills should be practised until mistakes are no longer made.

The training described will take place before the survey is started in the community.

During the survey the supervisor should accompany surveyors until they are confident and accurate.

After the survey the supervisor should check through the survey cards. Any mistakes should be discussed with the surveyor. If accurate answers have not been obtained, the surveyor should be asked to resurvey the family in question.

Team members, unless carefully trained, will tend to make many mistakes in surveying. We should start by training several team and community members and then select those who show the greatest interest and ability to become future 'survey specialists'.

Carry out the survey

The stages are as follows:

1. First arrange a day well in advance, inform the people and coordinate with community partners.
2. Work in pairs, a team member and community volunteer working together.
3. Decide on a numbering system for the houses with the survey teams before starting. If this is

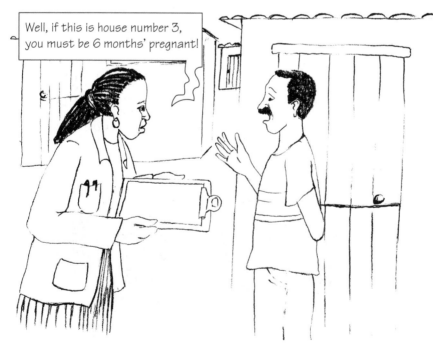

Figure 5.8   Numbering systems need to be checked before you start the survey.

forgotten, several houses can end up with the same code number.

Numbering often causes problems. Frequently houses have no numbers or else numbers change as extra houses are built. If a permanent numbering system exists, use that. If there is no such system devise one and make sure each family records and remembers its health survey number. Mark the number on the outside of the house (with the owner's permission) for the convenience of visiting health workers.

4. At the start allow at least five minutes per family member. This may be shortened later.
5. Then do the survey.

The model described here can be used or shortened. Each project should adapt methods and forms to suit its own situation.

Data to be gathered

The following information is recorded (letters in text headings correspond to those on the sample folder in Appendix F and in Figures 5.9, 5.10 and 5.11). Note: this is just one example developed by a particular project and we need to adapt or construct a form entirely appropriate for our own area.

a) Name, address, etc.

1. Name, address, and occupation of the head of the family.
2. Code number of the family.
   A useful method is to construct a code with three sets of digits. The first set represents the health centre code, the second the community code and the third the house code. For example:

03/10/46. A fourth set can be added to define individuals. For example: 03/10/46/01 would be the code number of the head of the family of the forty-sixth house in the tenth community of the target area of the third health centre.

b) Felt problems

What are the main problems affecting your family? This is probably the best wording to use and is asked as the very first question of the survey before the answers have been influenced by other health-related questions.

c) Family profile

1. Names of family members.
   Enter these in a logical order by starting with the head of the family, his wife or partner, the oldest son, his wife and children, the second oldest son, etc. Elderly relatives can be added either at the beginning or the end.
   In many communities this can be surprisingly difficult. Children may be known by several different names, or only given a permanent name after a certain age.
2. Ages.
   Children under five years should have the month and year of their birth recorded accurately to help in preparing growth charts. Those over five years can simply have their age recorded.
   If ages cannot be easily remembered make a 'local events calendar' where seasons and annual events are marked to help parents remember the time of year their children were born. Check that the age the parents give broadly corresponds with the appearance of the child.

(c) FAMILY PROFILE

No.	Name	Age/DoB	Sex	Relation to head	Relation to each other
01	MOHAMMED	65	M		
02	HASSAN	34	M	Son	
03	FATIMA	25	F	Daughter in law	Wife of 02
04	ALI	4 Nov'05	M	Grandson	Eldest son of 02 + 03

Figure 5.9   Family profile section of survey form.

3. Sexes.
4. Relationships.

These can be written in two columns:
The first records the relationship to the head of the family.

The second need only be used for large or extended families. It records how different members are related to each other. *For example*: Which wife is married to which husband, or which child belongs to which parents, etc.

d) Diseases

1. Suspected infection with TB, leprosy.

Other locally serious diseases can be included. We will need tact where people are sensitive about a disease and should be careful not to offend. This is especially the case for people living with HIV/AIDS and this should be recorded only with permission and in areas where little stigma remains.

2. Nutritional status of under-fives.

This can be found out only by careful measuring. There is little value in simply asking questions or just looking at the child.

Children can either be weighed or have their mid-upper arm circumference (MUAC) measured with a measuring strip (see Chapter 9 pages 175–7).

e) Immunisation

This will usually include the original six diseases covered by WHO's Expanded Programme on Immunisation (EPI):

1. BCG (for TB), DPT (diphtheria, pertussis, tetanus), polio, measles – for children.
2. Tetanus toxoid – for women of childbearing age.

Other diseases for which immunisation is given locally can also be included, e.g. hepatitis B, typhoid, yellow fever, meningitis. With polio nearly eradicated, follow any national guidelines on whether polio immunisation is still needed and if so which type to use.

Only record positive answers if certain that the complete course has been given. It is helpful to record the year in which each immunisation was completed. BCG scars can be looked for.

Many parents will be unable to give accurate answers. Where immunisation has already been started by the project, the immunisation register, or other records, can be used to help fill in this part of the survey (see Chapter 10 page 205).

f) Family planning

This is often a sensitive subject, in which case it can be done later when trust has been established and a Family Planning Worker trained (see Chapter 13).

No.	Name	Age/DoB	(d) DISEASES				(e) IMMUNISATION			Measles	Tet tox
			TB	Lep	Eye	<5nutr.	BCG	DPT	Polio		
01	MOHAMMED	65	1	0	0	0	0	0	0	0	0
02	HASSAN	34	0	0	1	0	0	0	0	0	0
03	FATIMA	25	0	0	0	0	0	0	0	0	1
04	ALI	4 Nov'05	0	0	0	1	1	0	0	0	0

Figure 5.10   Disease and immunisation sections of survey form.

1. Record year of tubectomy or vasectomy.
2. Record whether oral contraceptive pill, coil, barrier or other method is being used now.
3. Record if currently pregnant.
   This is useful to know only if antenatal care is being offered. Sensitivity is obviously needed.
4. Record if eligible for family planning.
   Those eligible are usually defined as (married or partnered) women from 15 to 49 who have not had a tubectomy or whose regular partner has not had a vasectomy.

g) Addiction

This covers smoking, drinking, or other drug abuse. Define the lower age limit, e.g. 10 or 15 in rural areas, 6 or 10 in cities. Ask about every family member over that age. Again we will need tact in asking these questions and in some communities it will not be advisable.

h) Education

1. Adult literacy
   One common definition is those aged 15 or over who can read or write. Male and female will later be separated in the tally (see page 90).
2. School attendance
   This commonly applies to children between 5 and 19 inclusive. Record the grade attended at the time of the survey (or the highest grade attended if no longer at school).

The level of education, especially female literacy, has an important effect on health.

i) Deaths in the previous 12 months

Record age, sex and cause of death. This needs to be as accurate a cause or description as possible.

> Deaths in the past year are often underreported. The family may not want to talk about them; they may not consider deaths in the first few days of life worth mentioning or they may report only the deaths of sons.

This means that, if we are using verbal reports of deaths within the last year to calculate mortality rates before the project starts, we will need to ensure they are accurately reported. If underrecorded, the original state of health of the community will seem better than it really is, meaning that any improvements brought about through the project will be underestimated.

j) Use of existing services

1. Who and where does the family attend when sick?
2. Who delivers babies?

k) Water supply

1. Type, distance and number of months functioning in year of main water supply (and alternative).

No.	Name	Age/DoB	Tub	Vas	O/C pill	Coil	If preg nant	Eligible FP	Alcohol ↓ Tobacco		Adult literacy	School	Remarks
01	MOHAMMED	65	O	o	o	o	o	o	o	1	1	o	Stroke 2 years ago. can walk in house
02	HASSAN	34	O	o	o	O	O	o	o	1	1	o	
03	FATIMA	25	o	o	o	O	1	1	o	o	o	o	
04	ALI	4 Nov'05	O	o	o	O	o	o	o	o	o	1	Twin Brother died at birth

Figure 5.11 Family planning, addiction and education sections of survey form.

2. How much water collected daily per person or household.

l) Sanitation

Method of human waste disposal used by the family.

m) Diet

For each main food source:
1. Number of months eaten per year.
2. Number of months grown by family, and number of months bought by family from outside.

Estimated socioeconomic status

1 is the richest subgroup, 5 the poorest. Try to estimate this for each family, or ask questions such as:

1. Type of housing and number of rooms.
2. Types and numbers of animals.
3. Area and quality of land owned.

This information helps us later to target resources to those most in need and shows which families might be eligible for reduced clinic rates or subsidies.

For details on how to complete 'Vital Events Since Survey' see Chapter 8, page 159.

Symbols used in recording

There is no value in asking carefully worded questions unless the answers are also recorded accurately. Each surveyor must record with care and use the same symbols.

- 0 can be written for a negative answer.
- 1 can be written for a positive answer.
- ? can be written if an answer is not known or a family member was absent. This can be altered when the answer is known.
- n/a can be written where the question does not apply.

Numbers can be written, e.g. for school grade attained.

Dates can be written, e.g. for year tubectomy performed or year an immunisation was completed.

No space should be left blank as this can mean one of two things – either that the question could not be asked (e.g. because a family member was absent) or that the questioner forgot to fill in the answer. When blanks are left, statistics, such as those for child nutrition, quickly become inaccurate.

Where an answer is descriptive (as in 'Felt problems') the key words or ideas can be recorded.

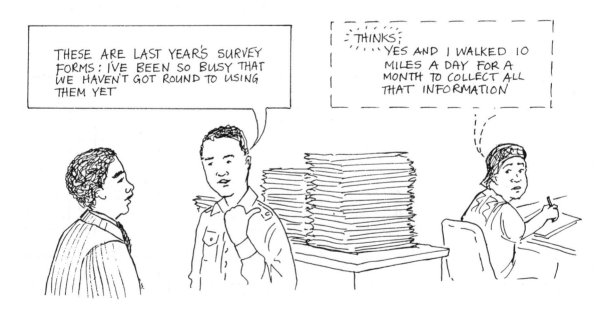

Figure 5.12

Use the results

Having completed the survey the results must now be used, not stored away and forgotten.

The results are analysed to make a community diagnosis (see the next section) and then discussed with the community to draw up a community plan (see Chapter 6).

COMMUNITY DIAGNOSIS

In this section we shall consider:
1. What we need to know
   - What community diagnosis means
   - Sources of information needed
2. What we need to do
   - Tally the results
   - Tabulate the results
   - Present the findings
   - List problems
   - Use of computers in data collection

What we need to know

What community diagnosis means

Just as we question and examine a patient to help find a diagnosis, so we can do the same for a community. In this way we can discover its main health problems, their underlying causes, and explore possible solutions with community members.

Sources of information needed

The main sources are:
1. The Participatory Appraisal, which provides descriptive or qualitative information.
2. The Community Survey, which gives numerical, quantitative or 'hard data' about the health of the community.

We may gain further information from previous reports and hospital or clinic records.

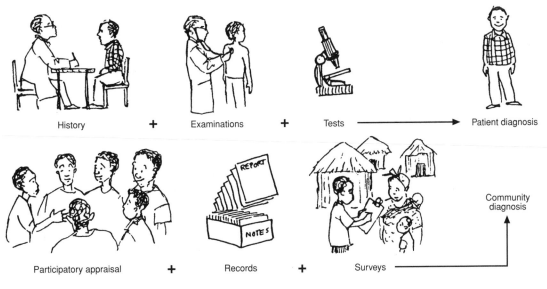

History   +   Examinations   +   Tests   ⟶   Patient diagnosis

Participatory appraisal   +   Records   +   Surveys ⟶ Community diagnosis

Figure 5.13   Community diagnosis.

What we need to do

Tally the results

A tally (see page 91) is a simple method of adding up. From each family folder, the totals for each subject are marked on the tally.
For example:
II means 2
IIII means 4
JHT means 5
JHT III means 8.

Tabulate the results

The totals from the tally are now tabulated on to a community diagnosis form. Figures 5.14 and 5.15 are examples used by one health programme but we need to ensure the design and contents are appropriate for our own programme

For example: For each community we will need to know the total number of malnourished children under five. This will be the numerator (N) or actual number.

We will also want to know the total number of children under five (both malnourished and well-nourished together). This will be the denominator (D) or eligible number.

Percentages (100 N/D) convey the most useful information. They give a picture of how serious a problem is at any one time. By comparing percentages over a period of time we are able to tell how much improvement has occurred. Often in practice the denominator is left out, which greatly reduces the value of any data and makes it harder to measure achievements.

Present the findings

We will soon need to present information to others such as community members, donors or government. This can be done through graphs, bar charts, pictograms and pie charts.

Literate community members may understand percentages, bar charts and graphs. See the Further reading and resources list for books that explain how to do this. However, it is important to make sure that illiterate members also understand the results of the survey. *For example*:

Percentages can be described as cents in the dollar or pennies in the pound, etc. Pictograms can be used (see Figure 5.16).

List problems

This involves drawing up a list of serious problems for each community surveyed. This is best done by the surveyor(s) in discussion with the team leader.

The Community Diagnosis form contains space both for figures from the tally, and written observations from the surveyor. Both are taken into account when drawing up the problem list.

Once we have gathered information from the PA and/or from a community survey, we have the basic information with which to start drawing up plans with the community. This is the subject of Chapter 6.

Use of computers in data collection

We need to be fully aware of the advantages and disadvantages before rushing into computerising our project statistics.

Advantages:
- They can process large amounts of information quickly and efficiently.
- They can generate effective reports.
- They can provide a range of support to the programme as listed under 'useful activities' (see page 93).
- Paperwork needed for community activities can be matched with data fields on the computer, making it possible to print off report forms, due lists, etc. for field work. On return from the field, data can be easily entered from the paper record back onto the identical data field.

Disadvantages:
- They can dominate the working of a programme. Team members can become more interested in computers than village paths, or slum alleys, with bad effects on community partnership.

TALLY SHEET

Name of village   Date of survey   Name of surveyor

....

				First Total	This column for later adjustments	Final Total

Total population .... M .... F ....

			First Total	This column for later adjustments	Final Total
AGE OF POPULATION	0 – 1	M / F			
	1 – 4	M / F			
	5 – 9	M / F			
	10 – 19	M / F			
	20 – 29	M / F			
	30 – 39	M / F			
	40 – 49	M / F			
	50 – 59	M / F			
	60 – 69	M / F			
	70 – 79	M / F			
	80 – 89	M / F			
DISEASES & UNDER 5 NUTRITION	TB				
	Leprosy				
	Eyes				
	M Don't know				
	U Green				
	A Yellow				
	C Red				
IMMUNI-SATION	BCG				
	DPT/Polio				
	Measles				
	Tet Tox				
FAMILY PLANNING	Tub.				
	Vas.				
	o/c Pill				
	Coil				
	Pregnant				
	Eligible FP				
ADDIC-TION	Alcohol	M			
		F			
	Tobacco	M			
		F			
EDUCATION	Adult	M			
	Literacy	F			
	School	M			
	Attendance	F			

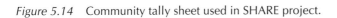

Figure 5.14   Community tally sheet used in SHARE project.

COMMUNITY DIAGNOSIS FORM

Name of village ....   Name of CHW ....

Name of supervisor ....   Name of Chief ....

Names of VHC members ....

....

INFORMATION FORM FIRST HOUSE TO HOUSE SURVEY   DATE _____

(a) Basic statistics

	Actual	Numbers Eligible	Percentage
Total population _____			
No. male _____			
No. female _____			
Total number of families _____			
Suspected tuberculosis _____			
Suspected leprosy _____			
Current eye problems _____			
Under 5 malnutrition (Red MUAC) _____			
(Yellow MUAC) _____			
No. BCG _____			
No. Completed DPT, Polio _____			
No. measles _____			
No. completed Tet Tox _____			
No. Tubectomy _____			
No. vasectomy _____			
No. o/c pill _____			
No. coil _____			
No. pregnant _____			
No. Eligible for family planning _____			
No. drinking (8 and over) _____			
No. smoking (8 and over) _____			
Total number literate (15 and over) _____			
No. male literate (15 and over) _____			
No. female literate (15 and over) _____			
Total number at school (5-19) _____			
No. boys at school (5-19) _____			
No. girls at school (5-19) _____			

Deaths in the last 12 months   Age   Cause

1. _____
2. _____
3. _____
4. _____
5. _____

(b) Problems mentioned by villagers   Number who mention

1. _____
2. _____
3. _____
4. _____
5. _____
6. _____
7. _____

(c) Surveyor's observations

_____
_____
_____
_____
_____
_____
_____
_____

Figure 5.15   Community diagnosis form used in SHARE project.

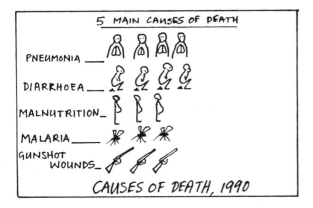

Figure 5.16   Pictogram to show causes of death.

- They tend to remove control of key information and function from the community to the project, thus limiting participation and community involvement.
- They depend on a reliable power supply.
- They need at least two project or community members trained both in how to use them and how to troubleshoot.
- They require finance to buy hardware, update software, train project members, and provide systems support from outside specialists.
- Computers can crash, lose data or develop viruses. Information can easily be lost or corrupted, meaning that data also has to be kept manually.
- Unless introduced as a carefully planned process with clear guidelines and training, computers can waste large amounts of time and cause much frustration.

Useful activities that computers can carry out
- To track and store large amounts of data on CBHC activities, including immunisation status of all eligible children, compliance of confirmed TB patients, maternity care and vital events.
- To provide 'due lists' of inputs needed at community and family level, e.g. who needs which immunisation in which village, who is due for antenatal care, what TB patients are due sputum tests, etc.
- To help CBHC to be efficient and comprehensive; to enable gaps in care to be identified and acted upon.

- To present information using graphs, bar charts and other graphics.
- To generate information for managers, donors and government.
- Statistical analysis, tracking of infectious diseases and research.

Hand-held computers allowing immediate data entry are proving increasingly useful.

Types of software needed
Without computers each programme develops its own systems for service delivery, reporting, data storage and community partnership. These systems are based on what works best for the project and the community, given the special circumstances of each. It is also determined by national systems used for collecting health data.

Introducing computers, even the most flexible, will require changes in the handling of data and in the management of the project. An ideal solution is to design a computer programme that largely fits in with how data is handled and the project functions. However, this is expensive and needs skilled computer programmers.

More flexible software is now being produced that can respond specifically to the needs of projects.

In summary, programmes should computerise only if they have reached a certain size, have robust management systems, have successfully developed community partnerships, have adequate power supply, trained personnel and expert backup to make systems dependable.

Summary

Before starting any health programme, we need to understand the communities we will be working with. Having established trust and friendship we can carry out Participatory Appraisal (PA) using combined project and community teams of observers. Training should be given to all involved and practical arrangements made that will work for the community. The main methods of PA include semi-structured interviews, focus group discussions, community mapping and other sources of local information.

All information gathered must be carefully recorded and analysed. One of PA's main values is to strengthen community partnership at an early stage in the development of a programme.

The main purpose of the community survey is to gather numerical information for a community diagnosis. It can also be used to discover all community members whose health is at risk for subsequent targeting of health care, and it provides a baseline for evaluating the project at a later date.

The community diagnosis reveals the main problems affecting a community and is based largely on information from the survey and the observations of team and community members, including information from the PA.

Further reading and resources

1. *Guidelines for Rapid Participatory Appraisal to Assess Community Health Needs*, H. Annett and S. Rifkin, WHO, Geneva, 1995.
Available from: WHO. See Appendix E.

2. *Community Assessment: Guidelines for Developing Countries*, D. Stockman. IT Publications, 1994.
Useful background and practical tips on assessing the health and development needs of communities. Available from: IT Publications. See Appendix E.
3. *Partners in Evaluation*, M. Feuerstein, Macmillan, 1986.
An excellent book covering the subject of this chapter as well as monitoring and evaluation. As valuable now as when it was written.
Available from: TALC. See Appendix E.

Epi Info Computer Software, WHO.
This is a public domain package with facilities for word processing, questionnaire design, data entry and analysis, and graphics. It is regularly updated and, though accompanied with excellent instructions, takes time and expertise for field programmes to use effectively.
Available from: WHO. See Appendix E.

Further information on PA techniques is available from www.praxisindia.org, the website of The Institute for Participatory Practices.

See Further references and guidelines, page 412.

6

Drawing up Plans

This chapter assumes we have formed strong links with the community, have gathered information, either through participatory appraisal, community survey or both and that we are now ready to plan with the community.

We will first look at how to draw up plans with the community and then how to translate these into a development plan for a one- to three-year period. This is best done through using a simple Logical Framework (logframe).

COMMUNITY PLAN

What we need to do

Prepare with the team

Before discussing the survey results with the whole community, the health team and all those involved in the survey will need to consult together. The purpose is to:

1. **Understand the results.**

> Spend time with all the survey team explaining what has been discovered about the health of the community. Help them to understand the significance of the findings. This enables each person to be informed, involved and interested.

2. **Prioritise or rank the problems.**
   This means rewriting the problem list already made in order of priority with the most important health problems at the top.
   To do this we can ask four different questions about each problem:
   - How serious is the problem?
   - How widespread is the problem?
   - How important is the problem to the community?
   - How suitable is it for joint project/community action?

   The team can now rate answers to each of the above questions from 1 to 3 making a maximum possible total of 12. Problems are then prioritised in order of their score (see Table 6.1). In the example shown, the resulting order of priority is: water 11, tetanus 10, alcohol abuse 8, malaria 6.
   This is a method of informing and preparing the team before they explain to the community. It is not a list to be imposed on the community by the team.

3. **Decide how much the project should take the lead in planning.**
   It will certainly be our hope that planning can be a joint activity and that the community itself can help to lead or shape the process. In

Table 6.1   Prioritising or ranking problems

Problem	How serious	How widespread	How important to community	How suitable joint action	Total
Lack of clean water	3	3	2	3	11
Occasional malaria in wet season	2	1	1	2	6
Many deaths from neonatal tetanus	3	2	2	3	10
Heavy drinking of alcohol	2	3	1	2	8

some communities there may be few people sufficiently well informed or educated to do this; the project may therefore need to take the lead in the early stages. In such situations project members should be trained to mentor and encourage members of the community in the skills and attitudes they will need, so that they can play an effective part in planning and management as soon as possible.

Discuss with the community

It is helpful first to meet with the whole community in order to share results and ideas, and then with a VHC or planning group to draw up specific action plans.

Meeting with the whole community

We may already have had meetings with the whole community, for example, when we were first invited to start a programme or to explain the results of Participatory Appraisal (PA).

Reporting back the survey results can follow a similar style and agenda as the PA presentation. If PA and survey have been done close together, the meeting can combine both.

It is important to report back both PA or survey findings as soon as possible after the work is completed. Matters will still be fresh in people's minds, their interest is aroused, and suspicion caused by a long delay has not developed.

Project and community members involved in PA or the survey can make a joint presentation.

Here is a suggested agenda.

Present the findings

The community will want to know the results of the questions they were asked during the survey.

Keep this simple. Explain the main problems found in a way that can be easily understood. The more talk-back and questions the better. Our purpose is not merely to inform but to raise awareness and motivate community members so that they both understand and feel the seriousness of their problems and the urgency to find solutions.

For example: One of the main findings commonly found is malnutrition in under-fives. The community may not even believe there is serious malnutrition, because all the children look much the same. Explain that weighing and measuring is the only accurate way to discover most cases of moderate malnutrition.

Tell them how doctors have found that children with moderate malnutrition are many times more likely to die from common illnesses such as diarrhoea, measles and pneumonia than those who are well nourished and on the correct part of the Growth Chart (often known as the Road to Health). Help them to understand that the correct feeding of children is the best way to stop them becoming seriously ill or dying.

Agree priority problems for joint action

During the meeting we will talk about serious problems suitable for working on together. We will already have prepared our priority list (see Table 6.1) but we must be flexible and ready to change if other priorities emerge.

Make sure that any problems chosen for joint action are:

1. within the resources of the project (both budget and expertise);
2. suitable for a joint community/project approach;
3. likely to bring early (and successful) results (see also Chapter 2).

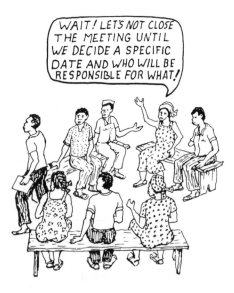

Figure 6.1   Before the meeting closes, make sure everyone knows what is to be done and who is to do it.

Practical planning with the Village Health Committee (VHC) or Community Action Group (CAG)

For each problem discussed and selected with the whole community, we must now draw up a detailed action plan. This is best done by the VHC or CAG, which will include members of the community. It is probably best for project staff not to be members, but they can usefully attend meetings as resource people or advisors.

In some new projects or in remote, backward, communities, initial planning may have to be done mainly by the health team members. Figure 6.2 shows ways in which planning and other activities range from being largely community owned (right side of diagram) to donor or programme driven (left side of diagram). We should always try to work as far to the right as possible in all programme activities

Because ways of planning will vary widely between projects, this chapter will not describe a stepwise guide to the process. However, four different techniques described below can be very helpful in drawing up a plan for any problem we have agreed to tackle.

Problem trees

A problem tree helps us to understand the causes and effects of problems we wish to address so as to guide us towards solutions.

For each problem identified we construct a problem tree as follows:

Step 1. We identify the causes of the problem by asking 'But Why?' until we can go no further: these can be thought of as the roots of the tree.
Step 2. We identify the effects of the problem by asking 'So what?' until we can go no further: These can be thought of as the branches and fruits of a problem tree.

In the example in Figure 6.3 the community identified lack of income, i.e. poverty as the main problem.

Constructing a problem tree helps us to understand the root causes of a problem. These may be difficult to deal with but, if we are successful, our work can have a major impact. It also shows us the effects of a problem, which are often easier for us to address at the beginning.

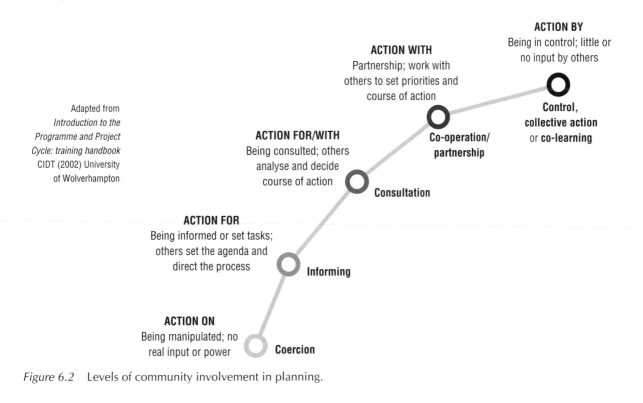

Figure 6.2 Levels of community involvement in planning.

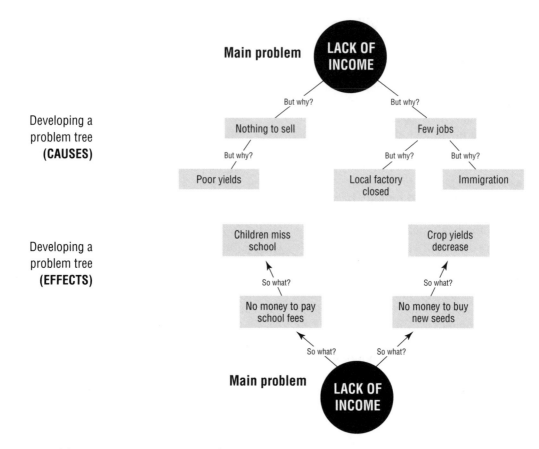

Figure 6.3   Problem trees. Source: *Project Cycle Management*, Roots 5, Tearfund, 2003.

A SWOT Analysis

A SWOT analysis helps us to plan a project activity. SWOT stands for Strengths, Weaknesses, Opportunities and Threats. It is a tool to help us examine available resources and potential obstacles. The S and W are the internal strengths and weaknesses of the community or action group; the O and T describe the external factors that may help or hinder a project in reaching its objective.

Table 6.2 gives an example of using a SWOT analysis in helping to draw up an action plan for building a community latrine complex.

SMART objectives

SMART is a technique that helps us to ensure that our objectives are clear. If we know what we are aiming for, we are more likely to achieve it. In fact, very clear objectives are essential for success. SMART stands for Specific, Measurable, Achievable, Results-orientated (or Relevant) and Time-bound.

Table 6.3 gives an example of constructing an objective using this technique. The example refers to an increasingly essential part of community health programmes: improving the home care of people living with HIV/AIDS.

What?How?Who?When?Where?

This can be a helpful technique as we try to work out the broad action plans we need to construct for each problem.

This approach helps us to think clearly about the problem before we record it in more detail on the logframe (see below).

For examples of two problems and how they might be solved, see Tables 6.4 and 6.5.

Key steps in this technique are to decide: What should be done? Who does it? How is it done? When is it done? Where is it done?

Table 6.2   A SWOT analysis for a proposed community latrine complex

SWOT	Strategy	Plan
Strength: Community has several divorced or widowed women who are doing unskilled construction work	• Train women in skills needed for latrine construction	• Identify women • Arrange training • Use them as resources when building latrines
Weakness: Land is too marshy so pit latrines cannot be used	• Persuade government to permit connection to municipal system • Determine site that is close to municipal sewer lines	• Visit government officials, agencies and politicians • Locate places where the sewer system runs closest to the community
Opportunity: International funding agency is willing to provide training for making latrine slabs from locally available materials	• Empower women's groups to be responsible for making low-cost slabs for sale to community	• Motivate women's groups • Find production space
Threat: Latrines will become dirty and then people will stop using them if government appoints and poorly supervises outside agency to maintain latrines	• Community will hire cleaners, attendant and supervisor • CAG will supervise • Small user fee will be charged to cover expenses	• Inform community; increase awareness of need for income to pay for cleaners, etc. • Hire latrine staff • Train latrine staff • Monitor that latrines are clean and working

From Booth et al., *Urban Health and Development*, Macmillan, TALC and Tearfund, Table 4.2, p. 62

Therefore, before a meeting that uses this technique closes, make sure that:

1. Any action decided on has been understood, agreed and recorded (with a summary circulated as soon as possible to all participants). This summary is sometimes known by the term Action Minutes. Key decisions are summarised and action needed recorded in a column at the side with the person responsible and date by which it must be done.
2. Everyone involved knows what they are meant to do next, and when the next meeting or joint activity is planned.

Some common situations

1. Health problems are not a community priority: non-health problems often are.

We must decide at an early stage whether we are able to offer help in other development sectors such as micro-credit, literacy, forestry or agriculture. If we ourselves cannot help, it may still be possible to link the community with those who can, so stimulating an 'intersectoral approach'.

In either case, the community must know to what extent we will be able to respond to the needs they voice. If our expertise is primarily health based, we will probably restrict ourselves at the start to health-related problems.

2. Gifts and skills of community members need to be used.

> Normally we start with community needs and think of solutions. Sometimes it is better to start with the gifts or abilities in a community or individual and see how they can be used in health care.

Table 6.3   *Steps to construct a SMART objective*

Step	Example
1. Restate the negative problem as a positive objective.	**Problem:** Some people with AIDS are not getting good home care. **Objective:** To provide home care for people with AIDS.
2. Make sure the objective is **SPECIFIC**.	**Objective:** To provide home care for people with AIDS *in our community*.
3. Make sure there is a **MEASURABLE** indicator in the objective.	**Objective:** To provide home care for *30* people with AIDS.
4. Make sure the project is **ACHIEVABLE**.	Consider: Do we have enough staff to provide care to 30 patients? Are there at least 30 people with AIDS who will require and request care from us?
5. Make sure the objective is **RELEVANT**.	Is AIDS a serious problem in the community and is the community concerned about it?
6. Make the objective **TIME-BOUND**.	**Objective:** To provide home care for 30 people with AIDS in our community *in the next year*.

From Booth et al., *Urban Health and Development*, Macmillan, TALC and Tearfund, Table 4.3, p. 65

Table 6.4   *Problem: 25 per cent children with moderate malnutrition*

	What causes	How solved	Who will solve	When to start
1	Lack of knowledge about correct feeding practices	House to house health teaching Teaching in clinic	CHWs and health team members	Immediately in community In clinic when it opens in 3 months
2	Irrigation channels broken and blocked leading to poor crop yields	Repair of channels	Community health committee with government development officer	Liaise with government office now Start repairs after harvest

Examples might include gifts in drama, singing, teaching, caring for the handicapped or organising youth activities.

3. Activities in different project areas need to be coordinated.

   After a short time we may be working with several different communities at the same time, each of which has its own list of needs and priorities.

This calls for careful forward planning to make sure that plans and promises made are always followed up. Constructing a Logical Framework for each community programme is an effective way of doing this (see the second half of this chapter).

Table 6.5   Problem: 5 per cent of population with possible tuberculosis

What causes	How solved	Who will solve	When to start
1 Lack of understanding	Health education	CHWs Folk-drama group	When CHWs have completed basic training
2 No medicine available or affordable	Ensure regular low-cost drugs	Project director liaising with District Medical Officer	At once
3 Smoke from cigarettes and cooking hearths	Health education Install simple chimneys	Representative from each house with instruction from health team member Community leaders	Prepare now for community-wide project after rainy season

LOGICAL FRAMEWORK (LOGFRAME)

Programme planning using a Logical Framework

We will now have identified problems in discussions with the community, and broadly agreed on plans for tackling them, probably using one or more of the techniques described in the previous section.

We now need to put these into a more detailed written format that will help us to plan effectively over a one- to three-year period. The tool that does this the best, and which many agencies now expect us to use, is known as the Logical Framework or logframe.

Why is a logframe used?

The logframe is a system widely used by agencies and popular with donors. It helps us to do four main things: design a project well, describe a project objectively, structure a project clearly and evaluate a project more easily.

A logframe also acts like a compass: it gives us information to help us know what we are doing and where we are going, which can be easily read and understood.

What are its advantages?

It is systematic, helps to focus team members in shared goals, provides a way of monitoring progress, and allows adaptations to be added as the programme evolves. It also helps us to think logically and it reveals any weakness in the design of the project, which we can then address.

What are its disadvantages?

- A degree of complexity. **It requires time, skill and training to use it effectively.**
- The danger of rigidity. The team must understand this should be seen as a flexible management tool, not an unchangeable record of facts.
- It can reinforce a top-down approach. However we can get round this. *For example*: Ideas and input from the community can be incorporated into each part of the logframe at regular intervals, such as when setting our original objectives, and in yearly monitoring.
  The logframe should be displayed as a working tool on a board in the project office, not just stored in the director's filing cabinet.

What does a logframe tell us?

A logframe tells us all the major things we need to know about a project in order to plan successfully, within a given time period. These include:

- What the project will achieve.
- What activities will be carried out.
- What resources (inputs) are required.
- What the potential problems and risks are likely to be.
- How progress can be measured.

What does a logframe consist of?

A logframe is a grid with four columns going across the top and four columns going down the side. There are some differences in the way people name and use these columns, but the example given in Table 6.6 shows a commonly used format. The description below adds some alternative wording which is sometimes used to describe the same things

Down the left-hand side are four columns:

First column – **Goal:** this is the wider problem we are trying to address.

Second column – **Purpose:** this is the specific change we wish to make to achieve the goal.

Third column – **Outputs:** these are the immediate results we want to see from our activities.

Fourth column – **Activities:** these are the tasks we will carry out .

Across the top are four columns

First column – **Summary:** this answers the question: What does the project want to achieve?

Second column – **Indicators:** these are the measurements of our performance *or* How can we tell if we have achieved our purpose(s)?

Third column – **Evidence:** this is the source of information to measure performance *or* Where can we get information that will tell us if we have achieved?

Fourth column – **Assumptions:** these are important conditions that could affect our progress *or* What (external) factors are needed for success or what threats are there to success?

We can use simpler or modified logframes if these tie in more accurately with the scale and approach of our programme. An example is given in Table 6.7. This was constructed in its present form as this fitted in more naturally with the particular project being undertaken and the abilities of those needing to complete it.

How should we fill in the logframe?

We can do this in different ways but here is a method that many people find the easiest:

1. We work down the summary column. This helps us to define our goal and then list increasingly detailed ways in which we will actually try to achieve this.

2. We next work across each row either starting at the bottom of the chart or the top, depending on which we find is easier. People good at thinking of concepts or the big picture may find it easier to start at the top; those who are good at thinking of practical details as found in the field, at the bottom.

How can we check the logframe?

This is one useful test. Start at the bottom (activities) and ask: 'If we carry out this activity and assuming our assumptions are valid, will we achieve this output?'. We can do the same for each activity and make changes if the statements do not tally or we feel anything does not fit or has been missed out.

We must also check that the wording and the various descriptions are clearly stated and not open to confusion.

An alternative to using a logframe

Some programmes will be too small, or have insufficient time or experience in filling out logframes especially in the early phase of a project.

We can use alternatives such as Donor or Community application forms that have questions constructed to produce much of the information that would be needed for a logframe. An example used by one agency is given on page 65.

Summary

The success of our project will depend partly on how effectively we draw up plans with the community and turn these into a workable format to guide our progress over a three-year period.

Planning with the community uses material from either a community survey and diagnosis, or a Participatory Appraisal or both. We must feed back information to the community in a way they can both understand and own. The main aim is to decide with them which problems to work on together.

Table 6.6   Example of a Logical Framework (logframe)

	Summary	Indicators	Evidence	Assumptions
Goal	Decreased incidence and impact of diarrhoeal disease	Mortality rate due to diarrhoeal disease reduced by 5% by end of year 3 Incidence of diarrhoeal disease in diocese reduced by 50% by end of year 3	Government statistics Local/health centre statistics	
Purpose	Improved access to, and use of, safe water in diocese	All households accessing at least 15 litres water per person per day by end of year 3 Average distance of households to nearest safe water less than 500 m by end of year 3	Household survey report Household survey report	Health care does not decline Diarrhoeal disease is due to unsafe water and hygiene practices
Outputs	1 Participatory management systems set up for needs identification, planning and monitoring	Diocese and community joint plans and budgets in place by end of month 9 At least 90% of WUCs raise local contributions by end of year 1	Plans and budgets WUC* logbooks	Adequate quantity of water available People are not excluded from accessing improved sources
	2 Improved sources of safe water	At least 90 improved or new sources of safe water established and in operation by end of year 2	WUC logbooks Water quality test reports	Access not for potentially polluting uses Hygiene practices are culturally acceptable
	3 Raised community awareness of good hygiene practices	Number of people washing hands after defecating increased to 75% of target population by end of month 30	Survey of knowledge, attitudes and practice	

*Water use committees

Table 6.6   Example of a Logical Framework (continued)

	Summary	Indicators	Evidence	Assumptions
Activities	1.1 Established water user committees (WUCs)	30 WUCs established in five diocesan regions by end of month 3 Once established, WUC meetings held once a month	Constitutions of WUCs Minutes of meetings Membership list	Groundwater is free of arsenic Communities have confidence that water sources can be improved Committee membership will take responsibility to work for community Water user committees continue to function in everyone's interests
	1.2 Provide training for WUC members in surveying, planning, monitoring and proposal writing	All WUC members trained by end of month 5	Training records	
	1.3 Communities carry out baseline and monitoring surveys of water use and needs and submit proposals	All WUCs complete baseline surveys and submit proposals by month 7	Survey reports and proposals	Community prepared to work with WUCs
	1.4 Hold joint Diocese, District Water Department and WUC regional planning meetings	Agreement reached with Water Department and all WUCs by end of month 9	Minutes of meetings Letters of agreement	
	2.1 WUCs select Community Water Workers (CWWs) and agree incentives	Two CWWs selected by each community by end of month 9	Minutes of meetings	Incentive arrangements for CWWs are sufficient and sustained
	2.2 Train CWWs to dig and cover wells and to maintain and repair handpumps	All CWWs attend training by end of year 1	Training reports including participants' evaluation	Effective supply chain for spare parts

*Water use committees

Table 6.6   Example of a Logical Framework (continued)

	Summary	Indicators	Evidence	Assumptions
Activities	2.3 Upgrade current wells and establish new wells	Sixty current wells deepened, covered and functioning at end of month 21 Thirty news wells established and in operation by end of month 21	Field survey WUC logbooks	District Water Department to be allocated enough resources to carry out water testing, alternative testing possible if not
	2.4 Arrange for District Water Department to test water quality	All sources tested before use	Field survey WUC logbooks	
	2.5 CWWs repair and maintain handpumps	97% of handpumps in diocese function at end of year 2	Field survey WUC logbooks	
	3.1 Train existing Community Health Promoters (CHPs) to increase their knowledge of diarrhoeal disease and the need for good hygiene practice	Three CHPs per community attend training and score at least 90% in a post-training test by end of year 1	Attendance records Test results	Community members apply the training they have received
	3.2 CHPs train men, women and children in good hygiene practice	80% of community members trained by end of year 2	Attendance records	

Adapted from 'Project Cycle Management', *Roots 5*, Tearfund, 2003.

Having decided this, the project and community now work through a Community Action Group to draw up action plans for each problem identified. Various techniques can be used to do this such as problem trees, and constructing SMART objectives. The SWOT technique can help the project-community partnership analyse whether they have sufficient resources to undertake a planned activity.

The best format for documenting the action plan is a logframe, which helps to clarify our goal and the ways we can attain it. For projects unable to cope with a standard logframe, simpler versions can be adopted or forms constructed that draw out sufficient information to guide planning.

After a period of time we will need to evaluate with the community whether we have achieved the purposes we set out to achieve. The logframe

Table 6.7   Example of a simplified Logical Framework (logframe)

	1	2	3	4
	Project plan or structure	Indicators of progress	Risks and assumptions	Outcome and findings after 2 years
A Wider project aims	To eradicate measles from project area	Incidence of measles falling	Minimal civil strife Rains not prolonged	Incidence of measles falls by 50%
B Immediate objectives	To immunise 30% of children under 12 months in year 1, 70% in year 2 in 10 villages	Percentage of children under 12 months immunised per year per village	Villages will cooperate. No staff strikes	Targets reached for 7 villages, (3 still have coverage below 50%)
C Tasks or activities	Train team to immunise	Health workers trained	Training effective	Team effectively trained to extend coverage
	Train Village Health Committee	VHC members actively participate	VHC members have time and willingness	VHC needing new challenge to avert boredom
	Gain understanding of villagers	Percentage of villages participating	Villages overcome suspicion of measles vaccine	7 villages well sensitised, 3 still resistant to change
	Set 4 immunisation days per village per year	Percentage attendance of eligibles per village per day	No unpredicted holidays and festivals on immunisation days	One out of four immunisation days ruined by festival hangovers
	Train CHWs to visit each child within one week of injection	Percentage of immunised children visited	Partners of CHWs do not object to extra work	Most families appreciated CHWs' concern
D Resources or inputs	Salaries for staff	Salaries paid	Funding continues	New funds needed for extending to new area
	Project vehicle	Vehicle in working order	No serious lack of fuel	Bicycles could be used for five villages
	Visual aids	Visual aids bought and used	Visual aids will be appropriate	Visual aids used were wrong culture for village
	Refrigerators and cold box	Fridge reliable, cold chain established	Kerosene supply stable	Solar fridge donated and maintained by other NGO
	Needles, syringes, vaccine	Disposables purchased Vaccine source secured	Price reasonable EPI supplies available	Disposable syringes available locally Time wasted as vaccine supply distant

gives us an opportunity to track our progress and make yearly adjustments to the project plan.

Further reading and resources

1. *Project Cycle Management*, R. Blackman, Roots Resources No. 5, Tearfund, 2003. Available from Tearfund. An extremely helpful practical manual on all aspects of project design.

2. *Toolkits Development Manual No 5*, L. Gosling and M. Edwards, Save the Children,1995. A very useful section on the use of the logframe and other ways of planning. Available from Save the Children.

3. *Logical Framework Analysis: Guidance Notes*, L. Taylor, N. Thin and J. Sartain, BOND, 2003, A step by step guide. See www.bond.org.uk/pubs/ipw.htm.

7

The Community Health Worker

In this chapter we will try to answer the following questions:

1. What is a Community Health Worker (CHW)?
2. What are the roles and functions of the CHW?
3. How is a CHW selected?
4. How is a CHW trained?
5. The CHW's health kit
6. How does a CHW keep records?
7. How is a CHW supported?
8. Should a CHW be paid?
9. How should the CHW be paid?
10. How much should a CHW be paid?
11. Practical hints if payment is essential.
12. Common reasons why CHW programmes fail.

What is a community health worker?

A community health worker (CHW) is a local person trained to respond to the health needs within his or her immediate community. As Community Based Health Care (CBHC) remains the basis for so many effective health programmes, the role of the CHW is as important as ever, and effective CHWs are usually essential to the success of the programme.

But we must think carefully about the need for CHWs to adapt to changing circumstances so they continue to be relevant and effective. In many poor or remote communities traditional CHWs will continue to act as the main front-line workers. Often there will be no choice. Hospitals and primary health centres may be scarcely functioning, especially where HIV is overwhelming the health system. But in other areas, as incomes improve, people will be increasingly drawn to

hospitals, private practitioners and other forms of health care as their point of first contact. In these situations, CHWs will need a higher educational background and more comprehensive training if they are going to meet the increased expectations of the people they serve.

Some CHW programmes have not lived up to their original objectives, often because of inadequate training, poor management and little or no support and supervision. Bearing this in mind and remembering the huge variety of health needs in different parts of the world, we must do everything possible to 'get it right' when we start a new programme or scale up an existing one.

One example of a successful CHW programme is in Bangladesh: the Bangladesh Rural Advancement Committee (BRAC) has been involved in grass roots programmes for over three decades and fully understands the needs of poor communities. This group alone has trained 30 000 community health workers covering 60 000 villages. As just one of their functions, these CHWs have trained 13 million households in the use of oral rehydration therapy (see Further reading and resources at the end of the chapter).

CHWs are known by a bewildering number of different names, of which Village Health Worker is probably the commonest. The term urban health worker is often used in cities. CHWs may be either men or women. In this chapter for the sake of convenience we shall refer to the CHW as female.

Features of a traditional CHW

The CHW is selected by the community and is ideally trained in the community. She lives in the community, serves the community and may be paid by the community. She 'belongs' primarily to the community and not to the project or the government.

The CHW has several advantages over other primary health workers:

1. She is accepted by the community because they have chosen her.
2. She is available to the community because she lives in it.
3. She understands the local language, culture and the norms of everyday life.
4. She is usually cost effective to health programmes, because she is inexpensive to train and can do many of the tasks traditionally done by doctors, nurses and social workers.
5. She covers populations where other health workers are often unwilling or unable to serve.

A CHW can, however, have certain disadvantages:

1. She may be drawn by money or status to separate herself from the people she is serving.
2. She may (quite reasonably) have expectations of promotion and future employment leading her to distance herself from working as a locally based volunteer.
3. She may provide inadequate care unless she is well trained and well supervised.

4. Any payment she receives may be hard to maintain, unless the community itself is involved in ensuring she is paid for her services.
5. She may be wrongly selected and therefore be ineffective.
6. She may be insufficiently educated, though with appropriate training this can usually be overcome.

This means in practice:

> A CHW programme that is well set up and well maintained can be highly successful, but a programme with poor planning and supervision is of little value. The future usefulness of any CHW will depend on how well she is selected, trained, supervised and supported.

What are the roles and functions of the CHW?

The roles of the CHW

The CHW usually has a triple role in her community as health promoter, health provider and agent of change.

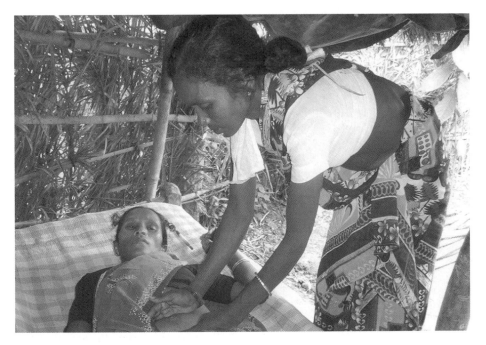

Figure 7.1   Antenatal care is just one part of a CHW's role.

As *health promoter* she will teach the whole community how to improve health and prevent illness.

As *health provider* she will treat common illnesses early, before they become serious. She may also be expected to give care and medication to the chronically ill

As *agent of change* she will help community members change their knowledge, attitudes and practice so that they lead healthier lives.

The functions of the CHW

The functions or job description of the CHW will vary greatly depending on:

- the needs of the community;
- the availability of other health care nearby;
- the plans and policy of the government;
- the aims of the project.

The following is a comprehensive list of a CHW's functions and **each project will need to adapt, and probably shorten, this for its own use.** It shows the huge range of activities that can be carried out by a well trained local community member.

A CHW will:

1. **Be available.**
   She must be willing to give appropriate care and advice to any community member, regardless of wealth, tribe, caste, or religion, whenever she is needed.

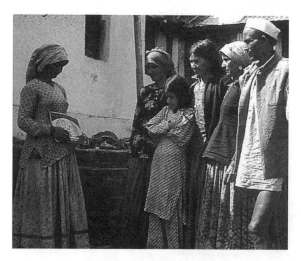

Figure 7.2 The CHWs will teach at every opportunity.

2. **Be a teacher.**
   She must be continually passing on knowledge in a practical and helpful way whenever the opportunity arises, both to individuals and to groups.
3. **Care for children.**
   a) By promoting good nutrition.
      The CHW can measure the weight (or mid-upper arm circumference) of under-five children once per month, filling in a growth chart, or other record card.
      She can give practical feeding advice to parents, emphasising the value of breast-feeding and appropriate weaning. She may help to arrange feeding programmes or set up kitchen gardens.
   b) By demonstrating the use of oral rehydration solution (ORS) so that all community members know how and when to use this in the treatment of diarrhoea.
   c) By promoting the immunisation of all children.
   d) By distributing Vitamin A and worm medicine (anti-helminthics) to young children where these are health priorities.
   e) By ensuring the supply of cotrimoxazole in children who are HIV positive.
4. **Care for mothers.**
   a) By encouraging antenatal care.
      The CHW will motivate women to attend clinics or will carry out checks herself. She may distribute preventive treatment such as iron and folic acid to pregnant and lactating women, and, where relevant, antimalarials. She will promote tetanus immunisation.
   b) By carrying out deliveries.
      The CHW may do this herself or work alongside the Traditional Birth Attendant (TBA) using clean and safe methods of delivery. She will refer women likely to have delivery problems, before any problems occur.
   c) By giving postnatal advice and care.
5. **Promote child spacing and family planning** and the prevention and treatment of sexually transmitted infections.
6. **Care for those with chronic infectious diseases** including those with AIDS, leprosy and other locally important illnesses. She may

have a key role in identifying cases of TB, and supervising 'DOTS' treatment schedules both for TB and for people living with HIV/AIDS who are taking antiretroviral therapy (see pages 280–1 and 299–300). She can help to remove the stigma of people living with HIV/AIDS by her attitude and her teaching.

7. **Care in the community** for those with non-communicable diseases such as high blood pressure and diabetes.

8. **Care for the blind**, the physically and mentally disabled, the elderly at home needing support and palliative care, and be involved in community rehabilitation.

9. **Treat simple illnesses and give first aid.**
Most CHWs will keep a stock of simple, effective medicines, using them to treat common illnesses or severe symptoms, under the supervision of the community health team. Where medicines are readily available, she may need to advise community members what medical treatment they need, including the dose and duration of treatment.

10. **Know when to refer.**
The CHW will learn to recognise and refer serious illnesses and those she cannot treat herself. She will be aware of those discharged from hospital and provide basic aftercare if this is required.

11. **Develop public health activities.**
With the support of the health team or committee, the CHW may promote waste disposal, safe water, smokeless cooking hearths

and other valid improvements to home and environment.

12. **Keep records** that are needed or useful for the health programme.

13. **Work alongside her supervisor** or other members of the health team. This may include taking part in surveys, immunisation programmes, care of school children, teaching and supervision, health centre activities and community projects.

14. **Form community clubs.**
Female CHWs may help to set up women's groups or teach female literacy. Male CHWs can set up young farmers' clubs or adolescent or youth activities. CHWs may play a role in micro-credit schemes.

15. **Encourage parents** to send children to school.

16. **Carry out other activities** as discussed between her, the community and the health team.

As new programmes are set up to target specific diseases, CHWs can be trained to play a central role in these programmes.

For example: In Ghana, where the eye disease trachoma is common, CHWs have been trained to distribute the antibiotic azithromycin to both adults and children and have encouraged face and handwashing. In Zanzibar, CHWs already trained in other community activities such as the polio eradication programme can switch their skills to new priorities such as treating filariasis: 400 CHWs have been trained to distribute ivermectin or albendazole.

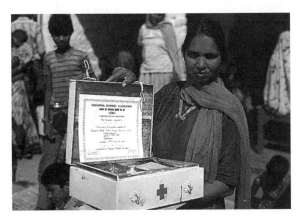

Figure 7.3   The community often judges a CHW by how well her medicines seem to work.

Differing CHW models
Some projects and countries are using new models for CHWs to fit in with specific needs. *For example*: in Bolivia and Paraguay, some of the military have taken on a role as health workers. However, this is controversial as there are good reasons why the role of the military and that of aid workers should be kept separate. In Malawi, 250 000 people attended health centres for orthopaedic problems in 1998. A new programme is training orthopaedic clinical officers (OCOs) who can manage 9 out of 10 of these injuries at community level.

How is a CHW selected?

It is common to see programmes where some villages or slum areas make great improvements while others seem to stand still. This may be because one community has a more effective CHW than another.

> The correct selection of a CHW is of critical importance to the whole future success of a community programme.

Who should choose the CHW?

The CHW should be chosen by the community. This can happen only if the whole community thoroughly understands what functions a CHW will carry out, and therefore what personality and gifts she needs to have. In order for the community leaders and members to grasp these issues, two or even three meetings or discussions may be necessary.

For example: several programmes in Malawi have come to realise that the criteria for selection as well as the choice of the volunteers themselves must be done with the community's involvement. This requires meetings and discussion until the community fully understands the value and function of the CHW,

For example: in one Himalayan project, community members assumed that, because the CHW would be involved in basic health care, she would serve as a low-grade health aide and that her level of education would be unimportant. As a result, inappropriate people were put forward for selection.

> Time taken in explanation is never time wasted. The more community members understand the role and function of their CHW, the more they will give her support and use her services.

Each community has its own way of reaching a decision. Although the health team should not

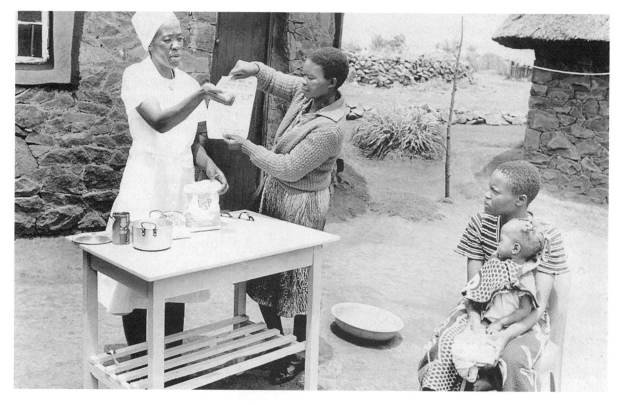

Figure 7.4   An effective CHW often holds the secret to a community's progress.

usually interfere in this, it must ensure that the CHW is acceptable to the majority of community members, including women and the marginalised.

Communities should be discouraged from suggesting a relative or friend of the local chief be appointed as CHW in order to gain power, money or influence.

Sometimes a community or Village Health Committee will put forward several candidates and allow the health team to make the final choice after seeing which one(s) prove to be the most effective.

In some instances, the health team may notice and suggest a community member who appears very appropriate.

Depending on the housing density of the area, a part-time CHW can cover at the most 50 families and ideally not more than 25, unless she concentrates on a few more specific functions. There is often value in choosing two CHWs to work in pairs, especially where they are working as unpaid volunteers or where communities are very scattered.

We must remember:

> Both NGOs and government programmes must take special care to allow the people themselves to choose their own CHWs and not force candidates on the community against their wishes.

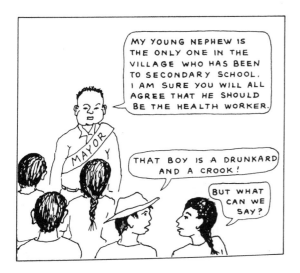

Figure 7.5

What type of person should be selected?

Male or female?

There are no absolute rules. Men are more appropriate in some communities, women in others. Some communities will expect men to care for men, and women for women. Here are some principles that will help us to decide:

Advantages of choosing men:

- They may be less busy than women.
- They may be better educated.
- They may find it easier to liaise with government officials and with other agencies.
- They may be less hesitant at the beginning and more willing to take initiatives.
- Some societies may insist that health workers are male.
- They can more effectively prevent and treat sexually transmitted diseases in men.
- They may be more appropriate where security problems and personal safety cause concern.

Advantages of choosing women:

- They may be more appropriate in mother and child health care.
- They are often less eager to make money or to set up as private practitioners.
- They are more likely to be resident and available in the community.
- They may be more compassionate and sensitive to people's needs.
- Some societies may insist that only women look after the health needs of other women and children.

A well respected community member

A CHW should ideally be:

- friendly;
- concerned for the welfare of others;
- able to keep confidence and avoid gossip;
- not primarily motivated by status or money;
- intelligent and eager to learn;
- hard-working;
- respected as a good parent and/or community member;

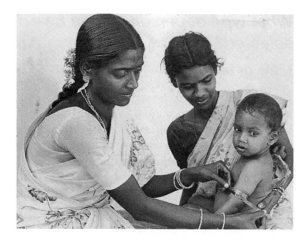

Figure 7.6   A CHW in south India measures a mid-upper arm circumference.

- willing to visit any who ask her, safety and security allowing.

The CHW should offer care to any community member irrespective of religion, caste, tribe or status.

This does not necessarily mean that CHWs need to be literate or educated. However, in most communities basic education is seen as increasingly important because of the range and complexity of tasks carried out by CHWs. Depending on the level of local education, the completion of eight years of schooling is often recommended.

CHWs will be expected to learn fresh ideas and gain new skills. Older CHWs, or those with little formal education, may find this more difficult.

Interested in the job

> CHWs need to have both a genuine interest in the work and an unselfish desire to serve.

In adequate health

CHWs generally need to be healthy and strong in body and mind. They will usually continue their other jobs at home or in the community, in addition to serving as CHWs.

Those suffering from infectious TB should not be chosen until the infection has cleared, though cured TB and leprosy patients are often suitable as may be those with a degree of disability. There are no valid reasons why people who are HIV positive but otherwise well should not be chosen as CHWs, whether or not they are being treated with antiretroviral therapy.

Mature in age and outlook

Younger people are quicker to learn. They are, however, more likely to marry and move away, or have young children, which will make them less available. They may also lack maturity or command less respect. Community members with previous experience as volunteers in another capacity may be suitable candidates

Backed up by her family

It is important, especially for female CHWs, that they have family support for their work. Husbands, mothers-in-law and other family members must understand their role and be able to encourage them.

Already engaged in health work

Traditional birth attendants (TBAs, Dais) often make good CHWs, providing they are ready to learn new ways. Their communities already know them and use their services. They are usually respected.

Other traditional practitioners can become effective health workers but there is a risk that after training they may use their new knowledge to increase their earnings, or be so interested in curative care that they take little interest in other health activities.

> An ideal choice? A man or woman, aged between 20 and 45, preferably married, and with at least eight to ten years of schooling.

How is a CHW trained?

Many good books and guidelines have been written on the training of CHWs and some are listed at the end of the chapter. Try to obtain one that is appropriate for the area or which is published nationally or regionally.

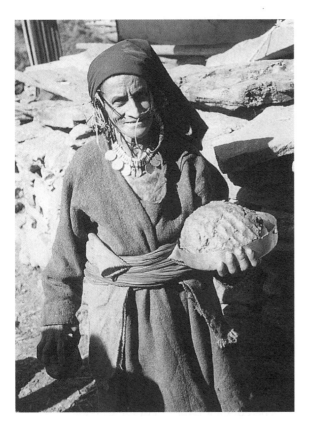

Figure 7.7   TBA in a remote mountain village. Such women, when appropriately trained, may make effective CHWs.

In this section we shall be considering:

1. The personal development of the CHW.
2. Where should the training be held?
3. How long should the training continue?
4. Who should do the training?
5. How should the training be done?
6. What should the curriculum include?
7. What supervision should be carried out?

The personal development of the CHW

CHWs often come from poor backgrounds. When first chosen they may lack self-confidence. This is especially true for women in male-dominated societies.

These same people, after a few brief months, will be expected to treat illnesses, give health talks, and alter their community's health patterns.

Great changes will be necessary within the CHW herself for this to be possible.

> The single most important part of CHW training is her personal development so that she becomes confident in her manner and caring in her approach. This transformation will come about largely by the attitude of the health team and the respect with which she is treated.

There is no place in CHW teaching for the harsh and insensitive attitudes sometimes seen from overworked hospital staff. Such attitudes may frighten and stifle CHWs, who in turn learn to treat their patients in the same manner.

All health team members, but especially the trainer and supervisor, will need to be accepting and appreciative of the CHW.

They should accept her the way she is, her personality, her beliefs and her fears. They should never despise or judge her for any ideas that may be wrong or different, or for customs and habits she may follow.

They should appreciate the CHW and take an interest in her family, her community and her traditions. This will involve learning from her and adopting good ideas from her own traditions, values and background.

They should affirm the CHW, always looking for ways to encourage her.

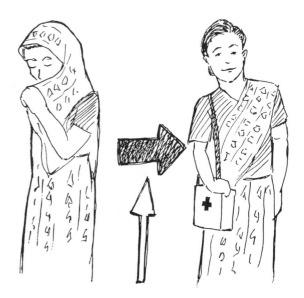

Figure 7.8   Effects of transformation.

This process of conferring dignity will happen both in lessons and in the community. The health team must always show the CHW respect, especially in front of others. She must not be ordered to do menial tasks such as sweeping floors or be expected to act as the unpaid personal servant of team members.

Where should the training be held?

Different programmes will choose different places. A few will choose hospitals or central training sites, which may be convenient but are probably not the most suitable environments; most will prefer local health centres or community rooms.

Although it may be less convenient for trainers, there are many advantages in training CHWs as near as possible to their own communities:

1. **It is more convenient for the CHWs.**
   In poor rural areas it may be hard for busy women to leave home for training. They may not be permitted by their husband or family to sleep away from their community.
2. **CHWs can relate what they have learnt** to actual problems in their community. They can take part in a community survey as part of their training.

3. **Trainers themselves can learn** about the CHW's lifestyle and the day-to-day problems she is likely to face.
4. **Practical work and supervision** in the field can be done more easily.
5. **The community recognises the training** being given to the worker.

There are also important reasons why rural CHWs should not be taken for residential teaching to towns and cities, where problems may arise following training.

These problems are often seen with male trainees. The more they learn in town-based training programmes, the more distant they feel from their villages. As one health educator wrote: 'All that is achieved in the end is just another set of unproductive workers in government service.'

How long should the training continue?

This will depend on:
1. The educational level of the CHW.
   Illiterate, uneducated or older CHWs may take a long time to learn basic knowledge and skills.
2. The time the CHW has available.

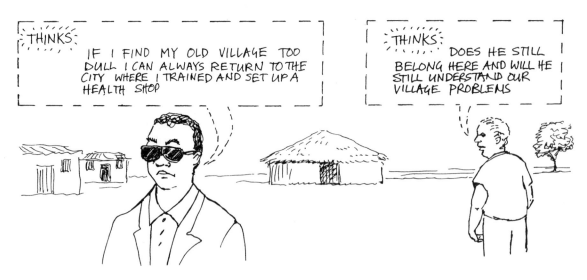

Figure 7.9   Disadvantages of training health workers away from their own communities.

Most female CHWs from rural areas are also mothers and farmers. Urban CHWs may need to have part-time employment in order to care for the needs of the family. The length of training must fit in with their home commitments.

Each programme should design its own timescale and pattern of training. Here are examples of two commonly used training models:

Block training

Teaching initially occurs each day for a period of from one week to three months. Three to six weeks is often an appropriate length. Regular lessons then continue once a week or once every two weeks until the full course is completed.

This method helps trainees develop fresh attitudes and gain new knowledge that is reinforced every day.

When this system is used, training often takes place in a hospital or central training site, convenient for teachers, but often inconvenient for CHWs.

Intermittent training

Teaching occurs one or two days or half days a week until the course is complete. Although convenient for rural CHWs, learning is slower and knowledge more easily forgotten between lessons.

With block training, CHWs may be able to start working in their communities within three months. With intermittent training, it may take six months to a year before the CHW can be useful. By this time the community may be losing its interest.

Regardless of which of these time models is used, training and update must continue for as long as the CHW is working. This culture of continuous learning is essential. It helps the CHW to remain motivated. It is also needed as new forms of treatment become available, and as new programmes are implemented by the government, such as Roll Back Malaria, Stop TB and the use of ART in the treatment of people living with HIV/AIDS.

Who should do the training?

The answer in practice is often 'whoever is available'. However, trainers will need appropriate qualities, appropriate qualifications and appropriate training themselves.

Ideal trainers should have these **qualities**:

1. **Appropriate gifts.**
   They should be friendly, lively, humorous, enthusiastic and good at explaining and encouraging participation.
2. **An appropriate cultural background.**
   The smaller the language and cultural gap between trainer and trainees, the more effective will be the teaching.

For example: In many mountainous areas of the world, hill people are taught by those from the lowlands with higher qualifications. Although such trainers may be very knowledgeable, they often make poor teachers because they are unable to understand the lifestyle and thought patterns of those living in the hills. In such situations hill people themselves with simple, appropriate training often prove to be better teachers than more highly qualified people from the plains.

Ideal trainers should have these **qualifications**:

- practical experience in community health;
- nursing, paramedical or teachers' training.

In practice, trainers will come from a great variety of backgrounds and will include doctors, nurses, lab technicians, teachers, medical assistants, multi-purpose health workers (MPWs) and social workers.

All trainers will need appropriate training themselves. Those at the top of the training tree will influence all those whom they themselves teach (the CHWs). Indirectly of course they will also influence those whom the CHWs teach. This makes it essential that CHW trainers are themselves carefully trained. They will need to have afffirming and positive attitudes towards those they teach, and learn interactive, interesting and varied methods of teaching.

The importance of learning has given rise to a whole new form of teaching, the training of trainers (TOT). Discover if there are any Training of Trainers courses that teachers could attend. If there are not, it may be necessary to arrange a training course, ideally by working together with other local NGOs or government programmes that may have the same training needs.

How should the training be done?

We will consider this under method and plan.

Method

Our method should be:

Pupil-centred

Traditional teaching is often done by dominant teachers, who stand at the front, look down on the class, and teach facts to their pupils. Such pupils learn by rote, often fail to understand, rarely participate and are scared to ask questions. The training of community health workers should be the opposite of this.

All sit in a circle. The teacher learns from the pupils and the pupils learn from the teacher, and all learn from each other. 'Teaching is not a one-way, nor a two-way but an all-way process.' Each class member is encouraged to take part, share ideas and ask questions. No one's ideas are mocked.

Problem solving

Lessons will often start, not with the teacher's knowledge, but with the pupil's problems and the community's concerns.

For example: Many teachers traditionally start their health course with a lesson on human anatomy. But the CHWs may be wondering what they can do about the latest outbreak of eye infection or recent deaths from malaria. A good teacher will choose a lesson that is relevant to the CHWs' current concerns, and not simply follow a curriculum from the first lesson through to the last.

> In the context of community health, the purpose of knowledge is to help find effective answers to practical problems.

Starting with the trainee's own knowledge

Before starting to teach a subject we first discover what the pupils or trainees know already, what their attitude is towards it and what they normally do about it. Discussing Knowledge, Attitude and Practice (KAP) can be rewarding both for trainees and for the trainer.

For example: In many parts of the world pregnant women believe they should eat less food so that their babies will be small. In this way delivery is easier and the baby is less likely to get stuck during delivery.

For example: In parts of rural Nepal many people believe that a vital worm resides in every person's stomach from birth and must not be killed. Until this is understood and discussed it will be hard to introduce a deworming programme.

Good teachers will respect these beliefs and gently correct any wrong ideas on which they are based, and which make an important difference to health. Many incorrect beliefs can be left, for example one where mothers are prevented from eating eggs during pregnancy, providing the diet is made up in some other way.

> Correct ideas are approved and built upon.
> Neutral ideas are left alone.
> Wrong ideas are corrected and altered.
> All ideas are listened to and respected.

Encouraging, friendly and enjoyable

We should encourage, not criticise, in our teaching, especially when CHWs may be unwilling to accept ideas that go against their own beliefs and traditions. The more CHWs enjoy the lesson the more they will learn, and the more likely they are to make their own teaching to the community enjoyable and interesting.

Repetitive

A large tree is more quickly felled by three axes falling at different angles than by one axe always hitting at the same angle. We should teach each subject using different methods and different examples.

At the end of each lesson, ask the pupils to give a summary of what they have learnt. Make sure

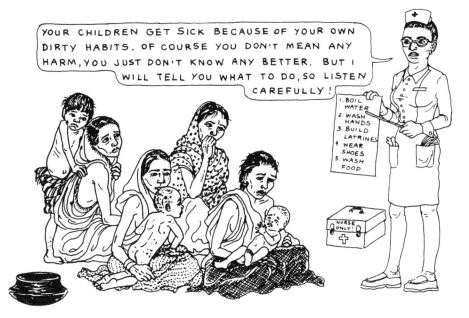

Figure 7.10   Teaching should *not* be like this.

they really know and understand one subject before going on to the next.

Use different senses so that trainees can:

- hear what is being said;
- see what is being shown;
- touch what is being presented.

Plan

Our plan for each lesson should include:

1. Greetings, welcome and introductions. Sometimes it is helpful to start with prayer or devotions.
2. Discussion on problems CHWs have recently come across in the community. Minor points can be discussed at the time, more major ones can form the basis of the day's lesson or be postponed till later.
3. Review of the previous lesson.
4. Introduction of the day's subject.
   Trainees should first share their own knowledge, attitude and practice (KAP) on the topic for the day's lesson.
5. Consolidation of the day's topic.
   This is the main part of the lesson. Use imaginative methods so the topic is really understood and learnt. Repeat-back, role play,

storytelling, drama, song, quiz, interview, etc. can be used (see Chapter 3).
6. Practical use of the day's topic.
   A skill may be learnt in the classroom such as bandaging or weighing. There may be a practical assignment to do in the community such as teaching a lesson or checking for a symptom like night blindness or chronic cough.
7. Review and giving of reminder cards.
   After reviewing the main points of the lesson, the CHWs are given special cards. These reminder cards summarise the main points – in words if the trainees can read, in pictures if they are unable to.

What should the curriculum include?

Try to obtain a training manual or outline curriculum either through the government, a voluntary health association or from a hospital. Make sure any manual has a correct approach and appropriate contents for the CHWs and their communities.

Most projects will be able to adopt and adapt existing manuals. Consider field-testing any

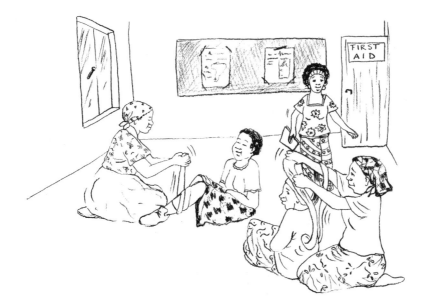

Figure 7.11   Each lesson should include time to try out practical skills.

manual before adopting it widely. Projects working in remote areas may need to write their own.

Trainers will know the important subjects to cover according to the manual and their own experience. Trainees will have ideas about the most useful things to know for their communities.

> The exact curriculum is best worked out by trainer and trainees discussing together at the start of the course.

As trainers use the manual they should be continually adding to it both new ideas and new information. In this way the manual becomes increasingly useful for each new group of trainees.

A suggested syllabus is shown in Table 7.1.

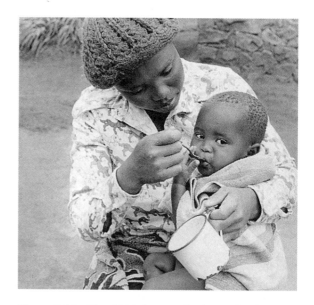

Figure 7.12   The CHW has taught the mother how to use oral rehydration solution.

Notes on the curriculum (See Table 7.1)

1. **Subjects included.**
   This list is a guide only and each project will develop its own curriculum.
2. **Order of lessons.**
   It is not necessary to follow a strict order as found in this list or in a training manual.

Start with subjects of interest to the trainees or relevant to the community. Mix teaching on diseases (often enjoyed most by the trainees) with other subjects, to keep the course balanced.

Table 7.1   Suggested syllabus for CHW training

Care of under-fives
1. How to recognise a sick child.
2. How to care for a sick child.
3. How to weigh children and use growth charts: how to measure the mid-upper arm circumference (MUAC).
4. Malnutrition: types, causes and prevention.
5. Malnutrition: supplementary and therapeutic feeding.
6. Hygiene.
7. Immunisations.
8. Diarrhoea and the use of oral rehydration salts (ORS).
9. Acute respiratory infection (ARI) and its treatment.
10. AIDS: its recognition and management. Mother to child transmission.

Care of pregnant mothers
1. Human reproduction.
2. Antenatal care: normal and abnormal signs: food supplements: preparation for delivery.
3. Birth of the child: stages of labour, normal and abnormal deliveries, use of delivery kit.
4. Postnatal care.
5. Care of newborn: breastfeeding.
6. Family planning and child spacing.

Parts of the body and how they work (anatomy and physiology)

Prevention and treatment of common illnesses
1. Diarrhoea and worms.
2. Abdominal pain.
3. Chest infections.
4. Tuberculosis.
5. Malaria.
6. Typhoid and cholera.
7. Measles.
8. Leprosy.
9. Sexually transmitted infections (STIs).
10. HIV/AIDS: prevention, voluntary counselling and testing (VCT), home-based care and use of antiretroviral therapy.
11. Anaemia.
12. Eye diseases.
13. Ear diseases.
14. Mouth and tooth problems.
15. Problems of menstruation.
16. Urinary infections.
17. Skin problems.
18. Other locally important diseases, symptoms.
19. Mental illness.
20. Non-communicable diseases: high blood pressure, diabetes, stroke and cancer.
21. Care of the handicapped, disabled, blind and hearing impaired.
22. Care of the elderly: palliative care.

First aid
1. Cuts and bruises: bandaging.
2. Burns.
3. Bone injuries.
4. Serious soft tissue injuries: shock.
5. Animal bites and injuries.
6. Snake and scorpion bites.
7. Drowning.
8. Poisoning.
9. The unconscious patient.
10. Cardiopulmonary resuscitation.
11. Prevention of common accidents in home, community and the workplace. Reducing the risk of road accidents
12. Treatment of drug reactions, and collapse after injection.

Environmental health
1. Clean water.
2. Sanitation and waste disposal.
3. Clean house and clean community.
4. Housing improvements: smokeless hearths.
5. Tobacco, alcohol and drug abuse.
6. Kitchen gardens.
7. Appropriate development.

General
1. The role and function of the CHW.
2. How a hospital works.
3. How and when to refer patients.
4. Record keeping and simple accounting.
5. Healthy living.
6. Keeping and using a medical kit.
7. Methods of teaching and communicating.
8. Leading discussion groups: raising awareness.
9. Details of the health project to which they belong.
10. National health problems and programmes.
11. Cooperating with others.
12. Millennium Development Goals: WHO and UNICEF.
13. Food security/disaster preparedness.

3. **Number of lessons per subject.**
   Some subjects can be easily covered in one lesson, others, such as antenatal care, may need several.
4. **Length of lessons.**
   Aim for about two to three hours per lesson providing there is plenty of variety of teaching techniques and that the trainees participate. Arrange breaks during the lesson for chat, refreshments or games.

> Learn to recognise boredom. If pupils get bored, we should stop the lesson, change our approach or set up an activity. Bored people don't learn.

5. **Hospital experience.**
   Whether or not a hospital or health centre is used as the teaching centre, CHWs will need to understand what a hospital does, and how a hospital works. This is best done by introducing them in turn to each department and its staff. As well as benefiting CHWs, this will have several helpful results for patients in the community:
   - They can be given useful, informed advice by CHWs before being referred to hospital.
   - They will receive better care in the hospital because staff will have met their CHW.
   - A transfer system can be set up between the CHW and hospital or health centre, which encourages continuity of care.
6. **Further training.**
   After the basic curriculum has been covered, CHWs will need further teaching including:
   - Revision and update on important subjects.
   - Teaching on new health topics.
   - Introduction to wider development issues.
   - Training so that CHWs themselves can become trainers, supervisors, or eventually trainers of trainers.
7. **Examinations.**
   CHWs should have regular oral and practical tests to make sure their skills and knowledge are accurate and up to date.
   Before they receive health kits, arrange a more thorough examination. *For example*: We could call in an outside 'examiner' familiar with the community, who can test each candidate both fairly and thoroughly.

Key topics are how to recognise common illnesses and the correct uses of medicines. Where CHWs are supplied with health kits, the more skilfully they use them, the greater will be their acceptance by the community.

What supervision should be carried out?

There is no value in training a CHW, sending her back to the community and forgetting her. The real value of a CHW to the community will depend on how well she is encouraged and supervised.

Supervisors should visit at least once a week in the first year of the programme, unless communities are remote, scattered or there is political insecurity. Later, when a CHW is established and confident, supervisors can visit less frequently, providing there is regular contact in other ways such as in the health centre, hospital or training centre, or when submitting monthly reports.

The supervisor will often be the same person as the trainer or teacher. Main jobs will include:

1. **Encouragement, support and training.**
   This is the supervisor's main purpose.
2. **Pastoral care.**
   The CHW will value her supervisor's advice about practical problems she faces in the community. She may need help with personal troubles also, especially if these arise from her work as the CHW. The supervisor must be willing to support and advise but be careful not to encourage dependence.
3. **Discipline.**

> If the CHW needs correcting, disciplining or warning, the supervisor should do this, gently, privately and fairly. There should be ten words of praise for every one word of criticism.

   CHWs should never be disciplined in front of community members.
4. **Payments.**
   When appropriate, the supervisor should make sure each CHW receives the correct payment on time.

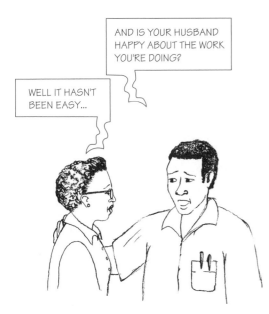

Figure 7.13 The supervisor must be willing to support and advise.

A point to emphasise:

> A supervisor's job is not simply to 'tell off and pay off'. Supervisors should make frequent community visits both to understand its needs and to support CHWs in their work.

The CHW's health kit

Although some CHWs will be involved only in health promotion, the offer of curative care helps to make a CHW more popular and more effective as a health promoter.

In some areas there will be no need for CHWs to carry health kits because there will be alternative supplies such as pharmacies, private practitioners or primary health centres. In other areas there is such a shortage of trained health workers and of medicines in local health centres that a CHW able to treat illness at village level is of great value.

However, CHWs should only be issued with health kits if two conditions are in place. First, they must be adequately trained and the community must believe this is the case. Second, they must be reliably supplied by the programme or government with a supply of essential medicines

so the community knows they can depend on their CHW.

What should a kit contain?

Medicines

Choice of medicines is a top-level decision and a doctor should advise on contents. We will need to be sure about national regulations on prescribing medicines, and whether CHWs are allowed to do this. If an error occurs and a legal case is brought, it will be essential that the drug prescribed has been recorded by name, dose and date, and the reason it was given clearly stated. CHWs will need to be trained to do this, even if simple symbols are used.

Medicines chosen should be effective, simple, safe, cheap, and easy to obtain. It is important to follow any national guidelines or rational drug policy. See also Chapter 17 and Appendix C.

A suggested list is shown in Table 7.2.

Notes on medicines

1. Medicines should be carefully packed into secure, damp-proof, containers. Liquid medicines such as gentian violet must be stored in leakproof bottles.
2. Medicines must be clearly labelled. If CHWs are illiterate this can be done through symbols or pictures. *For example*: Tablets to treat malaria can be labelled with the drawing of a mosquito. Normal doses can be recorded as a reminder.
3. Supplies must be regularly restocked. When seeing a sick villager, the CHW should never have to confess that her stocks have run out.
4. The kit should be safely stored. It should be kept locked and in a safe place.
5. Re-ordering. A system should be set up with the supervisor (see also pages 66–9 and 156–7).

Equipment

Keep this simple. It might include:

- bandages, tape and cotton wool;
- scissors and safety pins;
- envelopes for pills (can be home-made from magazines);

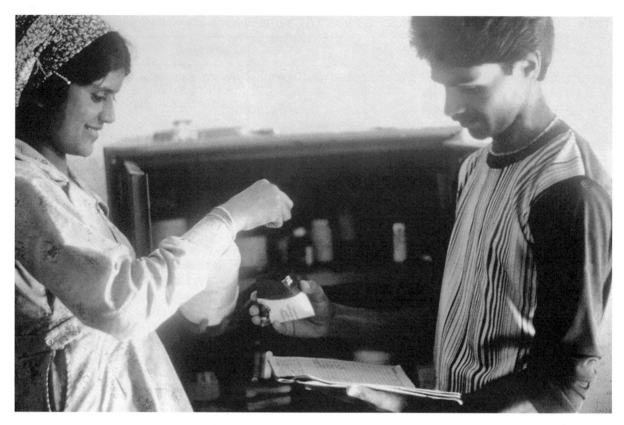

Figure 7.14   CHWs need to become expert in the use of simple medicines.

- mid-upper arm circumference measurer and/or portable weighing scale;
- simple health booklets and flashcards or teaching aids;
- delivery kits if used (see Chapter 12);
- record book and ball point pens.

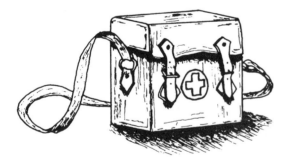

Figure 7.15   The CHW's box.

Both medicines and equipment can be kept in a box, which should be:

- large enough to contain all supplies;
- small enough to carry;
- strong enough for constant use;
- waterproof in wet climates;
- divided into two or three sections, either arranged side by side, or one on top of the other;
- marked with a red cross or crescent;
- fitted with a handle and shoulder strap;
- lockable.

How should the kit be given?

The health kit should be handed over to the CHW in a special presentation or passing out ceremony. The CHW is encouraged and affirmed in front of her people; the community has an opportunity to learn more about health care; the project has a chance to teach and raise community awareness.

Table 7.2   Suggested list of medicines for CHW's health kit

Disease/symptom	Medicine†	Comments
1. Pain, fever	Paracetamol (500 mg/100 mg) Aspirin (300 mg)	Aspirin not suitable if stomach ulcers common, and not to be used in children under 16.
2. Stomach ache/ indigestion	Aluminium hydroxide (500 mg)	
3. Worms	Mebendazole (100 mg/500 mg) Albendazole (400 mg)	Treatment of choice for pinworm, roundworm, hookworm, whipworm.
4. Diarrhoea, dehydration	Oral Rehydration Salts	Use cheapest available. Also, teach community how to make up, or use local liquid foods.
5. Malaria	Nationally recommended malaria treatment	Areas with high resistance need specialised advice. Ensure insecticide impregnated bed-nets are being bought and used.
6. Anaemia and for use in pregnant and lactating mothers	Ferrous salt (equiv. 60 mg Fe) alone or with Folic Acid (0.40 mg)	Warn that stools may turn black. Use iron with folic acid during pregnancy.
7. Serious bacterial infections*	Amoxycillin (250 mg) or Erythromycin (250 mg) or Cotrimoxazole (400/80 mg) (esp. for ARI)	Life-saving in Acute Respiratory Infections (ARI). Valuable in many situations. Careful protocols needed for prescribing.
8. Allergy and itching: insect bites	Chlorphenamine (4 mg)	Warn about drowsiness.
9. Vitamin A deficiency	Vitamin A tabs or syrup	Use only if deficiency locally present. For correct use see page 184.
10. Eye infections	Tetracycline eye ointment 1% or gentamicin 0.3% drops	Cures most eye infections. Tetracycline or azithromycin cures trachoma if used early and correctly.
11. Scabies	Benzyl benzoate (25% lotion) or permethrin cream (5%) or lotion (1%)	May be alternative local remedy.
12. Sores, cuts, skin infections	Gentian violet	Some communities won't accept.
13. Rub for muscles, bruises, headache, etc.	Local liniment or balm, e.g. Vicks, menthol	Usually popular.
14. Antiseptic for cleansing skin	Chlorhexidine or local equivalent: soap	For cleaning skin infections/wounds.

* These include chest infections such as acute respiratory infection, e.g. pneumonia and bronchitis, severe ear and skin infections, tooth abscess, severe sore throat or sinusitis, urinary infection, dysentery with fever and some forms of sexually transmitted infection.
† Other commonly used drugs include: aminophylline (asthma); griseofulvin tabs or Whitfield ointment (fungal skin infections); ergometrine (blood loss after abortion or delivery); laxative preparation (constipation); metronidazole (Amoeba, Giardia, Trichomonas); multivitamins (famine conditions only); phenobarbital (epilepsy).
Note: this is a fairly comprehensive list and many programmes may wish to shorten this depending on their situation, especially when CHWs first start using medicines.

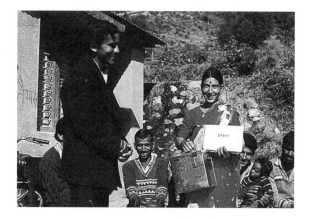

Figure 7.16   A CHW receiving her box.

Before the presentation, make careful plans with the community. Encourage them to choose a respected leader or official to be guest of honour, and to invite the whole community.

The presentation itself should be festive, and can include cultural items such as health songs or a short drama. Community leaders can say a few words (preferably not political speeches). A guest of honour can present both the boxes and certificates, each CHW being photographed in turn.

The health committee chairperson or Programme Director can help the community understand more about the work of the CHW, explaining what she can and cannot do. *The speaker can ask the community to give her encouragement and forgive any mistakes she makes when she first starts work.*

How does a CHW keep records?

This needs to be kept as simple as possible with minimum duplication.

The system described is appropriate if a CHW is literate or can work with a literate friend or col-

league. Where this is not possible, a book with pictograms or symbols can be designed.

The following information can be recorded:

A list of patients seen and treatment given

A possible layout on a double page is shown in Table 7.3.

Under 'Treatment' always record the name of any medicine used along with dose and total number of pills given.

An updated list of all 'at-risk' patients or families who need regular visiting

This is the CHW's list of those for whom she needs to take special care and who need regular visiting. It includes:

• under-five malnourished children;
• under-five children with any acute or chronic illness, and those who have not completed immunisations;
• pregnant and postnatal women;
• patients with TB, leprosy and people living with HIV/AIDS requiring home care;
• those with chronic 'non-communicable' illnesses such as diabetes, raised blood pressure, or requiring regular medication;
• the disabled, very old or socially outcast;
• those recently discharged from hospital.

It can also include those needing regular birth control supplies.

A separate section can be kept for each category or they can be lumped together. Whichever system is used, include the details as in Table 7.4.

An alternative system is to use a diary, recording patients' names on the date they are due to be seen. The two systems can be used together.

Table 7.3

Date	Patient's Name & No	Age	Problem	Treatment	Outcome	Money taken
January 4th 2006	Jose Lopez 01/04/19/05	46	Acute respiratory infection	Amoxycillin 250 mg 21 tablets	Much improved 48 hours later	30 cents

Table 7.4

Date	Patient's Name & No	Age	Risk Category	Treatment	Date next visit
Nov 22nd 2005	Mary 12/03/84/06	28	Pregnant 32 weeks	Revisit or check in clinic	29th November

Vital events record (Table 7.5)

Births, deaths and permanent movement in and out of the community (e.g. following marriage).

Daily activity list

Some CHWs also keep a list of daily activities carried out, both for their own interest and to show their supervisor.

Books used should be strong with tough bindings, and should fit into the CHW's box. Each of these records can be kept in different sections of the same book. The supervisor can help to prepare this.

Monthly report form

Most CHWs will also fill in a monthly report form containing key data already mentioned. The purpose of this is largely for transferring data from community to project office, or to provide government returns, for example, to the district medical officer.

This form should be as simple as possible, easy to complete from her other records and designed to be used alongside any computerised record system that may be planned. In this case it should be identical to the data input screen, and forms could be computer generated, making data entry simple.

Alternatively, computers can be programmed to generate simple forms on which the CHW records all information, and which act as a reminder to her of which people she needs to visit, for which purpose and on which date (known as the 'due list'). This might seem an efficient system but, unless care is taken, it can shift programme focus from community to office, and may disempower the CHW.

If the CHW is also carrying out functions under any special programme, she should use record forms required for that programme and be trained in their use. Examples are TB programmes using DOTS (see pages 280–8), the distribution of ivermectin in river blindness control, or praziquantel in bilharzia.

How is a CHW supported?

In this section support means personal support not financial support.

Table 7.5

For **births** include:

Date of birth	Name	Head of family	House No	Live, still	Name of midwife

For **deaths** include:

Date of birth	Name	Head of family	House No	Age	Probable cause

For **movements** (permanent) in and out of the community include:

Name	Head of family	House No	Age	In or out	Reason

In order for the CHW to become effective she will need both confidence in herself, and credibility in her community. She will only succeed or survive if she has an effective support system.

This support will come from various sources:

The health team

When first trained, the CHW will rely heavily on the health team and on her supervisor. The community may not have confidence in her, her family may misunderstand her, she may scarcely believe in herself.

The CHW will continue to receive regular lessons where questions and worries can be dealt with, and encouragement given. She can receive advice on how to deal with difficult people or puzzling cases.

The supervisor or other health team members must visit the CHW in her community, ideally once a week initially and in any case at least once a month.

Other CHWs

'A problem shared is a problem halved'.

By meeting together regularly, CHWs can share their problems and come to see that others are facing similar situations. More mature CHWs can give encouragement and practical advice.

The CHW's own family

The family may feel proud that one of its own members has been chosen by the community. However, family members may resent the time she spends away and the extra work that others have to do when she is absent.

It is important to encourage and involve the family so that they in turn can support the CHW. The husband's or partner's support is especially important. The supervisor should aim to build friendships with members of the CHW's family.

The community

At the beginning, the community may seem more of a threat than a support. As the CHW gains confidence and her treatment and advice are seen to work, the community will usually come to respect and support her. *For example*: Members of the health committee can accompany her to remote homes or at night; they or her husband or partner can help her to keep records.

Women's clubs, young farmers' clubs or youth clubs can play an active role in giving support. They can give practical help in her work and stand with her when others criticise or complain.

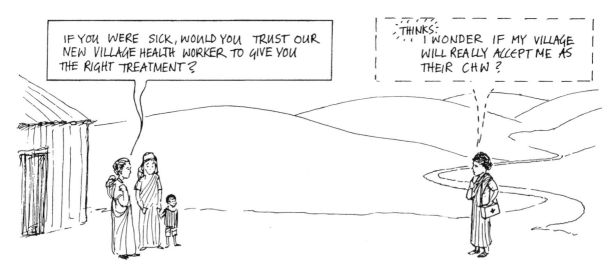

Figure 7.17   Newly qualified CHWs face big challenges.

Table 7.6   CHW's support points

	Health team	Other CHWs	Family	Community	Self	Total
1st month After 1 year	++++ +	+++ ++	+ +	+ +++	+ +++	10 10

The CHW herself

As she gains in maturity and knowledge, the CHW will learn self-dependence, and outside support systems will become less necessary.

It is helpful to consider each CHW as needing ten support points in order to develop as an effective health worker. Table 7.6 shows two examples of how they may add up.

Should a CHW be paid?

Please see also Chapter 21: How a Programme Can Become Sustainable.

This is one of the hardest questions to answer in community based health care and the future of the CHW model depends partly on finding practical answers.

The dilemma is this: health programmes using CHWs need to be financially self-sufficient so

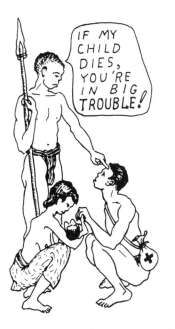

Figure 7.18   The CHW has less protection than most doctors and thus needs more support.

they can be sustained into the future. CHWs often demand to be paid. Programmes faced with increasing CHW salaries become unsustainable.

Unsatisfactory planning and agreement over CHW salaries and excessive payment demands are one of the commonest causes of failure in CBHC programmes.

Wherever possible, we should aim to set up CHW programmes in partnership with the community where CHWs are unpaid.

Although difficult to achieve, this may be possible under the following circumstances:

1. Where CHWs work a maximum of two days per week, ideally half to one day per week.
   This means each CHW will be able to care for about 25 families. Programmes based on unpaid volunteers will therefore use a larger number of part-time CHWs rather than a smaller number of full-timers.

2. Where CHWs possess a strong sense of social service or religious motivation. *For example*: In the Bodji area of Ethiopia over 100 church deacons serve as unpaid community health volunteers. Often churches and religious organisations are known to have fewer funds available than health programmes, meaning that faith-based programmes can sometimes be more easily sustainable.

3. Where CHWs receive their support and encouragement in ways other than through payment. *For example*: In the Adrokor Rural Clinic in Ghana, neither CHWs nor TBAs receive salaries. Being highly valued by the community, they are often brought gifts to supplement their income.

4. Where at the start of the programme everyone – both community and CHWs – understand that payments will not be provided and that CHWs will work out of service to their community.
   Two more examples:
   (1) A recent report from Malawi lists a variety of rewards that reduce the need for CHWs to

receive financial incentives. These include: recognition and praise, exemption from user-fees at the local health facility, gaining useful free training and experience that may later help job prospects, the interest of volunteering as an alternative to hard work at home or in some cases boredom with domestic routines.

(2) An urban CHW from Delhi recently wrote as follows: 'my family is much healthier now. None of us has become sick since I became a CHW. I also have more confidence in myself. I feel like a valued member of my community because people come to me for help and advice because they respect me.'

Such rewards can be emphasised to CHWs and their families when they are being trained.

> It needs to be made clear that appointment as a CHW is not a path to fame and fortune either for the CHW or her family.

How should the CHW be paid?

If payment appears to be essential, funding may be obtainable through the community, or from the government.

The community itself

Possible methods include: through a health committee, through an insurance scheme and payment by individuals.

Payment through a health committee

This will work only if:
1. The community so values its CHW that it is willing to pay her.
2. The community is able to work out a fair, honest and efficient way of collecting the money.

Few poor communities are able to do this at the start but may be able to later on as faith in the CHW grows and community organisation improves.

For example: Such a change has been made by the Comprehensive Rural Health Programme in

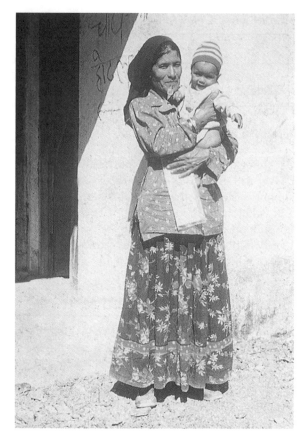

Figure 7.19   This CHW is popular, but is she so popular that the community is willing to pay her?

Jamkhed, western India. CHWs were initially paid by the programme but have become so widely appreciated that the community now provides their support.

Payment through an insurance scheme

Community members each pay a fixed amount into a fund and receive certain health services free in return. The CHW is paid out of this fund.

Schemes of this sort demand a good level of local organisation in order to be effective, and in particular require a sensitised and trustworthy health committee.

Payment from individuals as they are treated

This is the system often used by TBAs, traditional practitioners and village doctors in China, who are paid in cash or kind for the services they provide. The local community is often familiar with this approach and can apply it to its new CHW.

For example: The CHW can charge a fixed amount per consultation or per medicine given, as agreed with the project or health committee. She can then keep part or all of this as payment, or return it to a pool from which fixed payments are made monthly to CHWs.

There is one disadvantage to this approach (see Figure 7.20). The more medicines a CHW uses, the more she earns. This conflicts with one of the chief roles of the CHW – to be an agent of change in the community so that illnesses become less common and medicines become less necessary.

The government

Many NGO programmes will be run in close association with the government. In some, the government will be the lead partner, as in emerging programmes in the People's Republic of China. In others, government will 'contract out' CHW training and supervision to the NGO.

In both these models, government funding for CHWs may be available. There are, however, two problems that often arise in practice. First, the CHW may be seen primarily as a government employee, rather than a community member. Quality of care may suffer as a result. Second, government funding may be unreliable or subject to delay, thus leading to demotivation.

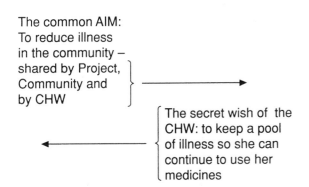

The common AIM:
To reduce illness in the community – shared by Project, Community and by CHW

The secret wish of the CHW: to keep a pool of illness so she can continue to use her medicines

Figure 7.20 Conflict of aims when CHWs are paid by patients for each medicine dispensed.

A sound principle is that we should use government funds where available, request that these be paid as block grants with minimum conditions attached, and keep other funding options open.

Funding agencies

This may seem the simplest or indeed the only solution at the start.

The danger resembles that of a car running downhill out of control. It keeps going faster and faster and becomes increasingly hard to stop.

Quite apart from the agency having ever larger bills to pay, there is a further disadvantage. The CHW may be seen as an employee of the project or agency rather than as a community member answerable to a health committee. We must also remember that, once a programme starts paying CHWs, it is extremely difficult to stop this

How much should a CHW be paid?

This is worked out in discussion with the community.

The amount paid depends on:

The expectation of the CHW, her family and the community

Effective CHWs often serve because of their social concern, interest in the job and personal commitment. On the other hand, CHWs usually come from poor backgrounds and their families may depend on the work they do at home, in the field or as job earners. It may seem unreasonable for such CHWs to serve for more than one or two days per week and receive nothing tangible in return.

We must therefore find a balance between paying a CHW too much on the one hand and too little on the other, both of which may take away her sense of service.

If too much is paid this sequence occurs:
1. The CHW's family starts thinking of her simply as another wage-earner.

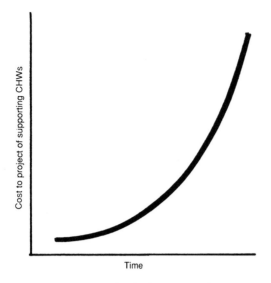

Cost to project of supporting CHWs

Time

Figure 7.21   Projects that both increase their coverage and give regular pay rises to CHWs become unsustainable.

2. Comparisons are made with salaries received by others. Higher wages may then be demanded and 'unionisation' may occur.
3. Money now replaces service as the reason for working. The quality of care starts to fall. The programme (or government) is unable to pay the salaries.

If too little is paid this sequence occurs:
1. The CHW and her family become discouraged or resentful.
2. The CHW spends less time in the community and more time doing jobs in the home.
3. The CHW starts charging (or overcharging) for her services. Quality of care again starts to fall.

For example: In one central African project, volunteers were reported as saying: 'people are asking us what sort of a job is this, that we do not get paid at the end of the month.'

Commonly, CHWs compare the amounts being received by their colleagues in neighbouring programmes and become discouraged or angry if they seem to be receiving less.

The amount of money available

We should not pay high salaries that can't be maintained. There are too many programmes where CHWs were paid well from the start and have now stopped working because the programme has run out of money. It is better for no or low wages to be paid rather than higher wages that are not sustainable.

Government policy

There may be agreed levels in the country or district, which we should follow. Some countries recommend that CHWs should not be paid, others expect that they should.

Practical hints if payment is essential

1. Avoid the term wages, salaries or income.
   Use instead the name or idea of an honorarium, contribution, or compensation for time lost. Make sure that the payment method used does not break national labour laws.
2. Payments must be punctual.
   If CHWs are to be paid, make sure payments are paid in full and on time.
3. CHWs should sign for payments received.
   This saves argument later and will be needed by the programme auditor or health committee accountant.
4. Training expenses and transport costs for training sessions can be reimbursed.
5. Modest pay increases can gradually be given as agreed with the health committee.
6. Equivalent grades of CHW are paid the same amount.
   Where possible, use similar rates to those paid by neighbouring programmes.
7. Encourage the health committee to make the payments as soon as it is able to take on this key responsibility.

Common reasons why CHW programmes fail

Most of these have been mentioned in the course of the chapter. Many cases of failure can be prevented with good programme planning or through recognising a problem early and taking action.

Volunteers' needs must be recognised and addressed adequately if a project is to succeed.

Here are some common reasons for failure:

- **Inadequate time to create awareness in the community**
  For example: We go too fast, impose our ideas on the community and then struggle to persuade them that CHWs are what they need. We must spend time in the community, carry out Participatory Appraisal and allow the people themselves to suggest and own any CHW programme.

- **Selection of inappropriate CHWs**
  For example: We fail to explain to the community just what a wide range of useful tasks a CHW can carry out. People fail to grasp the significance of her role and the qualities needed in those they select. Again, this is a matter of taking time to create awareness and working together with the community in the early phases of our CBHC programme.

- **Family members do not support the CHW in her role**
  For example: They may not understand what she is meant to do. Partners of female CHWs may feel threatened or become suspicious. There may be resentment that the CHW spends less time as mother, cook, water-gatherer and farmer. Most of these problems can be prevented if we spend time with family members at the beginning, helping them to understand that the family will benefit through the CHW's knowledge, status and any remuneration she may receive. We can identify and correct any false ideas that may have arisen.

- **Training is inadequate**
  For example: We may have given too little practical experience for CHWs to recognise and treat common illnesses. They may make mistakes in diagnosis and use wrong medicines. This can quickly cause the community to lose confidence, and it may take a long time to regain it. CHWs may have been taught or treated inappropriately. In turn they may lack confidence, or teach others health practices that are irrelevant for their community. This again can reduce their respect.

It is also important that CHWs continue to learn new skills and to carry out different tasks. Otherwise they may become bored, or be unable to meet the changing health needs in their community.

- **Supervision and backup are inadequate**
  For example: CHWs do not receive the support they need. Their supervisors fail to visit them, their health kits run out, they become confused by the records they are expected to keep.
  Irregular or inadequate supervision is a common reason why many projects start well but fail after two or three years.
  We need to plan for the long-term support and supervision of the CHW, and we need to train the health committee to take over a progressive role in her support and management.

- **Problems with payment**
  Disagreements about pay are one of the commonest reasons why CHW programmes fail. Usually CHWs (or their family) feel they are not paid enough. Issues about pay may not have been talked through at the start. *For example*: CHWs assumed they would be paid; the programme assumed they would be working as volunteers. Resentment will always be caused if payment is agreed but is then delayed or reduced. Funding may simply dry up, leaving everyone bewildered and demotivated.
  Make sure these issues are discussed in detail at the start of the project and, if any problems develop, deal with them at once before dissatisfaction spreads. Experience has shown that, even when CHWs clearly understand they will not be receiving payment, they may later forget this or be persuaded by others they should expect to be paid.

- **CHWs expect inappropriate promotion**
  For example: In programmes with strong government links, CHWs may be seen as the first level of health worker who later become promoted to nurse aides or go on to nurses' training. This may be fine for the CHW but can undermine the CHW programme, unless we develop a good strategy to overcome this.

- **CHWs drop out from the programme for personal reasons**

  For example: Young female CHWs may leave the village to get married, may become full-time mothers, may suffer from a breakdown in family relationships or have a tragedy to cope with. Male CHWs may be drawn to a nearby town or set up independently when they have gained sufficient health knowledge.

  For example: In many parts of the world CHWs die prematurely from AIDS, especially where antiretroviral treatment is not available. Also, CHWs and their families become overwhelmed by caring for friends and relatives, leaving little time for other duties.

- **Famine, war or disaster may affect the project area**

  If this happens, it may still be possible for CHWs to meet and members of the programme to remain in contact. Sometimes the CHW can take on additional roles, such as helping at feeding centres or having a health care role in a refugee camp.

  Even though there may be turmoil at national or regional level, grass roots programmes may still be able to continue. Programme leaders and supervisors should show leadership to try to make this happen. Programmes that have to be temporarily stopped should be restarted as soon as possible.

  Even under the worst conditions, CHWs who have gained knowledge and confidence may often find a valuable role in whatever situations they find themselves. They can help to care for those around them, start health classes and link with others to start new informal programmes.

  For example: In southern Sudan, in a situation with recent long-term war and instability, many health facilities are more than ten hours away and unsafe to reach. CHWs carefully trained to use specific field-tested materials improved the health of their communities, especially under-five children.

Summary

In many countries CHWs are becoming the key health workers in community based programmes.

CHWs should be well respected members of a community, often but not always women aged between 20 and 45, who are chosen by the community itself. They are trained appropriately using a comprehensive and practical syllabus in centres as near to their homes as possible.

When basic training is completed, CHWs are given an examination and may then be presented with a health kit. They now start serving in the community where their tasks include giving health teaching, acting as agents of change and, in many programmes, providing curative care. They also care for all community members whose health is at risk, liaising with the health team, to whom they refer serious cases. They are encouraged to keep accurate records.

When CHWs start work they need much encouragement and support from the project, from the community and from fellow CHWs.

CHWs ideally serve out of social concern, through religious motivation, or for other rewards apart from payment. Only if payment is the sole way in which CHWs can be recruited and retained should it be given, and then usually only if CHWs work more than one or two days per week. If payment is necessary, the best sources are usually the community or government, not NGOS or outside agencies.

There are several common reasons why CHW programmes fail. By understanding what these are we can help to avoid them, and when problems do arise we can take quick action to deal with them.

The future of the CHW model will be assured as it develops ways of being sustainable and as CHWs are sufficiently well chosen, trained and supervised so that community members have confidence in their services.

Further reading and resources

1. *Helping Health Workers Learn*, D. Werner and B. Bower, Hesperian Foundation, latest reprint 1995. This classic guide is unsurpassed and has been translated into numerous languages.
   Available from: TALC. See Appendix E.
2. *Teaching Health-care Workers*, 2nd edn, F. Abbatt and R. McMahon, Macmillan, 1993. Valuable ideas on appropriate training.
   Available from: TALC. See Appendix E.

3. *Jamkhed: A Comprehensive Rural Health Project*, M. and R. Arole, Macmillan, 1994.
   This classic contains detailed descriptions of how one outstanding CHW programme works in practice.
   Available from: TALC. See Appendix E.
4. *Community Health Workers' Manual*, 2nd edn, E. Wood, AMREF, 1999.
   A very useful book, especially for Africa.
   Available from: AMREF. See Appendix E.
5. *Community Health Workers: The way forward*, H. Kahssay, M. Taylor and P. Berman, WHO, 1998.
   A very useful review with areas to focus on for the future.
   Available from: WHO. See Appendix E.
6. 'How and what BRAC learns in health', J. Rohde, the website of BRAC, the Bangladesh rural advancement committee 2005, www.brac.net.

See Further references and guidelines, page 412.

PART III
Specific Programmes

8

Setting up a Community Health Clinic

In this chapter we shall consider:
1. What we need to know
   - What health services already exist?
   - Why develop a clinic?
   - What type of clinic should be set up?
   - Who will use the clinic?
   - How many people should the clinic serve?
   - Where should the clinic be held?
   - When should the clinic start?
2. What we need to do:
   - Design the centre
   - Set up the clinic stations
   - Keep and transfer clinic records
   - Decide on a system of payment
   - Set up a referral system
   - Concentrate on teaching and health promotion
   - Ensure that health centres are prepared for serious illness
   - Understand the role of mobile clinics

What we need to know

What health services already exist?

Before starting any new clinic or health centre we must do two things. First, find out what services already exist in our project area, and second, decide how any health centre we start integrates with what already exists.

We must also be sure we have the capacity to set up a clinic and to manage it successfully over a period of time.

Finding out what health services exist

We need to enquire about the following:
- **How are government health centres arranged in our country, region and area?**

Countries are usually divided into different health 'districts', or an equivalent term, e.g. Municipio in many South American countries, Département in many French-speaking countries. Districts are then subdivided into smaller administrative areas, often called subdistricts, and usually into smaller zones below that. *For example*: In India there are Districts, Tehsils, Blocks and Panchayats, the latter consisting of one or more villages. In the People's Republic of China there are Prefectures (the equivalent of Districts), Counties, 'Districts', Townships and Villages.

Where sufficient resources exist, districts will have a district hospital, usually run by the government, but sometimes handed over to a voluntary, private or religious agency to manage and support. Subdistricts and their equivalents usually aim to have primary health centres with basic inpatient and maternity facilities. They serve an approximate population number, or a defined geographical area. *For example*: In Tanzania, health centres were originally set up to cover a population of 50 000 or a radius of 10 kilometres.

At more peripheral levels there will be dispensaries or health posts, usually with few or no overnight beds. There may be mobile clinics. (See also Chapter 20, pages 376–7.)

- **How effectively are government health facilities functioning?**

Obviously, this will vary greatly not only between countries but between districts. There are many factors making it difficult for governments to keep up standards of health care.

High demand: Growing populations, civil war with displaced persons, a greater burden of illness, e.g. HIV/AIDS, malaria and TB, aging populations, an increasing load from non-communicable diseases such as diabetes and hypertension.

Low resources: Large debt repayments, loss of personnel because of low pay and morale, loss of trained staff because of outside recruitment and in many African countries AIDS-related illness leading to the premature death of health personnel.

As a result of these and other reasons, resources will be very stretched, staff morale often low and buildings unmaintained. Staff may be unpaid or absent and drug supplies will often be in short supply. In some areas there may be an almost complete close-down of any effective health care.

- **What other health-related programmes are functioning in the project area?**

There may be other NGOs, providing health or related services, e.g. Mission Hospitals. There may be 'vertical programmes' organised by the government or a multilateral agency, which concentrate on specific tasks, e.g. childhood immunisation, the Integrated Management of Childhood Illness (IMCI), or on one particular illness of global importance such as Stop TB and Roll Back Malaria, or the control of locally important illnesses such as filaria, bilharzia or river blindness. There may be overlap, duplication and confusion between these programmes making an integrated community based approach even more important.

Other agencies may be concentrating on health development, e.g. sanitation or water, or on other sectors involved in literacy, control of soil erosion, micro-credit, and housing – all of which have a direct effect on health.

Deciding how we can integrate with existing services

Governments have the prime responsibility for the health care of their populations. However, they often have insufficient resources to provide these. NGOs on the other hand may offer innovative and successful ways of bringing good quality health care or setting up special programmes. It is important that government and NGO recognise the responsibilities and strengths of each other. That means building relationships and discussing these issues in detail.

NGOs will need to make sure they cooperate as fully as possible with government and integrate their services wherever possible. But they also need to make sure they don't lose their distinctive strengths as they do this. It is valuable also if NGOs seek to become partners in the scaling up of existing or successful services.

> **Ways of linking NGOs and government health services**
> - Thoughtfully consider the most appropriate way any new health centre could tie in with existing facilities.
> - Build relationships with government, at district and local levels, and also with any other NGOs working in the same area. In particular visit and discuss the situation with the District Medical Officer (DMO).
> - Decide whether it is possible to strengthen an existing health centre, e.g. by working in partnership with existing staff, or even offering to run it on their behalf.
> - Decide whether it is appropriate to start a new centre, in areas where there are no existing or functioning facilities.
> - Secure written permission, a contract or agreement from the government and/or the DMO for any new health facility or programme you plan to set up.
> - Arrange to collect and send statistics to the DMO in line with national guidelines.

This chapter describes the setting up of a clinic. The emphasis is on setting up a new community based clinic such as a health post, a 'dispensary', or equivalent where nothing effective exists. It does not include how to set up inpatient facilities, as in a hospital or Primary Health Centre, but some sections in this chapter will be useful in these situations.

The chapter can also be used for ideas on how to improve or scale up existing clinics, ranging from District Hospital Outpatients, through Primary Health Centres down to peripheral health posts. Our emphasis must always be to involve the community as much as possible so that their needs and ideas help to mould how the health centre develops; they must also become involved in managing it. We must regularly liaise with government officials.

> Our aim should be that the health centre functions with the three strands of project, government and community working together as closely as possible, based on CBHC principles.

Why develop a clinic?

The reason may seem simple: people are sick; health workers can make them better; the community requests it.

But we need to look at the reasons more carefully, and understand the different expectations between community members and health workers (see Figure 8.1). At this stage it is also helpful to be clear about the possible roles of doctors and how they often approach health care in a very different way than from a community health based model. (See Chapter 20, pages 372–4.)

If curative care alone is provided this situation occurs:

> The same patient with the same illness comes back to the same clinic to get the same medicine to return to the same environment to get the same illness ...

The community may in the long term be worse off than before, still just as sick and now newly dependent.

What type of clinic should be set up?

This should be decided in partnership with the community, and in discussion with the District Medical Officer or equivalent.

Some projects will develop general clinics, also sometimes known as multipurpose or polyclinics. Here any person can attend with any problem. Others will run separate clinics for different problems such as Mother and Child Health (MCH) clinics on one day of the week, TB clinics on another.

General clinics are usually more convenient for patients unless access is exceptionally easy. All patients can be dealt with at the same time – grandmother with toothache, father with indigestion, mother pregnant again, and the twins with malnutrition.

Moreover, each individual can use the same visit to have all problems seen on one single occasion. *For example*: A mother with sore eyes,

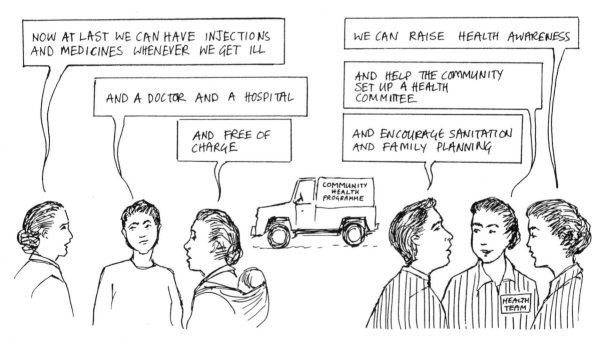

Figure 8.1   A case of differing expectations.

having a chronic cough, needing a final antenatal check, and requesting advice about family planning.

Separate clinics are sometimes appropriate, each being run on a different day of the week. These can be used where access is very easy, or patient numbers large, as when a clinic first starts, or when chronic poverty causes much illness. They can also be used in established refugee camps.

> Health team members must never develop clinics at the expense of being involved at the community level. It is usually more useful to spend half the week teaching CHWs or improving a community water supply than spending five days within the walls of the health centre.

Who will use the clinic?

Unless the clinic is part of a genuine community programme: the least needy may use it most, the most needy may use it least. This is known as the 'inverse care law'.

The least needy who use it most

These may include:
1. Those with minor health needs wanting injections and pills.
2. Those ill a long time who have already seen many doctors, and arrive clutching sheaves of reports.
3. Those living nearby who can easily attend.
4. Those well enough to reach the clinic or who have relatives able and willing to bring them.
5. Men, who in poor communities often have more time to attend, and are often less willing than women to tolerate pain.

The most needy who use it least

These may include:
1. The poor, the distant and the frightened.
2. Women unable to leave home.
3. Children too sick to walk, or with no one to carry them.
4. The very ill, the very old, the disabled.

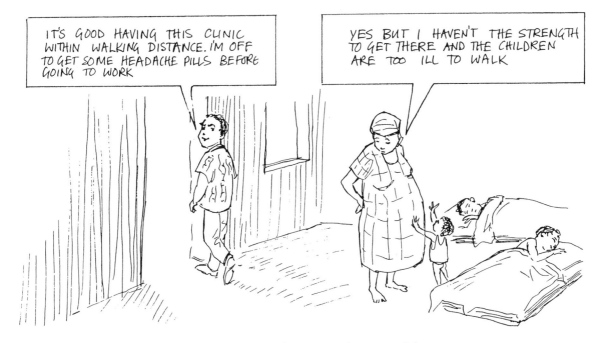

Figure 8.2   The least needy may use the clinic most, the most needy may use it least.

Our project must run clinics in such a way that the inverse care law is reversed. Clinics must therefore be priced sensibly and sited correctly, be user friendly, and run in partnership with the community.

At an early stage it will be useful to find out any reasons why people may not be using the health centre to the fullest extent, in other words to investigate access. Of course there may be a good reason, e.g. because effective CHWs are consulted by community members and deal with the majority of problems. But often there may be other reasons, not always obvious.

For example: A recent study in Uganda asking community members why they did not take sick children to the health unit were given the following answers (often there was more than one reason): lack of money was cited in 90 per cent of cases; transport problems (26 per cent); other children at home to care for (15 per cent). Also mentioned were: health services not good; father sick at home; husband absent so unable to give his opinion; child improved after first treatment; no alternative but to remain at home.

How many people should the clinic serve?

There are several factors to consider:

The 'natural community'

A clinic may serve one large village, one cluster of smaller villages, a plantation, a factory or a refugee camp. It may serve a certain section of a city slum.

Usually the clinic will tie in with our survey area, existing government facilities, our CHW training programme, and other community activities. It will serve the 'target' area and population.

The number of CHWs working effectively

The more CHWs that are trained and the more skilled they become the fewer the number of patients who will need to attend clinics (see Figure 8.3).

The length of time the clinic has been running

If our clinic is serving a definite target area and CHWs are working effectively, numbers attending may actually decline and we may later be able to reduce clinic frequency.

This effect is not seen in clinics open to anyone with no CHW backup, nor where people's expectations for health care have been raised, as

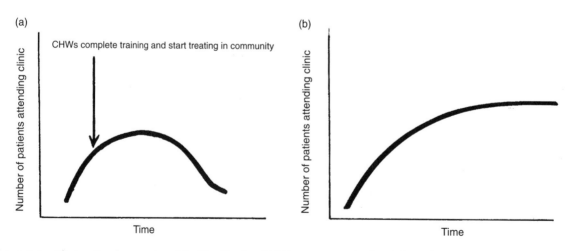

Figure 8.3   Clinic attendance rates: (a) with effective CHWs at community level (b) with no effective functioning CHWs.

through the media or commercial pressures. In such cases clinics may actually increase their numbers as others come to hear of good quality or inexpensive treatment available.

A very approximate guide for the population a clinic can serve might be as follows:

A team of five health workers able to spend adequate time with each patient can manage up to 50 or 100 patients per day. For a once-a-week clinic, this might represent a target population of about 5000 people. Later, as CHWs are trained and the community becomes healthier, larger populations can be served or clinics can be held less often.

Numbers attending clinics are very hard to predict and can vary greatly during the year. Climate, harvesting, the presence of an especially well liked (or rude) health worker, and levels of illness in a community make it hard to predict (or plan for) accurate numbers. Also important is whether the centre is perceived as being able to care for seriously ill community members and emergencies.

Where should the clinic be held?

1. Close to the community.

> Clinics should be set up within the community or as near to it as possible. No one should need to travel more than one hour's easy journey.

2. In an acceptable location for all.

If one clinic serves different villages, tribal groups, religions or castes, it must be in a 'neutral' place where all community members are happy to attend. A roadside or pathside building is often appropriate.

The clinic and its waiting area must be safe for children, and other vulnerable members of the community.

When should the clinic start?

This should be discussed with community leaders. It may have to be started before training CHWs or carrying out any other community activity. Remote or poor communities may have so much illness or so little understanding of community involvement that they are not prepared to work in partnership with us until basic health services are provided.

If possible, wait to start a clinic until after CHWs are trained. In this way the community understands that CHWs are the front-line health workers whom they go to see first.

> Once people become used to visiting a clinic for day-to-day health problems they may later ignore their newly trained CHW.

If we do delay starting a clinic there must be some nearby health centre or hospital where sick

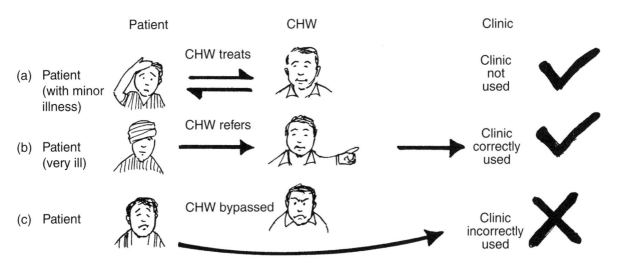

Figure 8.4   The correct (a) and (b) and incorrect (c) relationship of the CHW and clinic.

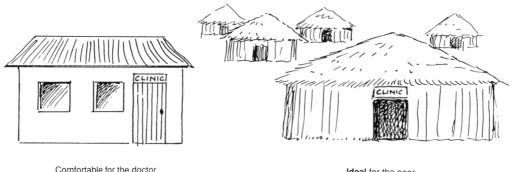

Comfortable for the doctor
Enjoyed by the well-off
Threatening to the poor

LESS APPROPRIATE

Ideal for the poor
Acceptable for the well-off
Adequate for the doctor

MORE APPROPRIATE

Figure 8.5

people can attend and to which serious cases can be referred.

What we need to do

Design the centre

Doctors, project directors and community leaders may want impressive and expensive health centres. The local community, especially the poor, may want a simple building, as much like home as possible, which they feel is their place rather than the doctor's palace.

For example: The Accord project in Tamil Nadu, India, planned and implemented an entire health system with full community involvement. In the health centre patients slept on mats not on beds, nurses spoke only the tribal language and most staff were trained vocationally from the community. After ten years, antenatal coverage reached 90 per cent, and childhood immunisation increased from 2 per cent to 75 per cent.

> We should rent or construct the simplest building that is able to support the services we are planning to give.

In doing this we must remember the main functions of a health centre building:

1. To enable patients to receive good quality health care.
2. To protect patients, health workers and equipment from the weather.

A well known community health doctor has written: 'There is nothing which so effectively prevents health workers from getting out into the community, as an expensive health centre building.'

In designing a centre we must carefully consider what facilities will be needed. This in turn will depend on:

• The number of people being served.
• The services being offered.
• The nearness to a referral centre.

At the largest level, a community health centre will need to be a permanent, purpose-designed building, with inpatient beds and a delivery room. It will serve the function of a typical primary health centre

At the smallest level, a room or the verandah of a CHW's house may be all that is needed.

At the middle level – appropriate for most small-scale projects – a simple building with three or four rooms and a careful 'flow pattern' will be adequate.

Regardless of the size or design of the clinic, there will need to be a room where confidential counselling or intimate examinations can be carried out.

> Health centres ideally should be made of local materials and should follow local building styles. They can be purpose-built by the project and community. Alternatively, an appropriate local building can be adapted and used.

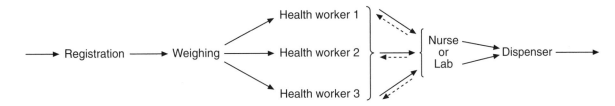

Figure 8.6   Flow pattern for a typical size clinic.

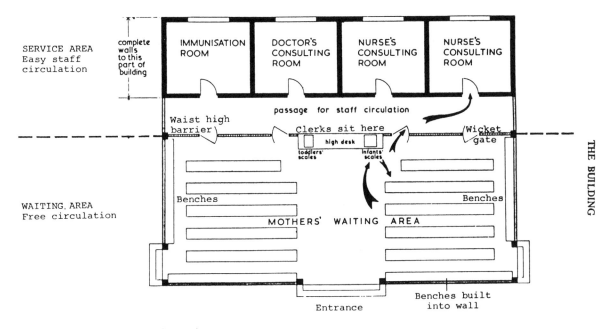

Figure 8.7   Plan of an under-fives' clinic.

Make sure the health centre is well labelled in the local language(s). On the outside include opening times and, where relevant, which clinics are held on which day. (This is for guidance only and we must still be willing to see seriously ill patients or those who have walked long distances, beyond normal clinic hours or on the 'wrong' day.) On the inside have clear but friendly notices explaining where people should sit, the functions of the various rooms and a simple arrow system. Make sure any health posters are easily understood and relevant for the majority of clinic users. Discuss with local people how notices can be designed with symbols as well as words for those unable to read.

A suggested flow pattern for a typical size clinic is given in Figure 8.6.

Enough waiting space out of the sun and out of the rain needs to be available, either centrally or next to each station.

A suggested design for an appropriate building is given in Figure 8.7.

Set up the clinic stations

Station 1: Registration

The registrar has two main jobs: to welcome and to register. Just as important is the registrar's attitude. It is essential that registrars develop a friendly and welcoming attitude and do not act in an arrogant or bossy way with the vulnerable people who will be attending the clinic.

To welcome

To do their job well registrars must also understand the way patients may be feeling. Imagine the situation of a mother who has never visited the centre before:

> She has got up early, walked a long way in the sun and is carrying a sick child. She is worried. She does not know what to expect, or how the clinic works. She is not sure if she can afford the charges. When she does arrive there are many people before her – all looking anxious. There is a notice giving information but she is unable to read it…

A friendly smile or a welcoming word from the registrar can be extremely reassuring to a sick or anxious patient.

The registrar looks out for very sick children or seriously ill patients and makes sure the health worker sees them as soon as possible.

To record details

Each project will need to work out an appropriate system. Here is a method that can be adapted:

1. Registrar arrives in plenty of time, and gets organised before patients arrive.

2. Patients arrive to register.
   Various methods can now be followed. Some examples:
   - either former patients place their self-retained record or previous registration card on the desk, sit down and wait until their name is called. New patients report to the registrar.
   - or all patients queue, standing or sitting.
   - or when large numbers attend, all patients take a number on arrival, sit down and wait until the registrar calls out their number.

3. Registrar records details:
   - In clinic register as follows:

Patient name	Name Head Fam.	Patient No	Age	Sex	Village or urban area	Money paid

   - On patients' card as follows:
     In case of former patients, registrar writes date and stamps card. In the case of new patients (or those who do not have their card with them), a new one is made out with details of patient's name, age, village/area of city, etc. being recorded in addition to date and stamp. The card is put into a protective plastic envelope.

4. Registrar takes money, if patients prepay a fixed amount.

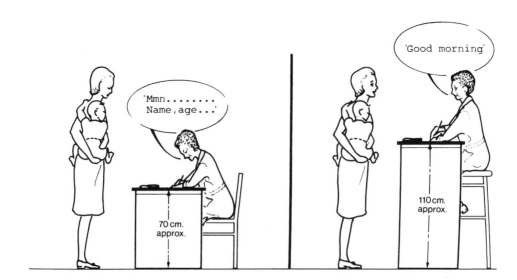

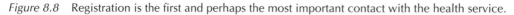

Figure 8.8   Registration is the first and perhaps the most important contact with the health service.

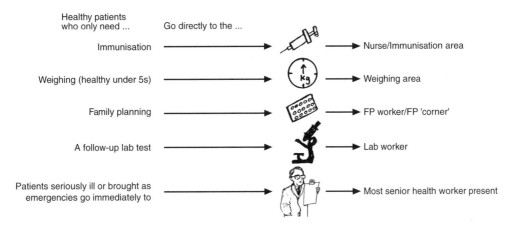

Healthy patients who only need ...	Go directly to the ...	
Immunisation	→	Nurse/Immunisation area
Weighing (healthy under 5s)	→	Weighing area
Family planning	→	FP worker/FP 'corner'
A follow-up lab test	→	Lab worker
Patients seriously ill or brought as emergencies go immediately to	→	Most senior health worker present

Figure 8.9   Saving everyone's time in a busy general clinic.

5. Registrar gives patient a number, placing this visibly within the plastic envelope that covers the self-retained card.
6. If a family folder is being used the registrar extracts this. (See page 158 and Appendix B.)
7. Self-retained record cards (plus family folder) are placed in a pile in order of arrival.
   If different health workers are seeing different patients (e.g. a nurse seeing pregnant women), separate piles are made for each health worker. The registrar takes care that where possible patients who have recently visited the clinic attend the same health worker they have seen before.
8. A clinic assistant, e.g. a CHW or Health Committee member, collects the pile of cards from the registrar's desk and places them on the health worker's desk, calling out names in turn.
9. Meanwhile patients sit down awaiting their turn except for certain categories (see Figure 8.9).
10. Registrar finalises entries after patients have stopped arriving, totals up money taken, hands this over to the person-in-charge, who checks and countersigns the register. Finally a check is made that there are sufficient cards, stationery, etc. for the next clinic.

All Multipurpose Workers (MPWs) should be trained to register patients. Any with special gifts can take on the job more permanently. Community members make good registrars providing they are fair, trustworthy and friendly; also

that they have been adequately trained to do the job.

Station 2: Weighing

Those who need weighing
- Children under five years;
- Pregnant women – this is traditionally done but is of limited value;
- TB patients;
- People living with HIV/AIDS providing that this does not risk their being stigmatised;
- Any malnourished patients in a feeding programme.

A suitable place for weighing
This can be a separate room, a convenient place near the registrar, a verandah or under a tree.

Suitable equipment
Good types for children include round-faced spring balances or tubular scales. New and experimental methods of weighing and recording are available from TALC (see Appendix A).
   Stirrups or trousers are needed for children under three years, baskets for newborn babies. Adults can use simple 'stand-on' scales.

A suitable person to do it
As in all community health activities, the least qualified person who can do the job well should be given the task.

With careful training family members such as parents or older siblings can do the weighing. MPWs and CHWs should be able to weigh accurately. Nurses can teach others but should not do it permanently themselves, as one of their tasks is to pass on their skills.

A suitable system for weighing children

1. The child sits on the parent's or guardian's lap and the weighing trousers are put on.
2. The parent lifts the child by the body, not by the straps, and hangs the child on the weighing scales.
3. The child hangs just long enough for an accurate weight to be measured, and is then lifted down.
4. The weight is plotted on the growth chart.
5. The card is explained to the parent. Feeding advice is given where necessary.
6. Any child making good progress can be shown as an example to waiting parents.

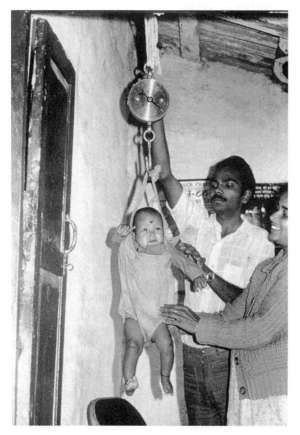

Figure 8.10 Family members weigh their own children, with guidance.

7. Children over three can hang with their hands.
8. Very young or very frightened children can be weighed with their mother on an adult scale, the mother's own weight then being subtracted: this method is less accurate.

Common mistakes in weighing

1. Many children are waiting but there is only one pair of trousers. Excess clothes are not removed.
2. Frightened children are left to hang while adults and onlookers unsuccessfully try to cheer them up.
3. Weights are misread through carelessness, because the child is bouncing, the scales are not at eye level or because the mother fails to let go. Weights that don't seem correct should be rechecked.
4. Growth charts are wrongly filled in (see pages 177–8).
5. The community culture is not understood.

For example: In some rural areas people think that weighing children is wrong or dangerous. Such beliefs should be understood and gently corrected.

Clinic weighing should not necessarily replace weighing in the home by mother or CHW.

If time is limited it may be more useful to give nutritional advice than spend time weighing and plotting this on a weight chart. A general rule is that advice should always be given and that weighing should be done whenever time allows, ideally using a weight chart.

Station 3: The consultation

One model of a health consultation, originally described by Stott and Davis, lists four key elements in any consultation between a health worker and a patient:

1. Dealing with the acute problem, i.e. the felt reason the patient attends.
2. Dealing with any underlying or chronic problems – often the most important reason the patient attends.
3. Helping the patient to change their health behaviour so in the future they are less likely to attend.
4. Helping to promote one aspect of good health related to the reason they attend.

Those people with the greatest health needs often live in areas where doctors are unwilling to provide primary care. For this reason many of the world's neediest people will continue to be seen by CHWs at community level, backed up by appropriately trained health workers at clinic level.

Health workers who see patients must be trained carefully and be supervised by doctors. (In some countries it is illegal for unregistered health workers to see patients.) They should also follow guidelines prepared by doctors, such as standing orders, treatment schedules or group protocols or directives, where the symptoms and treatment of common diseases are clearly set out.

The Integrated Management of Childhood Illness (IMCI) gives details on how to assess and manage sick children. We should use this where possible along with any national adaptations that may have been made.

Below is a general system that can be followed by any trained health worker who sees patients. Simplify this for your situation. Practice and efficiency will speed the process.

THE INTEGRATED CONSULTATION USED BY ONE PROJECT IN NEPAL

In   **I**nvestigate using the protocol
Every   **E**xplain the disease using the body diagram
Case   **C**ounsel about non-drug treatment
Follow   **F**ollow up/refer according to protocol
The   **T**reat according to protocol
Protocol **P**reventative health issues: discuss one
Source: Tropical Doctor, July 2004, 34:141.

---

1. **Health worker (HW) warmly greets the patient.**
2. **Health worker consults patient's records**, notes the patient's village, or city area and any other relevant family or ethnic information. HW looks for details of any previous illness or treatment.
   If a family folder is being used, HW takes note of the size, structure and socioeconomic status of the family.
3. **Health worker takes history.**
   a) HW asks the patient what the problem is – listening carefully without interrupting.
   b) For any important symptom HW now asks questions. Here are some examples:

- For diarrhoea:
  How many stools per day?
  How many days have you had it?
  Is there fever? blood? mucus? vomiting? excess flatus? significant pain?
- For pain:
  Where is the pain?
  How long have you had it?
  Have you ever had it before?
  What makes it better or worse?
- For cough:
  How long have you had it?
  Is there sputum, blood, fever or chest pain?
  Have you ever had TB treatment?
  Does anyone else in your family have a cough; or has anyone been recently treated for TB?
- For fever:
  How long have you had it?
  Is it continuous or does it come and go?
  Is there sweating, shivering, vomiting or headache?
- For cuts, bites, accidents:
  When did it happen?
  How did it happen?
  If an animal bite, is the animal alive, and where is it?
- For any other symptom:
  How long have you had it?
  Have you had it before?
  Any other suitable questions.
- For malnutrition: obtain full details (see Chapter 9).
- For antenatal patients: obtain full details (see Chapter 12).
- For women of childbearing age we should usually ask whether pregnant. This is both so we can offer antenatal care and also so we can know what medicines are safe to prescribe.
- Where TB is common we ask whether there has been cough for more than three weeks.
- Where HIV/AIDS is common we sensitively enquire whether the person is interested in voluntary counselling and testing (VCT) and if so explain where and when it is available.

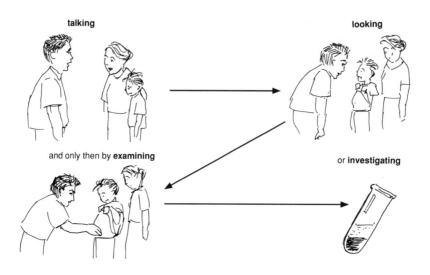

talking

looking

and only then by **examining**

or **investigating**

Figure 8.11   Learn to diagnose patients mainly by …

c) Other questions if diagnosis still unclear:
 • Has there been any weight loss?
 • Is there any sign of alcohol or drug abuse or persistent use of tobacco?
 • Ears: any pain or discharge?
 • Eyes: any pain or difficulty seeing?
 • Throat: any soreness or loss of voice?
 • Chest: any other symptoms?
 • Bowels: any other symptoms?
 • Urination: pain, frequency or trouble in passing? Any discharge?
 • Periods: pain, heavy loss, discharge, bleeding between periods?
 • Skin: any sores, itching, rash or swellings?
 • Genitals: any sores, ulcers or other problems? (In many cultures this is best asked by a HW of the same gender as the patient, and in private.)
 • Bones, joints, muscles: any swelling, pain or stiffness?
 • Mind: any sadness, agitation or fits?
 • Any other symptoms not mentioned?

4. **Health worker examines patient:**
 a) By looking:
 • General appearance: anything unusual?
 • Well or ill?
 • Thin or dehydrated?
 • Normal colour? Pale? Yellow? Flushed with fever?
 • Breathing normally? Child with breathing rate of 50 or more per minute? (If so, suspect pneumonia. See page 221.)
 • Eyes: Infection? Pale mucous membranes? Yellow? Vitamin A deficiency? Trachoma?
 • Tongue: Pale? Dry? Sore or smooth?
 • Part of body where symptom located: Anything to see?
 b) By touching and feeling.
 • Pulse: Rate? Regular? Strong?
 • Part of body where symptom located: any swelling, warmth, pain or tenderness?
 c) By listening if problem is in the chest.
 • Any unusual or added sounds over lung?
 • Any heart murmur?
 d) By measuring temperature and blood pressure if necessary.

5. **Health worker diagnoses the problem.**
 With the result of any tests (if the clinic has a field laboratory) and helped by the Standing Orders, or IMCI algorithms, HW makes the diagnosis.
 If HW is uncertain what the problem is or how serious it is, advice should be sought from a doctor, nurse, supervisor or colleague.

6. Having dealt with the patient's felt needs, HW now searches for any real need(s) of the patient.

Patients nearly always come because of felt needs – some pain, problem or irritation for which they want a cure.

Trying to find real needs is our most important task. A real need can be thought of as a problem, disease, or lack of health that seriously affects the long-term health of the patient, the family or the community.

Important real needs will include:

a) Malnutrition found by weighing or, if severe, by observation.

b) In the case of children, incomplete immunisation, and in women of childbearing age, incomplete tetanus immunisation.

c) Presence of serious illness such as TB, AIDS or leprosy – especially if patient undiagnosed or defaulted from treatment.

d) Pregnancy with the need for antenatal care.

e) The need for family planning.

f) Recent discharge from hospital especially if due to an infectious or serious disease.

g) Chronic illness, e.g. diabetes, hypertension.

The health worker can discover these real needs by:

• Questioning the patient.

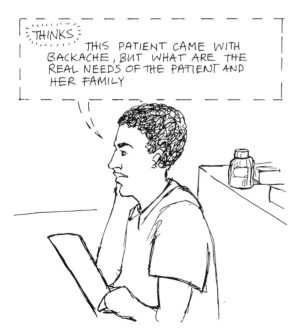

Figure 8.12

• Checking the patient's record card and in particular the family folder and insert cards. This gives a quick and easy way of discovering real needs.

• If patient records are computerised, using any 'due lists' generated for the day's clinic.

7. **If time, HW checks for any real need of any other family member.**

For example: If a child is accompanying the patient, HW makes sure that the child has been recently weighed and completed immunisations. If a mother is accompanying a patient, could she be pregnant and if so is she having antenatal care? If a coughing father is accompanying, has he himself been tested for TB?

The family folder and insert cards should be checked to make sure immunisations are complete and that any important follow-up to previous problems has been carried out.

Any family members needing to be seen can be brought to the next clinic.

When clinics first start or cover too large a population there may be such a rush of patients that there may be little time to search for real needs. Remember however:

Health projects should be set up in such a way that CHWs deal with routine problems in the community. This frees clinics for treating serious illness and caring for the real needs of patients. Unless this is prioritised, clinics spend all their time treating minor, felt needs and the real needs of the individual and community remain unmet.

8. **Health worker treats the patient.**

a) HW prescribes any medicine necessary, writing down the generic name, the dose, how often the medicine should be taken and how long it should be taken for, to guide the dispenser. HW mentions any precautions, special instructions or side effects.

Many HWs have a tendency to prescribe more than is needed. This wastes money, and creates wrong expectations.

For example: One survey showed that church hospitals in Uganda used between two and three medicines per outpatient, compared to more than five from a survey in Ecuador. We should keep the number of medicines prescribed to the minimum needed for adequate treatment, or to follow the relevant protocol.

Two other areas need care: the use of abbreviations for medicines, which may not be understood by all team members especially new recruits, and dosages for children, which are often incorrectly calculated.

b) HW advises the patient about how to help prevent the condition from recurring.
For example: A method that has proved successful in some projects is the use of 'health drills'. These are carefully worded summaries of health advice that are listed alphabetically for each common health problem. The health worker seeing patients, the nurse and dispenser all have copies.

HW explains the relevant health drill to the patient, then 'prescribes' it in the notes. When the patient later sees the nurse or dispenser this health drill, i.e. identical instructions, will be explained again.

c) HW arranges any procedure such as bandaging, tooth extraction or immunisation.

d) HW refers the patient to a more senior health worker if not sure of the diagnosis or treatment.

9. **HW makes sure the patient understands**, asking the patient to repeat back any important instructions.
For example: A project in Tansen, Nepal, uses body diagrams as part of the medical consultation, so that patients can better understand their health problems. Even though most patients are poorly educated or illiterate, the diagrams doubled the number of patients who gained understanding, and took only a small amount of extra time.

Finally, HW recognises if the patient does not seem satisfied and tries to discover the reason. HW tells the patient when to return to the clinic.

10. **Health worker records important information** on the patient's record card, the family folder insert card, and any relevant register (see later). If the programme is computerised, HW fills in the due list or any other computer-generated personal or family record produced for the clinic.

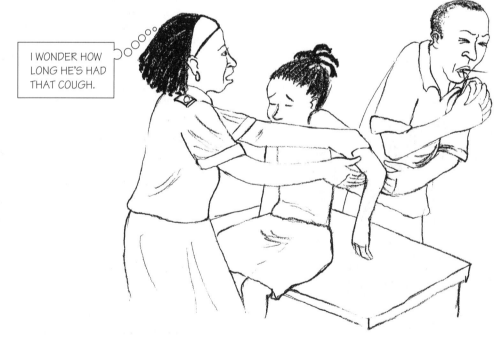

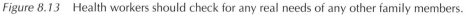

Figure 8.13   Health workers should check for any real needs of any other family members.

Practical suggestions when seeing patients:

1. **Patients learn as they wait.**
   In Mother and Child Health clinics patients can wait in the consultation room, or just outside it, so that they 'learn by overhearing'. CHWs can gather groups of waiting mothers and give appropriate teaching (see Chapter 3, page 43). This approach must be guided by how confidentiality is understood in the culture.
2. **Each one teach one.**
   Use the consultation as a time to teach other health workers, especially CHWs. Encourage other health team members to pass on their knowledge and skills whenever they have a chance.
3. **Respect patients' beliefs.**
   Patients may have ideas that seem strange or wrong to us. They may be more interested in who caused the disease than in what caused it. We should instruct gently without causing patients to lose their dignity, or feel offended.
4. **The same patient sees the same health worker.**
   The more a patient comes to know and trust one particular health worker the more likely advice will be followed and the patient will return for follow-up.
5. **Respect the need for privacy.**
   In many busy clinics patients are seen with others waiting or watching nearby. If this is the case, make sure there is strict privacy when necessary, for example when HIV/AIDS, STIs, TB, leprosy or other stigmatised conditions are commonly present. In most cultures, family planning is also a private matter.

Station 4: The field laboratory

A small field laboratory is quite easy to set up and greatly adds to the value of a community clinic:

Advantages:

1. It confirms the diagnosis, meaning that clinics can concentrate on curing illness rather than on treating symptoms.
2. It makes health care more accurate especially when health workers without formal qualifications are seeing patients.
3. It gives 'customer satisfaction'.

4. It is cost effective. By reducing the number of visits to hospital it saves the patient time, and saves the project money.

Types of test available

Here are examples of tests that can often be handled by a well managed field laboratory with simple equipment, and staffed by a carefully trained worker.

1. Blood tests: haemoglobin, white cell count and differential, erythrocyte sedimentation rate (ESR), malaria smear or dipstick test such as 'Parasight F', HIV testing in the context of VCT, with careful training and control.
2. Sputum tests: for acid-fast bacilli (AFB) in tuberculosis.
   This is the correct way to confirm TB. Treatment should not normally be started unless a patient is sputum positive, ideally after two positive tests (see Chapter 14, pages 278–80).
3. Stool tests: for worms (e.g. hook, round, whip, tape), protozoa (e.g. amoeba, *Giardia*) and *Schistosoma* ova.
4. Urine tests: microscopy for pus cells, bacteria and *Schistosoma* ova.
   Dipstick (or other method): for sugar, protein, bile and blood.
5. Skin tests: slit skin for leprosy, scrape for fungus.
6. Vaginal swabs: for gonococcus, Trichomonas, or Candida.

In many situations haemoglobin levels and malaria slides are the most valuable tests. Malaria is commonly underdiagnosed and overdiagnosed, each of which can be dangerous for patients.

The quality control of sputum testing for TB needs to be in line with national guidelines but on-site testing is very valuable especially if the project is integrated into the national TB programme.

VCT for HIV/AIDS is a valued service providing it follows good practice guidelines and is offered in such a way that clients feel comfortable to use it.

The laboratory worker

Tests can be done either by a qualified laboratory worker with basic training, or by a multipurpose

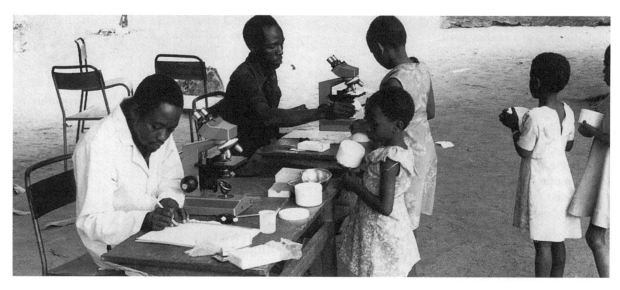

Figure 8.14   A simple field laboratory helps a clinic to treat causes rather than symptoms.

worker carefully trained in simple laboratory skills.

Laboratory workers must be:

- accurate, reliable and thorough;
- aware of their own limitations.

Unless carefully trained and supervised, workers may be tempted to 'fudge' results, especially if they are rushed for time or lacking confidence, or want to record a result that will please the doctor.

Equipment needed
Needles and syringes that are disposable or reliably sterile must be used and supervisors should make regular spot checks. A suggested list of general equipment appears in Appendix B. For further details on setting up a field lab and the equipment needed, see the Further reading and resources list.

Procedure for patients
Patients needing laboratory tests will be referred by the health worker. They will proceed to the laboratory, bringing either their self-retained card or a separate laboratory request slip, on which the lab worker will record the result.

Patients should wait their turn, both for the test and its result, preferably sitting in an area near the lab. They can then report back to the health worker they saw originally.

Station 5: The clinic nurse

The nurse's background
Larger clinics may have fully qualified nurses. Smaller clinics will often use nurse-aides, MPWs or fully trained CHWs.

> Nurses who have been trained in hospitals and then join community health projects will need a complete reorientation in their approach and outlook. In practice, MPWs trained on the job are often more suitable than trained nurses who wish they were back in the hospital.

The nurse's function
Here are some typical tasks:

- Giving injections (see Chapter 10, page 197).
- Dressing and bandaging.
- Cleaning skin infections and wounds.
- Lancing abscesses.
- Giving family planning advice and supplies.
- Running an ORS corner (see pages 211–16).
- Assisting the doctor or the health worker.
- Taking temperatures, weights, blood pressures.
- Teaching.
  Nurses may also be involved in consultation and trained nurses will often serve as the lead health worker or be in charge of the clinic.

Station 6: The dispenser or pharmacist

Any MPW with a particular gift or interest can be trained as a dispenser, be put in charge of the dispensary and teach others. Some countries have laws preventing those without formal qualifications from dispensing.

The dispenser is usually the last health worker whom the patient will see. A smile, or a sharp word, may linger in the patient's mind, affecting future compliance.

> It is good practice in smaller health centres for all MPWs to be trained in dispensing. In this way the job can be shared out so that no one person has to count pills and give instructions for hours at a time, leading to boredom and inaccuracy.

The dispenser's job can include both dispensing and stock-keeping. However, combining this role opens an easy route for corruption. There is value in a different team member, ideally a trustworthy person in a managerial role, checking and ordering stock, if the team is large enough for this to be possible.

Dispensing

This includes:

1. **Reading the doctor's or health worker's handwriting.** This may be difficult! If in doubt the dispenser should ask, not guess. If a medicine has run out or is not available, the health worker or doctor should be asked if an alternative can be used.
2. **Counting.** The exact number of pills must be given. This is especially important in TB DOTS programmes and where health centres provide antiretroviral treatment. Also when using antibiotics and anti-malarials.

   Any broken, dirty or discoloured medicines should be thrown away. Medicines past their expiry date should not normally be used unless there is a genuine shortage of supplies (see Chapter 17, pages 328–30).
3. **Explaining.** For each medicine the patient will need to know:
   - How many?
   - How often?

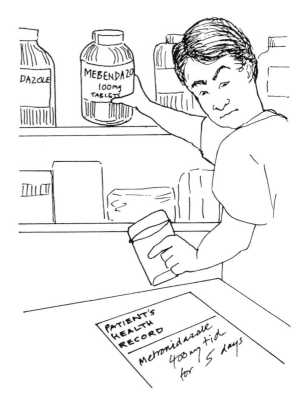

Figure 8.15   Mistakes are easy to make when a doctor's writing is unclear or a dispenser is overworked.

- How long for?
- How? With water, before or after food, etc?
- What side effects?
- What food, drink or activity needs to be avoided?

In the case of eye drops, ear drops, ORS packets, or capsules that have to be opened and mixed on a spoon for children, the dispenser should be ready to show how it is done, as well as giving verbal instructions.

Before leaving, patients should repeat back the instructions, to make sure they have understood.

> Many patients who leave clinics clutching pills and medicines will not take them as instructed. They may fail to understand the instructions given, forget what they have been told or think their own ideas are better than the health worker's instructions.

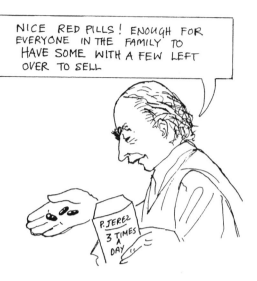

Figure 8.16

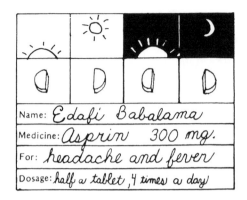

Figure 8.17   If patients cannot read, use pictures to explain amounts and timings of pills and medicines.

> The purpose of this system is to re-order in plenty of time so that stocks never run out unless there is a national shortage of drugs. Health centres must always keep in stock an adequate supply of essential drugs.

For example: A doctor greeted a leprosy patient by the roadside who one month previously had been diagnosed at a clinic and, as part of the treatment, been given 30 white dapsone tablets. The dispenser had instructed him to take one per day. Asked now how he was feeling, the patient replied: 'Fine, Doc. I took the tablets – all 30 together and now I feel well.' Other patients may not be so fortunate.

4. **Labelling the packet or bottle.**

   Any container or envelope must be well labelled. If the patient is illiterate, we should use symbols.

   For example: One aspirin to be taken four times a day can be represented as shown in Figure 8.17. Even these symbols must be explained.

5. **Repeating the health drill**.

Stock-keeping (see also pages 67–9)
This includes:

1. Checking levels
   The dispenser will need to:
   * check all drugs:
     * for quantity remaining, at least once monthly;
     * for expiry dates at least once quarterly.
   * Use a stock list (Figure 8.18) made out alphabetically, so that the check can be systematic.

2. Re-ordering supplies.
   The dispenser will need to use a re-order sheet. (Figure 8.18.)
   Two copies are made:
   Copy 1 is sent with the order. Central stores returns the form with the new supply, filling in (b). The dispenser then writes down the amount actually received in (c) (Figure 8.18).
   Copy 2 is put directly into the dispenser's file and is attached to Copy 1 when this is returned.

3. Labelling supplies.
   Drug names are confusing. Each drug may have several different brand names but only one generic name. The generic name should therefore always be used, even though it may be longer, harder to remember and can have minor variations in spelling. Avoid using abbreviations. The storekeeper in central supplies should always send out supplies with labels attached. The label can include the details indicated in Figure 8.19.
   Where supplies are sent out in bottles labelled by drug companies, a bold ring or circle can be made around the generic name instead of sticking a new label on to each bottle.
   When semi-literate CHWs help in counting out tablets, colour codes can be used, e.g. green labels for antibiotics, orange for anti-malarials, etc. The dispenser must check the CHW's work for any mistakes.

Stock list

Drug name	Code No	Unit of issue	Full stock level	Stock level when re-order necessary
Asprin	P 04	Bottle 100	2000	500

Re-order sheet

Name of health centre .... Date ordered .... Date received					
List of items needed	Code Nos	No ordered (a)	No sent (b)	No received (c)	Remarks

Figure 8.18   Stock list and reorder sheet.

Generic name of drug	Code No.	Number of tablets when container full

Figure 8.19   Drugs label.

4. Storing supplies in the clinic cupboard.
    Supplies should be arranged neatly, in alphabetical generic order with the newest supplies at the back of the shelf. The front of the shelf itself can be labelled either with the drug name or with a letter of the alphabet.

    In practice it is easy for new supplies to be put at the front and for old supplies to get pushed to the back and expire. Huge amounts of drugs can be wasted in this way.

    The following system can prevent this:

    For each drug, storage space is divided into two sections, side by side (see Table 8.1):

    Supplies also need to be stored at the right temperature, which in practice means avoiding buildings or rooms in full sun and having a good means of ventilation even when the building is closed.

    At the beginning, A is existing stock and B is empty. When the amount remaining in A reaches the re-order level, new supplies are requested and these are put in B. These new supplies are not used until all of A has been used up. Then when B gets low, new stock is put in A but not used until supplies in B are finished.

5. Prepacking.
    In busy clinics much time can be saved if standard courses of commonly used drugs are prepacked and prelabelled.

    Use bottles or plastic envelopes during the rainy season, or paper envelopes, e.g. folded from magazine paper, in dry climates.

Keep and transfer clinic records

Each project will develop its own system of records. Most centres can use patient-retained record cards, the family folder and insert cards, clinic registers and, where computerised, due lists and computer-generated record forms for completion by hand. In addition, they will usually need a system of transferring data from the clinic to the project headquarters.

Health projects should have one central location where key project data is stored either manually or on computer. Usually this will be in a project base or hospital, rather than in a Community Health Clinic. Key data therefore needs to be transferred as simply as possible from clinic to base.

Table 8.1   Arrangement of supplies in the clinic cupboard

A B	A B	A B	A B
Drug 1	Drug 2	Drug 3	Drug 4

Table 8.2   Examples of health worker's entries in patient's notes

Adult	6-year-old child
Symptoms and how long they have been present Cough with blood 3 months *Findings on examination* Patient very thin, crackles in both lungs. Temperature 38°C *Diagnosis* Suspected TB *Management* Sputum test today and on arrival next week Meanwhile amoxicillin 500 mg t.i.d. 5 days 'Cough drill' given	*Symptoms and how long they have been present* Diarrhoea with mucus 6 times daily for 8 days: no fever *Findings on examination* General condition good, lips dry, skin elastic *Diagnosis* Suspected amoebic dysentery with mild dehydration *Management* Demonstrate use of ORS (nurse) Metronidazole 200 mg t.i.d. for 5 days Return 1 week if no better

Here are examples of systems used by different projects:

- Adding to the clinic register (see page 146) a column for a chief diagnosis against each patient entry.
- Completing a clinic report form listing numbers of patients seen by gender, community, diagnosis, etc. An alternative is to make carbon copies of the pages used by the registrar and take these back to base after each clinic.

  Many projects will design their own forms or be using the reporting forms needed by nationwide programmes such as IMCI or stop TB.
- Calling in all registers from clinic to base either monthly, quarterly or half-yearly for key data to be transferred from clinic registers to an HQ Master Register or computer.
- Designing a computer-based system that can print off clinic stationery that is the equivalent of the various clinic records mentioned later in this section, e.g. register pages, family folders, insert cards, etc.

This stationery would be used for each clinic, taken back to base at the end of the clinic, then entered onto identical computer screens. This system means less duplication of records and is a method of keeping a regularly updated database of all community members and their needs. This may be the direction in which information systems are moving but this is experimental at present and requires a great deal of time for programming and training. Hand-held and 'wind up' computers are likely to be used increasingly.

Patient-retained record cards

There will be separate designs for adults, and for children under five, which will include a growth chart printed on one side. Those with chronic diseases, such as TB and leprosy, can in addition have a specially designed card. Those using ART can have specially designed cards.

Patients keep their cards in plastic envelopes (if available) and bring them whenever they come to any clinic, see the CHW or go to hospital.

Members of the team can make entries on these cards as follows:

- The registrar writes down the date (and where relevant) the amount of money paid.
- The person weighing children fills in the growth chart.
- The health worker seeing patients will make brief, accurate, legible notes.

Examples of notes that could be made for two different patients are shown in Table 8.2.

The family folder and insert card

This section applies only if a family folder system is being used.

INSERT CARD

Date	Problem	Action	Date to be seen again
4 February 2006	Cough with blood 3 months	Sputum test today and next visit Amoxycillin 500mg t.i.d. 5 days	11 February 2006

Figure 8.20   Example of an entry on an insert card. (Same patient as adult in Table 8.2.)

The family folder itself

With the exception given below, nothing is written on the family folder itself unless a mistake is discovered. The folder is a record of the state of health of the family on the day of the survey (see pages 84–88).

If the folder has a section 'Vital Events Since Survey' this can be filled in if any new family member has been born, if anyone has died, or if anyone has permanently joined or left the family.

The insert cards

These should only be used for patients 'at risk'. This includes all children under five, pregnant women, and those with serious or chronic illness such as TB and diabetes. For people living with HIV/AIDS, even if taking ART, cards should only be kept if confidentiality is secure and/or stigma is not a major issue.

Make brief strategic notes for the purpose of follow-up (see Figure 8.20). Insert cards are placed in the family folder and can be prepared either when the person in question attends the clinic or a member of their family comes. Some programmes fill out cards at the time of the community survey.

Self-limiting or trivial problems should not be recorded on the insert card, otherwise valuable time is wasted.

Clinic registers and report forms

These should be kept as simple as possible.

The health worker seeing patients fills in any special register or report form.

The nurse can fill in the immunisation or family planning register or report form (see page 265).

A note of patients referred will be kept (see page 161).

The registrar keeps a note of patients seen and money received.

Decide on a system of payment

How much should be charged?

A great deal of care needs to be taken in deciding this. In many countries, such as Uganda, which introduced user fees as part of health reforms, many of the poorest and most in need stopped using health centres. We need to make sure that any system we use does not discourage those most in need from attending. In other words we must not reinforce the inverse care law (see page 141).

Patients can usually pay at least some contribution for the services and medicines they receive.

This is in the interest of the patient, who values the treatment more and does not come to expect free handouts.

It is helpful for the project, which can help to cover its drug supply costs.

1. **If too much is charged:**
   • The poor cannot afford it and may not attend, indicating we are not providing a comprehensive service to those who need it most.

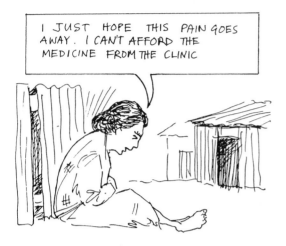

Figure 8.21   A problem of charging too much.

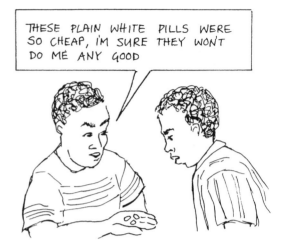

Figure 8.22   A problem of charging too little.

2. **If too little is charged:**
   • Patients may think the clinic or the medicine is poor quality.
   • People may suspect our motives, or abuse our services by demanding medicines for minor problems.
   • The project will be less sustainable.

Payment levels therefore need to be just, acceptable to most of the community and affordable by the poor.

Despite setting up an appropriate system, some patients may still claim they are unable to pay.

When this happens we have several options:

1. We can check the socioeconomic status on the family folder, and give a concession to those genuinely poor.
2. We can ask for advice from the CHW or Health Committee member helping in the clinic, who will probably know the patient's real situation.
3. We can encourage patients to pay as much as they are able, or to pay in kind. *For example*: by bringing grains, fruits, vegetables or poultry, which can be used or sold by the project. (See also Chapter 21.)

What system of payment should be used?

Fixed prepayment to the registrar

A fixed amount is paid to the registrar at the time of registration. Patients must understand this is to pay for services given, whether or not any medicine is prescribed. Children pay less than adults or can be seen free. Certain other categories can receive free care such as women attending for antenatal checks or family planning, and in many programmes TB patients and PLWHA on ART.

Two variations on this system can be used:

Example 1: Patients coming to a health centre from villages who have their own CHW pay a lower rate or 'A' rate. Patients coming from villages who have not sent CHWs for training pay a higher rate or 'B' rate. This encourages 'B' villages to send a CHW for training or, if the village is too distant, to request a health centre with CHW training for their area.

Example 2: In communities who have fully trained CHWs a 'B' rate is charged to any patient who has not first seen the CHW and brought a referral slip. This encourages patients to use CHWs for routine problems, and to attend the clinic only if referred.

When using a pre-payment system, the final four columns in the registration book can be prepared as follows (refer back to page 146):

Rate	Amount paid	Any Amount refunded	Total

Payment by item of service

This system is commonly used in hospital outpatients and can be adapted for larger clinics.

The registrar gives each patient a registration or payment slip. As the patient goes from one clinic station to the next, each service, medicine or test is written on this slip along with the cost. Before leaving the clinic, the patient hands this in to the cashier, dispenser or registrar, who totals the charges, takes the money from the patient, enters the amount received in the clinic register and gives a simple receipt to the patient.

In practice, charges per station often tend to work out higher, making it more difficult for the poor. It also takes more time. See pages 391–2 for details of insurance schemes.

Set up a referral system

Without a good referral system, CBHC can be dangerous and inefficient. In addition, patients can waste a huge amount of money and health workers a great deal of time.

> Unless a good referral system is set up, patients may wander from one doctor or health worker to another, collecting ever increasing amounts of medicine, advice and reports. Because patients receive partial treatment from many doctors, they often receive effective treatment from none.

Who should be referred?

1. Any seriously ill patient who needs expert advice or tests to find the cause of the illness.
2. Any patient needing treatment or surgery that cannot be done in the health centre.
3. Anyone demanding a 'second opinion'.
4. Emergencies.

How should patients be referred?

1. **They should be given a referral letter (see Figure 8.24).**
   One copy should be given to the patient, the other kept in a clinic file or the family folder. Alternatively, a note can be written on the self-retained card.
   In the case of patients unable to afford the cost of hospital referral and where subsidy may be available, this system can be used:
   Discover the maximum amount the patient is able to afford, agree this amount with the patient, record it at the foot of the referral letter, ask the patient to sign and a health worker to countersign.

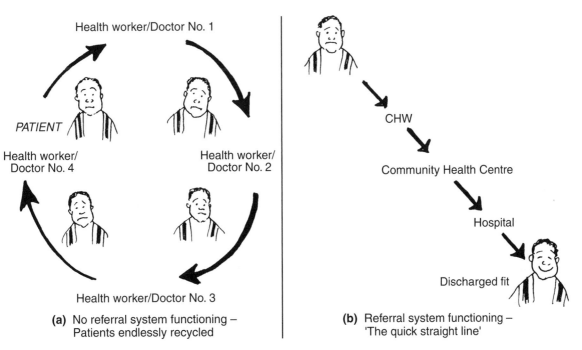

(a) No referral system functioning – Patients endlessly recycled

(b) Referral system functioning – 'The quick straight line'

Figure 8.23   (a) Recycling illness and (b) correct referral system.

HOSPITAL REFERRAL LETTER   Clinic:

Date:

Dear Doctor
Thank you for seeing this patient and if necessary admitting him/her to hospital.

Patient's Name .... Age .... Sex ....

Patient's Village/urban area .... Number ....

Reason for referral:

Relevant History and Clinical Findings:

Current Drug Therapy:

Known sensitivities

Financial status

Other relevant details

We would be glad if you could give the patient a discharge letter and tell him/her to report to the
health centre bringing the letter.
With thanks for your help.
Yours sincerely,

I ....(patient's name) agree to pay ....
direct to the Hospital.
The remainder will be paid by the project direct to the Hospital.
              Signature   (a) Project Medical officer ....

                          (b) Patient or patient's relative ....

Figure 8.24   Example of a referral letter used by one project.

2. **They should be given a careful explanation.**

> All health workers must be trained to recognise
> the patients they are unable to treat or diagnose
> themselves. Unless they learn to refer such
> patients, the community will lose confidence in
> the project and use other health facilities.

The health worker must take time to meet the
patient's fears and to answer his or her questions.

3. **When necessary, patients should be accompanied to hospital.**
In addition to being accompanied by relatives,
many patients need someone to go with them
who knows the system and can show solidarity
with them. This might be a project member, an
experienced CHW, or a member of a health
committee, who will help to guide the patient
through the frightening world of white coats,
queues and demand for illicit payment.

Projects with their own referral hospitals still
need to ensure that the poor are treated with
dignity and respect.

Seriously ill patients should be transported
in a project vehicle or accompanied
on public transport (or light aircraft) by a
project member.

> For the poor, sick or timid, going to a crowded
> hospital can be a terrifying experience. They will
> wonder: Can I afford it? What will they do to me?
> Will I need an operation? Supposing I die? Are the
> stories I have heard about this place really true?

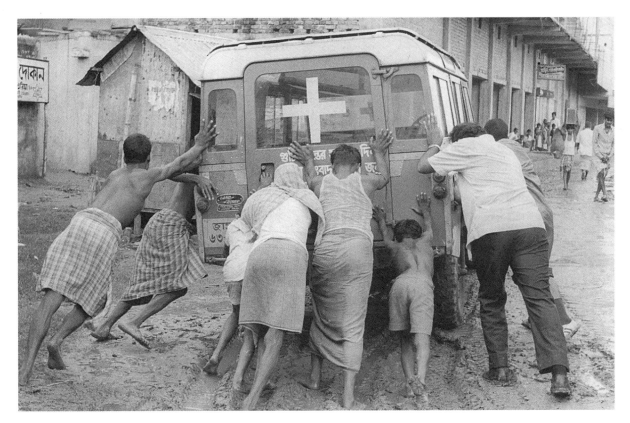

Figure 8.25   Partnership between the community and project in referring a patient to hospital.

Who should patients be referred to?

Many projects will have their own hospital to which most patients will be referred.

If this is not the case, the project director needs to set up links with suitable doctors, clinics and hospitals to which patients can be referred. Often this will be the district general hospital or an equivalent such as a mission or church based hospital. In practice the success of such a referral system will depend on making a network of social contacts and friendships outside the project.

Concentrate on teaching and health promotion

Clinics give great opportunities for health promotion. Patients who are either worried or unwell are often open to new ideas.

> When clinics are busy, health teaching is the first activity to get squeezed out, unless everyone knows that teaching is a priority and that a particular health worker, CHW or community member has been appointed to carry it out.

The following teaching methods are appropriate for clinics:

1. **Person to person.**
   This occurs at each station and 'health drills' can increase its effectiveness.
2. **Health talks, dialogues and demonstrations.**
3. **Learning through 'overhearing'.**
4. **Patient support groups.**
   TB patients, PLWHAs or those wanting to stop drinking or abusing drugs can be formed into support groups, with a health worker acting as facilitator.

5. **Demonstrations using patients.**
   A health worker can request a patient to underline a health message.
   For example: If an interesting or important case is seen by a health worker from which others would benefit by learning, clinic staff can be summoned and a teaching session held, similar to a hospital ward round.

6. **Patients teach other patients.**
   Cured TB patients can teach those newly diagnosed. Mothers of children once malnourished, now on the Road to Health, can share their experiences of how they successfully fed their children. Those who have been HIV positive for some time or are recovering through the use of ART can help lead self-help groups.

7. **CHWs can teach health songs.**
   For other examples, see Chapter 3.

8. **Use of videos and DVDs.**
   For example: One project in a mission hospital in Uganda made a video using local people and in the local language, which was shown while patients were waiting. This type of approach can cause intense interest and convey health messages very effectively.

Ensure that health centres are prepared for serious illness

There are three obvious reasons why this is necessary. The first is the need for a point of referral for each community when serious illness or accidents occur. The second is because clinics known to provide care in emergencies gain credibility and are used more by the community. The third is because communities expect a clinic to provide this.

For example: a survey amongst two communities in Sri Lanka showed that people expected to receive emergency care from the primary health system including treatment for their seriously ill children, but used traditional home remedies for more minor ailments.

These actions can save lives before we refer seriously ill patients:
1. First aid – the abc: airways, breathing, circulation.
2. Using naso-gastric tubes to rehydrate children severely dehydrated and unable to drink.
3. Injecting benyzl penicillin in children with suspected meningitis.
4. Using rectal diazepam in children with convulsions.
5. Using rectal artemether in those with cerebral malaria.

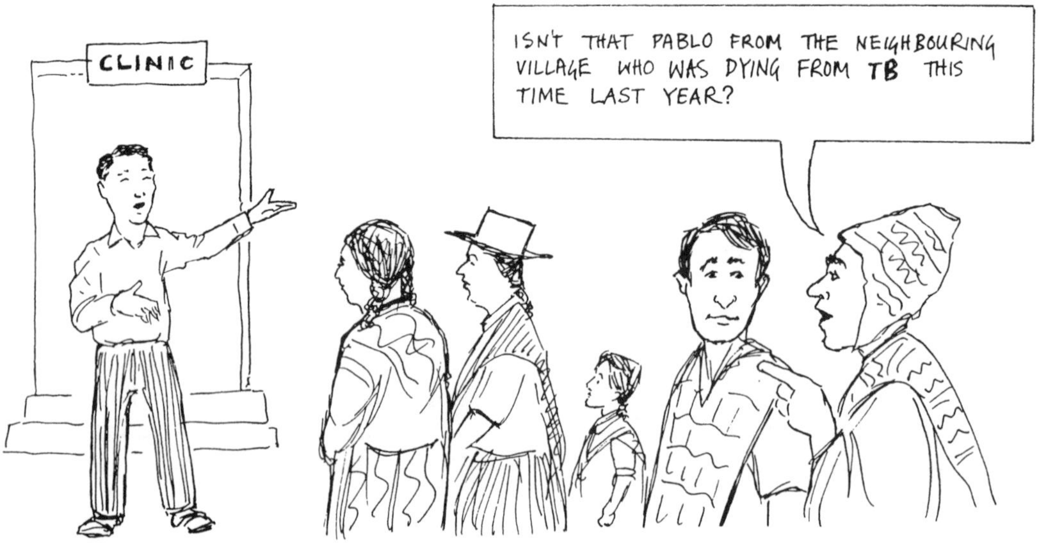

Figure 8.26   Cured patients make effective teachers.

To deal effectively with emergencies and serious illness, three things need to be in place at community level:

1. **Recognition of emergency conditions in the home.**

   Examples are early signs of serious illness in children and signs of life-threatening complications before or after delivery.

   For example: in a Mexican project the training of mothers and CHWs in recognising early postnatal blood loss, and breathing difficulties in children under one, almost halved death rates.

   This approach could easily be extended to managing an airway, controlling external bleeding and immobilising fractures.

2. **Availability of emergency transport.**

   For example: in one remote Himalayan valley community members owning or having access to a vehicle arranged to make these available to anyone in the valley requiring emergency transport to hospital. The journey would take two hours by jeep but usually a whole day by bus.

3. **Emergency medical care at the first contact health centre.**

   With simple equipment and basic training many conditions can be treated or first aid can be provided until referral can be arranged. Often unnecessary delays after reaching the clinic cause avoidable death especially in seriously ill children and in pregnant women. There need to be simple systems in place for immediate response when such patients are brought to the health centre.

   One way to reduce death rates in children is to use the syndromic approach to severe childhood illness. This simply means recognising a characteristic combination of symptoms, signs and investigations.

   For example: meningitis in children under two comprises fever, fits and prostration. All children with these features are immediately given a combination of chloramphenicol and benzyl penicillin before being referred. This will usually save their lives.

Finally, we need to have a plan outlined in case there is an outbreak of a serious infectious disease locally that puts health care staff at risk.

Examples include diseases such as Lassa fever, Marburg fever and Ebola in Africa, and any future outbreak of SARS or avian 'flu.

Understand the role of mobile clinics

Mobile clinics have been used for many years and are an important part of health care in remote or poor communities. Eye camps, family planning camps and surgical camps where mobile teams spend longer periods in one location are variations on this idea. We should actively consider whether this approach might be useful in the community we are working in.

Smaller community health clinics are in practice almost mobile clinics. Often there is a simple building or room that a visiting project team uses once per week or once per month. The team brings most of its supplies, though some equipment is often stored at the centre.

Mobile clinics are usually thought of as fully equipped vehicles (or occasionally small aircraft or hovercraft) with an appropriately trained team. They visit a sequence of remote villages on a regular basis at prearranged times and locations.

The advantages of mobile clinics are that patients with no other way of receiving health care can be examined, treated and if seriously ill brought back to a Primary Health Centre or hospital. They also enable many communities to receive basic health care, who would otherwise have no services at all. There are usually no buildings to maintain or rent, though there is usually the use of a community room.

Their disadvantages are that health care is often seen in terms of delivering a service rather than involving a community. The clinic can be little more than a hospital team plus medicines based in a vehicle, rather than in a hospital outpatient clinic. The mobile clinic usually concentrates on curative care and may make little impact on the underlying health problems of the community.

But there are ways of using the advantages, and avoiding the disadvantages. Here are some suggestions:

- Only visit communities with a mobile clinic if this is part of a Community Based Health

Programme. Get to know the community, carry out Participatory Appraisal (page 72), encourage them to identify needs and solutions, consider setting up a CHW training programme.

- Use the clinic for health promotion, teaching and involving community members, not just for curative care. The visit of the mobile clinic could be combined with village meetings, a CHW training session or helping with a community survey. Health committee members can be taught how to organise the site, remind the people when the clinic is due, and carry out tasks such as registration and crowd control. TBAs and other traditional health practitioners can attend and learn. This depth of programme would usually mean staying two or three days.

- Empower the community to build its own simple health post where CBHC activities can be carried out on a regular basis under the leadership of the community. The mobile clinic would continue to visit but the emphasis would be on support and training in a locally run health post. Any patients too sick for CHWs to manage would be seen when the mobile team visited.

Mobile clinics can also be used in urban areas

For example: ASHA project working in the slums of Delhi has recently bought a vehicle that has enabled the project to serve several slum colonies that currently have no buildings. However, this vehicle does not simply bring curative care. It helps to mobilise community members and is seen as a chance to build relationships, give health teaching, take the first steps to setting up CHW training, and forming community action groups.

Summary

Most projects will be asked to set up clinics. This should always be carried out in partnership with the community with the aim that the community should eventually manage it.

Buildings can be built or rented. They should be as simple as possible, well designed, with careful patient-flow plans, and sufficient waiting area.

Clinics comprise various stations, which patients visit in turn – registration, weighing, consulting, nursing, field laboratory and pharmacy. At each point patients are treated with respect and compassion. As well as offering curative care, health workers also discover and treat the real needs of patients and their families, in an attempt to cure causes of ill health and to promote health-affirming practices in the community. Clinics can be the local centres for national clinical programmes such as stop TB and the Integrated Management of Childhood Illness. Clinics should have systems in place to deal with simple emergencies.

Careful records are kept but registers and clinic reports should be few in number and easy to use. A fair method of payment needs to be set up so that the poor are not excluded. An effective referral system has to be established, with close links between the project and its referral hospitals. Finally, clinics provide an excellent opportunity both for teaching and creating health awareness. Mobile clinics can also become the focal point for community based health activities.

Further reading and resources

1. *Management Support for Primary Health Care*, P. Johnstone and J. Ranken, FSG Communications, ODA, 1994.
Chapters 2 and 3 are especially useful.
Available from: TALC. See Appendix E.
2. *Where There is No Doctor*, revised edition and African edition, D. Werner, 2003.
Available from: TALC, and more details at www.hesperian.org. See Appendix E.
3. *Where Women Have no Doctor: A Health Guide for Women*, A. Burns, R. Lovich, J. Maxwell and K. Shapiro, Macmillan, 1997.
A comprehensive guide to women's health problems and how to prevent and treat them.
Available from: TALC. See Appendix E.
4. *First Aid Manual*, St John's Ambulance, St Andrew's Ambulance and British Red Cross, 8th edn, 2002.
An excellent, well illustrated manual.
Available from: Tropical Health Technology. See Appendix E.

7. *District Laboratory Practice in Tropical Countries*, M. Cheesbrough, Tropical Health Technology, Part 1, 1998, Part 2, 2000.
A detailed guide, mainly for hospital use but with valuable information for labs in peripheral health centres.
Available from: Tropical Health Technology. See Appendix E.

8. 'Microscopical Diagnosis of Tropical Diseases'. A series of laminated brochures.
Extremely useful bench aids.
Available from: Tropical Health Technology. See Appendix E.
Please see also the Further reading section at the end of Chapter 16.

9. *Common Medical Problems in the Tropics*, C. Schull, Macmillan, 2nd edn, 1999.
Revised edition of an immensely useful book, ideal for primary health care level.
Available from: Macmillan. See Appendix E.

10. *Diagnosis and Treatment: A Training Manual for Primary Health Care Workers*, K. and G. Birrell, Macmillan, in association with VSO, 2000.
A very useful practical manual.
Available from: Macmillan. See Appendix E.

11. *Medical Supplies and Equipment for Primary Health Care*, M. Kaur and S. Hall, ed. K. Attawell, ECHO, 2001.
This is an immensely useful book, which all programmes are recommended to obtain.
Available from: ECHO. See Appendix A.

12. *Primary Diagnosis and Treatment: a manual for clinical and health centre staff in developing countries*, D. Fountain, 2nd edn, Macmillan, 2006.
An essential book for health centre staff.
Available from: Macmillan and TALC. See Appendix E.

13. *Practical Guide to Common Medical Problems*, M. von Blumroder, IAM and RCGP, 2005.
Available from: PO Box 1167, Peshawar, Pakistan.

Also see the Further reading lists at the end of chapters on specific health topics, Chapters 11–14 of this book. See also Further References and Guidelines, page 413.

Slides

A whole range of slides on identifying and treating common diseases is available from TALC. See Appendix E.

9

Improving Childhood Nutrition

In this chapter we shall consider:
1. What we need to know
   - Why adequate nutrition is important
   - The different types of malnutrition
   - The root causes of malnutrition
   - The common ages for malnutrition
2. What we need to do
   - Monitor (measure) malnutrition
   - Record malnutrition
   - Understand parents' response to advice
   - Prevent and cure malnutrition: the six rules of good nutrition
   - Consider special feeding programmes
   - Encourage micro-enterprise
   - Set up home food gardens
   - Consider mass deworming
   - Evaluate the programme

What we need to know

Why adequate nutrition is important

No loud emergency, no famine, no drought, no flood has ever killed 250 000 children in a week. Yet that is what a silent emergency is doing now – every week.

The chief killers in this silent emergency are pneumonia, diarrhoea, measles, malaria – and malnutrition.

A recent UNICEF report states that almost one third of all children in developing countries have malnutrition. Areas worst affected are south Asia and Africa.

Malnutrition contributes to more than half of all childhood deaths. Adequate nutrition is essential to help the body fight common childhood illnesses and is also important in TB and HIV/AIDS.

Tackling malnutrition at local level does not need a large number of doctors, huge sums of money or expensive equipment. What it does need is an enthusiastic health team and good management.

Of course, eradicating poverty and reducing civil conflict are the global challenges we must all help to overcome but …

> At the local level, malnutrition and its associated illnesses can best be prevented and treated through community-based health programmes.

Adequate childhood nutrition is important not only to prevent death but also to prevent mental and physical disability, improve the chances of finding a job and increase the quality of life.

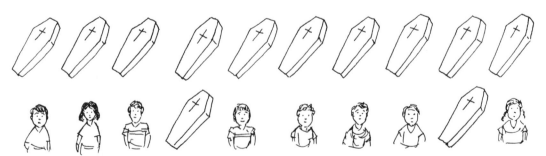

Figure 9.1   In poor communities, 8 out of every 10 deaths among under-fives can be prevented by effective community based health improvements.

Prevention of death

Well fed children get ill – sometimes – but usually recover on their own.

Malnourished children get ill – frequently – and die more often.

For example: Diarrhoea, measles and chest infections are not dangerous for most well nourished children, but those with malnutrition are many times more likely to die in childhood from these diseases.

Lack of nutrients can prevent children's brains from developing normally – and those most at risk often come from homes where there is little stimulation, which adds to this problem.

These challenges have given rise to a key programme directed at children, the IMCI (Integrated Management of Childhood Illness), which aims to deal with all these causes together.

Prevention of disability and increased quality of life

Malnourished children have impaired mental development. This means they usually grow up to become less intelligent adults, less likely to get good jobs and so less able to provide for their own children. If there is also iodine deficiency, this effect is multiplied.

A child with Vitamin A deficiency may become blind. A girl with vitamin D or calcium deficiency may develop rickets, leading to a malformed pelvis and extra dangers in giving birth. A woman with iodine deficiency may deliver a baby with severe mental disability.

Children receiving insufficient food over a long period of time may become stunted. They will grow up shorter and less strong than those who are well fed in childhood. They will become less productive farmers and less able workers.

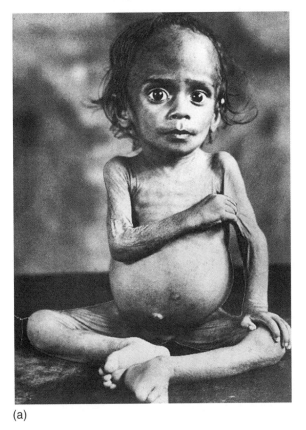

(a)

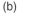

(b)

Figure 9.2   (a) Marasmus and (b) kwashiorkor: two extreme forms of malnutrition.

The different types of malnutrition

Malnutrition is usually a combination of both Protein-Energy Malnutrition (PEM) and a lack of one or more 'micronutrients', especially iron, Vitamin A, iodine and zinc.

A child has severe malnutrition if there is severe wasting and/or oedema.

Severe wasting means extreme thinness, which is most visible over the shoulders, ribs, upper arms, buttocks and thighs. The skin on the buttocks may look like 'baggy pants'.

Oedema (excess fluid in the tissues) usually occurs first in the lower legs and feet. To test for oedema, grasp each foot with thumb on top and press gently for ten seconds. The child has oedema if a dent remains after removing the thumb.

The terms marasmus (severe wasting) and kwashiorkor (wasting with oedema) are sometimes used to describe these severe forms of malnutrition. It is not fully understood why some children tend to develop one form rather than the other, but lack of protein as well as of energy foods is thought to be one cause of kwashiorkor.

Severe malnutrition in practice nearly always results from lack of energy foods and protein and so malnutrition is the preferred term we should normally use.

Children become malnourished because they eat less food than their bodies need. They may eat too little because there is a shortage of food at home, they are given too few meals or they are fed meals that are too watery (e.g. gruels). Children may not eat because they feel ill, or they may get insufficient breast milk. Poor growth is an early sign of malnutrition, and unless urgent action is taken, the child may become severely malnourished very quickly. This underlines the importance of regular weighing so malnutrition can be picked up earlier when it is easier to deal with.

Most cases of mild or moderate malnutrition are not obvious to the mother or even to the health worker. They often look like ordinary children. This 'hidden' group of malnourished children has higher than average health risks.

Anaemia or iron deficiency

This is nearly always present in undernourished children, and is often present in apparently well nourished children.

Children with marked anaemia have pale mucous membranes but may otherwise look quite normal. However, they will often be tired, catch infections more easily and perform less well at school.

For example: a study in Zanzibar found that children aged between one and four years given a small iron supplement daily had improved language development.

Anaemia is usually caused by insufficient iron in the diet but malaria, schistosomiasis, hookworm and whipworm can make it worse. Infections can block iron absorption and drinking tea and coffee with a meal reduces iron absorption.

Vitamin A deficiency or blinding malnutrition

This is the commonest cause of blindness in children, affecting 250 million in 80 countries. Eyes that are affected go through these stages: nightblindness, dislike of sunlight, and dryness of the conjunctiva with frothy white patches ('Bitot' spots). In addition the cornea becomes dry and cloudy and may ulcerate and burst.

Lack of Vitamin A also increases the dangers of diarrhoea, respiratory infections, measles, and probably malaria.

Nearly all cases of Vitamin A deficiency could be avoided if mothers simply knew that feeding their children green vegetables or yellow fruits usually available in their communities would fully prevent it.

For example: A recent study in India has shown that supplementing infants with Vitamin A reduces mortality.

Giving high dose Vitamin A to mothers at the time of delivery is a recommended intervention. See page 180.

Zinc deficiency is often associated with Vitamin A deficiency and increases the dangers of diarrhoea and acute respiratory infection.

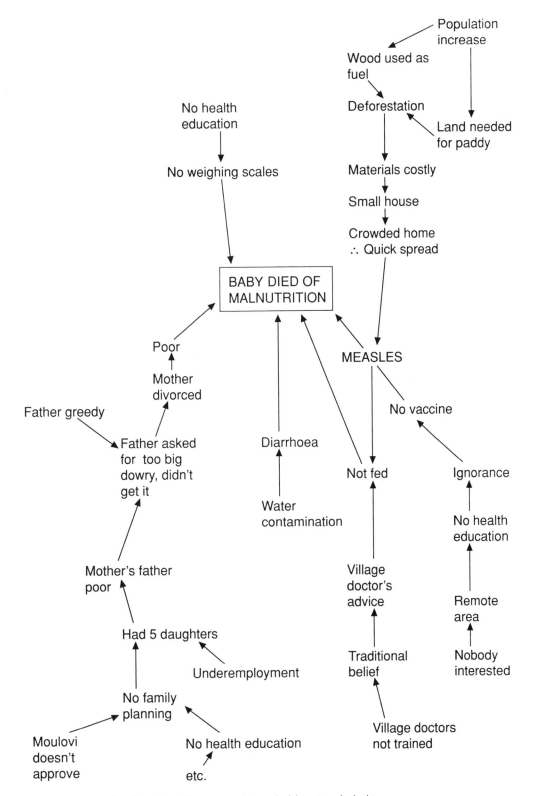

Figure 9.3   Some causes of malnutrition (from a workshop held in Bangladesh).

For example: One project in an Indian slum community found that daily zinc supplementation using 10 mg elemental zinc for infants and 20 mg for children reduced the number of children between 6 months and 3 years catching pneumonia, especially if they were also receiving Vitamin A.

There is evidence that 70 mg of zinc supplements given weekly can reduce pneumonia and mortality in young children.

Iodine deficiency

A report in 2003 from WHO showed that more than 1.9 billion individuals have inadequate iodine intake, of whom 285 million are school age children. People in many mountainous areas are especially likely to develop symptoms. However, the more widespread use of iodised salt is gradually reducing the number of people affected.

Goitre (a swollen thyroid gland) is the most obvious sign of iodine deficiency and is most commonly seen in women. The most dangerous effect is in children born to iodine-deficient mothers. These children will typically be deaf, dumb, slow, look puffy and tend to be constipated.

However, most iodine-deficient children may show very few signs, yet can still grow up to become less intelligent adults. Iodine deficiency is the most common cause of mental retardation, affecting almost 50 million people. Recent research has shown that a child with a thyroid lobe larger than the terminal phalanx of their thumb is likely to have a goitre.

Other deficiency diseases

These include:
- Lack of vitamin B leading to pellagra and beriberi.
- Lack of vitamin C leading to scurvy, often found in refugee camps.
- Lack of vitamin D or calcium leading to rickets – found mainly in women and girls where custom forbids exposing their skin to sunlight.

The root causes of malnutrition

The root causes of malnutrition are:
1. **Famine, war, and disasters** where food may be in short supply or impossible to obtain.

2. **Poverty and illness** – where community members:
   - are unable to grow or buy sufficient food.
   - lack adequate water supply and sanitation.
   - live in overcrowded conditions.
   - are unable to afford health care.
3. **Lack of appropriate knowledge** – where food is available but incorrectly used.

It is also helpful to look at specific causes to help us target our programmes (the 'spider chart', Figure 9.3 on page 171, includes many of these):

Causes in the child

- Low birth weight.
- Frequent infections such as diarrhoea, coughs and malaria leading to poor appetite, loss of weight and decreased resistance to further infection.
- Parasitic infections, e.g. hookworm, roundworm, *Giardia lamblia*, *Trichuris*.
- Poor relationship with mother.
- Bottle feeding, watery gruels, too few meals, no encouragement or assistance at meal times.
- AIDS – now the commonest cause in parts of Africa.

Causes in the mother

- Mother herself tired, ill or malnourished.
- Overwork in home, and through demands of other children.
- The daily need to collect fuel and water.
- Work outside home to help family income.
- Mother illiterate and uneducated, thus following incorrect practices, such as withholding food from an ill child and fluids in diarrhoea.
- Mother divorced, separated or widowed.
- Mother with HIV/AIDS and/or caring for orphans.

Causes in the family

- Husband or partner chronically unwell, uncaring, absent, drunk, addicted, unemployed, overworked, violent.
- Too many children to feed and care for, no family planning, no child spacing, twins.
- Tensions with mother-in-law.

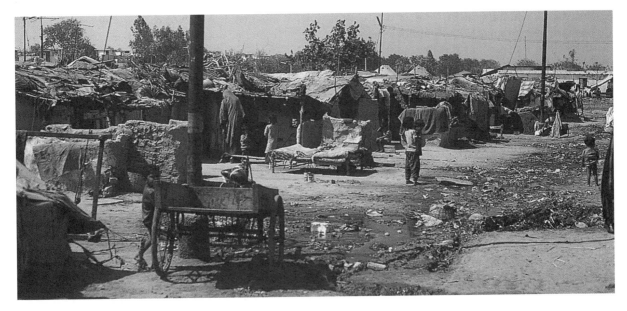

Figure 9.4   The circle of infection and malnutrition.

- Cash crops replacing food crops, meaning less food for children. Extra money wrongly spent on cigarettes and tonics rather than better food.
- Daughters not wanted.
- One or both parents with HIV/AIDS.

Causes in the community

- Insufficient land or employment.
- Poor farming practices, soil erosion and defor-estation; no irrigation, unproductive land, no land at all.
- Remote area with poor transport and little access to markets.
- Poor water supply and sanitation leading to diarrhoeal illnesses.
- Debt, bonded labour. Threats by landlords and moneylenders.
- Money, by tradition overspent on weddings, religious ceremonies and dowries.
- Tribal, class and religious conflicts.

Causes in the country

- War, civil unrest, famine, seasonal floods or drought.
- Depressed economy, national debt, lack of foreign exchange.

- Education and health not government priori-ties.
- Previous food aid leading now to attitude of dependence. Depressed prices for locally grown food and commodities and so no incen-tive to grow. Seed grain used up.
- Corrupt, inefficient or extreme political system causing the poor to suffer the most.
- Unjust trading laws that favour wealthy coun-tries.
- Structural readjustment programmes.
- High levels of HIV/AIDS or lack of access to antiretroviral therapy, leading to premature death and illness, in turn affecting the local and national economy.

The common ages for malnutrition

This partly depends on local customs, the season of the year and the types of food available in the community. The greatest risks usually occur at the following times:

1. **At birth.**
   In poor communities the child will usually be of low birth weight, and therefore at greatest risk in the first week (perinatal period), and the first month (neonatal period).

2. **Between 6 and 24 months.**

In many communities other liquids and foods are started too early or too late. Ideally, children should be fed on breast milk alone for the first six months except in special situations, e.g. where the mother is HIV positive (see page 182).

Weaning problems occur in this age range.

- Breastfeeding is often stopped. This may happen either gradually, or suddenly if the mother becomes pregnant or gives birth to another child.
- Food given may be inadequate in amount and it may be contaminated with germs, leading to diarrhoea, or by toxins in food especially in West Africa where aflatoxins from stored peanuts and other foods can affect health and nutrition. Toddlers may get infections by placing objects in their mouths and through unclean feeding bottles, or from infant formula that may itself be made up with unclean water.

3. **Whenever a new child is born.**

The mother will give her time, attention and breast milk to the newborn meaning that the next youngest child receives less of each. This effect is most important when the birth interval is less than three years.

4. **Any time of family crisis.**

What we need to do

Monitor (measure) malnutrition

Growth monitoring without teaching and involving parents does not improve nutrition. Many programmes spend a great deal of time weighing and using growth charts because this is often easier than careful explanations to parents about how they can better feed their children.

This chapter explains the two most commonly used ways of growth monitoring, but if time is limited and problems are severe, we should concentrate on educating and training mothers in clinic and home – i.e. on promoting growth rather than monitoring growth.

There are two ways of measuring malnutrition: by using weighing scales and by measuring the

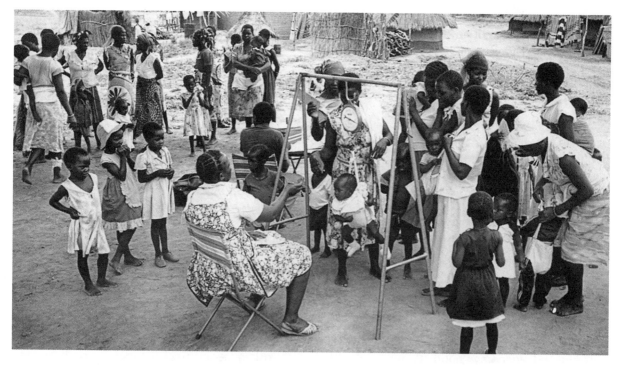

Figure 9.5   Community weighing session in Zimbabwe.

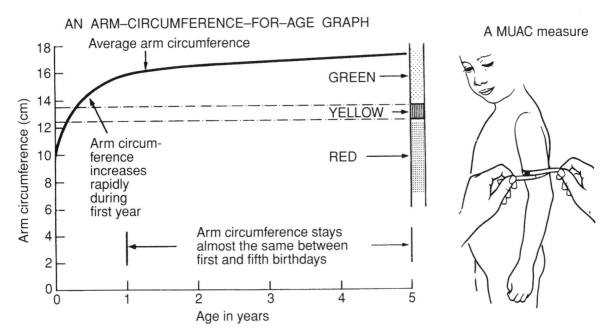

Figure 9.6   Measuring mid-upper arm circumference (MUAC).

Mid-Upper Arm Circumference (MUAC) in children between one and five years old.

Weighing scales

Advantages: used carefully, weighing shows us accurately the degrees of individual and community-wide malnutrition.

Disadvantages: scales are expensive, may be hard to obtain and many brands are heavy to carry.

Unless everyone is trained how to use them, mistakes can easily be made, especially in completing the Growth Chart.

The TALC Direct Recording Scales are recommended because they involve parents in the process of weighing. See Appendix E.

How often should weighing be done?

- Usually once per month in children under two years of age.
- With serious cases, once per week.
- Daily during treatment of severe malnutrition.

Where should it be done?

- In health centres, clinics or feeding centres.
- By mothers in small community-based groups.

- In homes, but if time is limited, home visits should concentrate on education rather than weighing.

Who should do it?

- At first, probably a nurse or other health worker who will teach
- the CHW, who will teach
- the mother, father or older sibling.
- Members of women's clubs or health committees can weigh children either from house to house or as a community activity, giving feeding advice at the same time.

All those involved in weighing will need careful teaching and supervision until they can do it quickly and accurately, so leaving time for identifying problems and explaining better ways of feeding.

How is it done?

- This is described in Chapter 8, pages 147–8.

Arm measurers

How do they work?

In children, the mid-upper arm circumference (MUAC) hardly changes at all between the ages of one and five years (see Figure 9.6).

Measurements are as follows:

- Well-nourished child: MUAC 13.5 cm or more
- Malnourished child:
  moderate: MUAC 12.5–13.5 cm
  severe: MUAC 12.5 cm or less.

In some areas a measuring tape with coloured zones is used, for example red for severe malnutrition, yellow for moderate and green for normal. Locally appropriate colours can be used instead. Tapes can either be bought, or made from strips of X-ray film.

How is it used?
- The child should be sitting or standing with the arm hanging unsupported from the shoulder.
- The tape should be wrapped firmly but not too tightly around the left mid-upper arm.
- The CHW, mother or older siblings can carry it out, but will need supervised practice, and be trained to identify problems and seek solutions.

Advantages of MUAC measuring:
- The strip is cheap and easy to carry.

- It is quicker and easier than scales, allowing more time for health education.
- It is ideal to use in homes, scattered communities and refugee camps.
- It can be used by those who are unable to read, write or understand numbers.

Disadvantages
- It is slightly less accurate than weighing. Growth charts cannot be used, but MUAC record cards can be designed (Figure 9.7).
- Mistakes can be made if the person measuring is in a hurry or if the child is fretful.
- It is less valid under one year of age, an important time to know a child's nutritional state.

Further use of the MUAC
MUAC measurements can be used at birth to assess if the newborn is malnourished.

A MUAC of 8.7 cm at the time of birth is approximately equivalent to a birth weight of 2500 grams. If a tape is marked at 8.7 cm, any measurement below that is considered low birth weight.

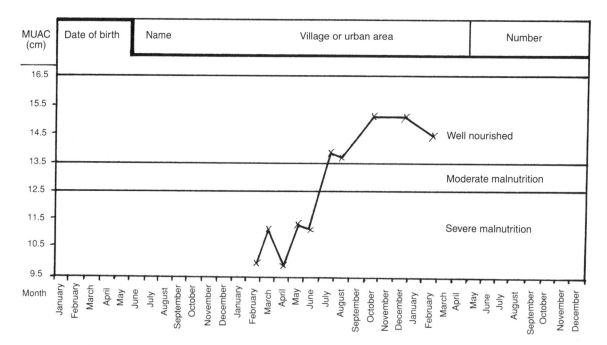

Figure 9.7   Mid-upper arm circumference record card.

Measuring the MUAC enables illiterate Traditional Birth Attendants (TBAs) or CHWs to discover low weight children at the time of birth and target care towards them.

Record malnutrition

MUAC measurements can be recorded on a MUAC Record Card (see Figure 9.7).

The best way of recording weights is on a growth chart. (sometimes known as a road to health chart). These are used in almost all countries of the world and are available in different languages and layouts. The basic design is the same.

We will need to follow these stages:

1. **Obtain and if necessary adapt growth charts** so they are suitable for our target population. We must ensure that the feeding advice on the card is relevant to the mothers in our community, and is written in the local language.
2. **Teach all team members (and CHWs where literate) how to use them.**

Many growth charts are completed incorrectly. Health workers should not start training others until they no longer make mistakes themselves.

When using a growth chart (see Figure 9.8):
a) Fill in the month and year of birth in the long box in the lower left corner.
b) Fill in the month and year each time the child is weighed.
c) Put a dot (and a ring), or a (x) for the measurement, checking and rechecking that it is in the right place, and linking it up with previous measurements using a pencil.
d) When using the TALC Direct Recording Scales, follow the instructions and involve the parent.
3. **Learn to interpret the findings, and explain these to the parents.**
The direction of the weight curve is the most crucial.
a) If it is rising – good – reinforce teaching.
b) If it is flat – this is a warning – find the cause, take action and give suitable teaching to the parents. If the line is flat for two months or more, this is known as growth

faltering. Recognising this and taking action is a main reason why we monitor weights.
c) If it is falling – there is a serious problem, which must be discovered and treated as soon as possible.
The actual weight itself is also important. We should not be satisfied until all weights are regularly on the Road to Health.
The most common causes of poor weight gain are:
- The child is not getting enough food.
- The child has an infection.
4. **Remember the purpose of the chart.**
a) It is an early warning system.

The growth chart tells us if things are going wrong before we (or the mother) would otherwise notice them. This means we can find and treat the cause at an early stage so preventing illness and disability later.

b) It helps us to evaluate whether parents have been following the nutrition teaching they have been given.
5. **Identify mistakes commonly made.**
These occur very frequently especially when the child is crying. Examples include:
a) Mother forgets the date of birth – often the month, sometimes the year.
- Buy or make a local events calendar. This has festivals, seasons, etc. marked on it, which serve as a reminder.
- Take time to work out the date with the mother. Always consider: does the child appear and behave the age the mother says?
b) Heath worker gets confused.
- Health workers need plenty of supervised practice.
- A ruler or straight edge helps in plotting the correct weight.
c) Mother doesn't understand the chart. It looks complicated and she thinks it must belong to the health worker.

Include the mother at every stage in weighing and recording, taking time to explain how the card works and how it shows the progress of her baby. She will soon start taking a pride not only in the card but in the weight gain of the child.

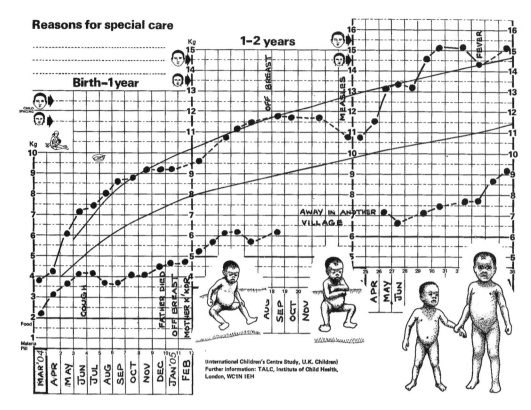

Reasons for special care

Figure 9.8   Growth chart for two children born in the same month in the same village.

- Most mothers, even those who are illiterate, will be able to understand a growth chart. Many will be able to weigh children themselves. However, if a mother is slow to understand, spend time in health education instead.
d) Mother forgets the card or has spoilt it.
   - A mother who takes pride in her children and their cards will usually remember to bring them.
   - Try to provide a protective plastic envelope.
e) Health worker gets angry: mother gets discouraged and stops coming.
   - Teach the team to be patient and to make sure that weighing is enjoyable.
   - Make sure that the mother is always commended for something she has done well.
6. **Ensure the mother keeps the card.**
   She should bring it whenever she visits the CHW, the clinic or the hospital.

Understand parents' response to advice

A mother or father will only improve feeding practices if they follow this 'chain of action'.

- Becoming aware that the child is malnourished. How? By our patient explanation, with or without a growth chart, and, where possible, also explaining to other family members.
- Being empowered to do something about it. How? By foods we recommend being available or affordable. By the family allowing the parent to take time, and to have flexibility in how and when to feed, even if this means altering family traditions. Older children may be able to give support in this.
- Possessing knowledge and skills to prepare and store food correctly, feed it appropriately and give it in sufficient amount. How? By our teaching being based on an exact understanding of community life, foods available and how

Table 9.1 Children aged 1–5 with mid-upper arm circumference of 12.5 cm or less

Village Name	April 1985		January 1988	
Parogi	4/16	25%	0/17	0%
Bell	7/21	33%	0/17	0%
U. Sarab	1/17	6%	0/17	0%
L. Sarab	13/30	43%	0/30	0%
U. Kandi	10/19	53%	2/19	11%
L. Kandi	6/24	5%	0/24	0%
Total	41/127	32%	2/128	2%

Source: SHARE Project, North India.

families function. By home visiting to fine-tune our advice and answer questions.

We must always ensure we listen to the mother and respond to her concerns and her particular situation. We will need to discuss action plans with her and make sure she understands, agrees and is able to carry them out.

Prevent and cure malnutrition

Before doing this we will need to understand both the general causes in the community and the special causes in the family we are caring for (see page 172).

Having discovered these, we will need to target our teaching in the clinic, community and the home.

For example (1): There is a well-known health programme in north India where many children attend local clinics and where their parents attend health talks. Yet studies here have shown that children who attend these clinics continue to have levels of malnutrition little different from those who do not attend.

For example (2): In a small Himalayan health project (SHARE) working among seven scattered villages, 32 per cent of children aged between one and five years were found to be severely malnourished by MUAC measurement when the project started. By training CHWs to give nutritional advice from house to house, using foods grown by each family, only two severely malnourished children remained two years later (Table 9.1).

From these examples we can learn this lesson:

> Where food supplies are adequate the key method of curing and preventing malnutrition is to train community health workers to make regular visits to each home. Here they give practical advice according to the exact needs of the family, and make sure this advice is put into practice.

There are six rules of good nutrition:
1. Ensure adequate nutrition for the pregnant mother.
2. Promote breastfeeding.
3. Introduce mixed feeding at six months.
4. Continue to feed ill children.
5. Prepare, cook and store food correctly.
6. Avoid harmful and inappropriate foods.

Rule 1. Ensure adequate nutrition for the pregnant mother

The baby's weight at birth and during the first few weeks of life depends mainly on the health of the mother.

> One quarter of all deaths in children under one year old occur in the first week of life, and one half occur in the first month. These deaths usually happen because the mother herself is ill, malnourished or poorly prepared.

In our antenatal care we should aim for birth weights of 2500 grams or more, or MUACs of 8.7 cm or more.

In order to achieve this:

1. **Encourage adequate weight gain in pregnancy.** Mothers should ideally gain about 5–8 kg during pregnancy.
   Adequate maternal nutrition depends on:
   • Eating enough food and eating well balanced food throughout pregnancy (and during lactation).
   • Taking enough rest, especially in the month before the baby is due.
2. **Prevent and treat anaemia.**
   Mothers should have a haemoglobin level of at least 11 g/dl at the time of the delivery. This will depend on:

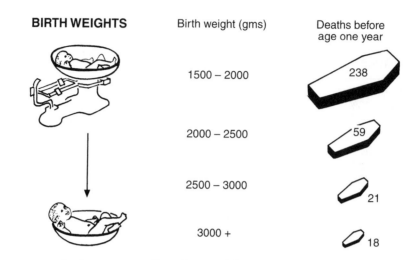

Figure 9.9   There are more deaths among smaller infants and those who survive are more likely to grow up short and undernourished. A major cause of low birth weight is short, undernourished mothers.

- Eating enough iron-rich foods such as green leafy vegetables, eggs and meat where locally available.
- Taking iron-folate tablets daily.
- Treating and preventing malaria (see page 232), hookworm and bilharzia, ideally before becoming pregnant.

3. **Prevent and treat Vitamin A deficiency in mothers and infants.**
   - The mother should eat foods rich in Vitamin A – green leafy vegetables; orange, red or yellow fruits or vegetables; or red palm oil.
   - If there is local Vitamin A deficiency (e.g. night blindness affects over one per cent of children aged one to five), she can be given a weekly supplement of 25 000 IU during pregnancy.
   - After delivery she can be given 200 000 IU within the first six weeks, if she has not received supplements during pregnancy.
   - The infant can be given 100 000 IU as a single dose between 9 and 12 months (with measles vaccine). See also page 195.

4. **Prevent and treat iodine deficiency.**
   Where iodine deficiency is known to occur (e.g. where any cases of goitre are observed):
   - Use only iodised salt.
   - During pregnancy give iodised oil either orally or as an injection, as early in pregnancy as possible.

   - Women of childbearing age can be given regular iodine supplements. For doses follow national guidelines, and use preparations available.

5. **Discourage smoking, alcohol and drug-taking.**
   If the mother smokes, or drinks heavily, the baby is born smaller and weaker and is more likely to die in the first months of life.

6. **Treat and prevent serious illness.**
   Tuberculosis, sexually transmitted illnesses, HIV/AIDS and other chronic illnesses can all seriously affect the baby's health.

7. **Ensure regular antenatal care** (see Chapter 12).

There is little value in teaching pregnant women about correct nutrition and regular antenatal care unless we encourage husbands and other family members to make available the extra time and support mothers need.

Rule 2. Promote breastfeeding

If a new vaccine became available that could prevent more than 1 million child deaths per year, was cheap, safe, could be given orally, had no side effects and needed no cold chain, it would be a public health triumph.

Breastfeeding can do all this and more.
Many mothers today are being wrongly persuaded to use the bottle instead of the breast.

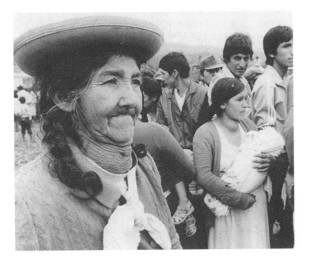

Figure 9.10   Iodine deficiency affecting three generations in the Bolivian Andes.

They may listen to the advertising of big companies who sell artificial milk, or think that wealthy and fashionable women use infant formula. They may start thinking that breastfeeding is dirty or old-fashioned. A sequence that often happens is that a mother tries to combine breastfeeding and formula, finds her supply of breast milk lessens, and the infant soon becomes wholly fed by formula.

Unless mothers are HIV positive, bottle-fed babies are several times more likely to die than breastfed babies. Our job is to make sure that our teaching in favour of breastfeeding is more powerful than the pressures on mothers to adopt bottle feeding.

Breast is best because:
1. It is the natural food for babies, having the perfect balance of nutrients and providing natural protection against illness.
2. It is free and easily available.
3. It is clean, meaning the baby is less likely to get diarrhoea; and is up to 14 times less likely to die from diarrhoea than bottle-fed babies.
4. Breastfeeding strengthens the bond between mother and child.
5. Breastfeeding, if regular and frequent, acts as a contraceptive and so helps child spacing.

Help mothers to understand:
1. The reasons listed why breast is best. Be imaginative. *For example*: Help mothers work out how much money they would save if they used breast milk instead of bottle milk. Families sometimes spend up to one quarter of their income on infant formula for their baby.

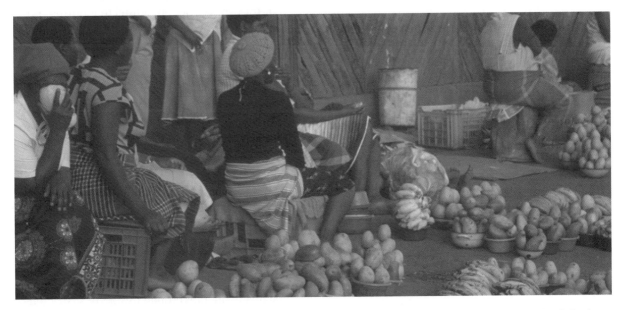

Figure 9.11   Vitamin A can be stored in a child's body for a few months, so encourage families to feed foods high in vitamin A as much as possible when available.

2. Colostrum is good!
   The thick yellowish milk produced in the first one or two days is not 'bad milk', but full of nutrients and antibodies that the child really needs.

> In many communities children are only put to the breast on the second or third day. Patiently encourage mothers to start breastfeeding within hours of birth.

3. Breastfeeding should be continued where possible for at least two years. WHO now recommends it should be used exclusively up to six months in most communities. Exclusive means breast milk alone – no water, teas or other foods or liquids.
4. Breastfeeding is usually possible. Mothers often incorrectly believe they cannot make enough milk. Where this is the case encourage them:
   • to allow the baby to suckle often, both day and night.
   • to drink more fluids.

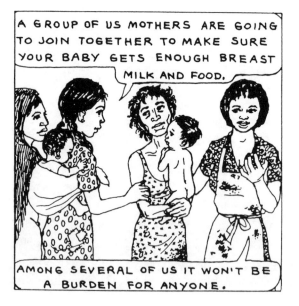

Figure 9.12   Members of a women's club help a recently widowed mother.

> The rules for breast milk substitutes:
> Mothers should use these only if they are:
> • acceptable to the child;
> • feasible for the mother;
> • affordable for the family;
> • sustainable in the circumstances;
> • safely prepared and used;
> • recommended because the mother is HIV positive.

> The more the baby suckles, the more milk is produced. This is especially important in the few days after birth when milk may not flow easily.

If the mother is really not able to breastfeed it may be possible to find an HIV negative 'wet nurse' in the community (both Moses and Muhammad were reputedly fed in this way). Other family women with children, and even grandmothers, may be able to provide breast milk, but this is acceptable in only some communities.

Note on breastfeeding and HIV

• Women known to be HIV positive have a significant risk of passing on HIV infection to their infants through breastfeeding, especially if they have become infected during pregnancy, during breastfeeding or have symptoms of AIDS. This risk is greatly reduced if they use antiretrovirals, see below.
• If women are known to be HIV positive, they should be counselled about the option of using breast milk substitutes, or of exclusive breastfeeding for the first six months. Research shows that partial breastfeeding is more likely than exclusive breastfeeding to cause mothers to pass on HIV to their children. Mothers using substitutes will need careful instruction in how to use these, and appropriate formulations must always be available for them. In some communities, using substitutes may imply HIV infection and cause the mother to be stigmatised.
• Women known to be HIV negative (or whose status is unknown unless strongly suspected of being HIV positive), should be encouraged to breastfeed. Breastfeeding must be continuously

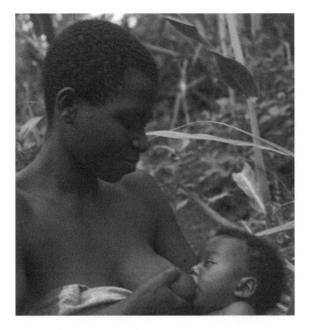

Figure 9.13   Children who are well fed during the first two years of life are likely to stay healthy for the rest of their childhood.

promoted as the safest option for the majority of children.

- In areas where HIV is common, encouraging mothers to go for voluntary counselling and testing (VCT) is important as this provides the only basis for offering the best advice. Antenatal clinics are an ideal location. Children cannot reliably be tested until 18 months old.
- Antiretrovirals substantially lower the risk of transmission in HIV positive women. Current recommendations are: zidovudine (AZT) 300 mg twice daily from 28 weeks of pregnancy to birth plus single dose nevirapine 200 mg during labour plus one week of zidovudine for the infant. A simpler and cheaper regimen is nevirapine 200 mg at onset of labour and single dose 2 mg/kg for babies within 72 hours of birth, but future development of resistance is a potential problem when a single drug is used. Other regimens are also approved by WHO. To use any of these regimens we will need to ensure careful training of health workers and well managed clinics and supplies; also readily available VCT, and full support services. Guidelines are fre-

quently changing. Check WHO or UNAIDS websites for latest recommendations. (See below.)

Rule 3. Introduce mixed feeding at about six months

If mixed feeding is started too early children lose the benefit of exclusive breastfeeding and pick up diarrhoeal disease more frequently. This may worry the parents, who then delay too long in trying to reintroduce mixed feeding.

If started too late the child will start falling off the Road to Health chart. This usually happens at about eight months.

Follow these guidelines:

1. **Find out local customs and beliefs.**
   Make sure that health workers encourage only the use of foods that are locally available and that the poor can afford.
   For example: This mistake is commonly made: health workers who come from a city or from a different part of the country will promote foods they are used to eating. These foods may be very expensive in the project area or not be used at all.
2. **Encourage appropriate foods.**
   Such foods should be:
   - easy to prepare;
   - rich in energy content, protein and micronutrients;
   - easy for the child to eat;
   - clean and safe;
   - locally available and affordable.
3. **Use correct foods for different ages.**
   Some general principles to follow

From 6 to 12 months:

- Feed a little at a time, twice a day, to start with, building up to at least four times a day.
- Foods should be soft and easy to digest.
- Include soft fruits and thick porridge mixes with milk or pounded groundnuts.
- Introduce new foods one at a time. Wait until the child is used to one food before offering it another. A good rule is to start a new food about every two weeks.
- Feed the child gently, never using force.

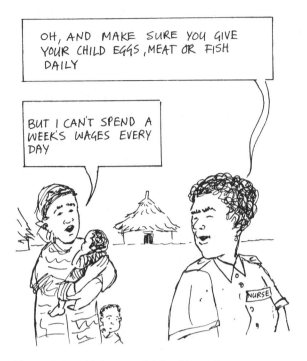

Figure 9.14   Make sure that health workers encourage only the use of foods that are available locally and are affordable by the poor.

- Give mixtures of mashed foods: include such foods as legumes, potatoes, roots such as cassava and yam, eggs, finely chopped meat or fish, as well as cereals and fruit. These can be prepared according to local custom.

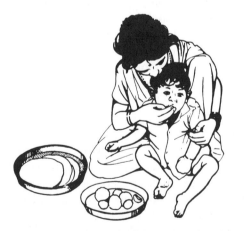

Figure 9.15   Until nutrition workers have tried to deal with the problem of the cranky child who refuses to eat whatever the mother prepares, they have not come to grips with the most essential element of applied nutrition.

For example: For many years in parts of Nepal, children have been fed with what is known as 'super-flour porridge' (see below).

Ingredients for super-flour porridge

The flour is made from:
- Two parts pulse – soybeans are best, but other small beans, grams and peas can also be used.
- One part whole grain cereal such as maize or rice.
- One part another whole grain cereal such as wheat, millet or buckwheat.

The pulses and grains need to be cleaned, roasted well (separately) and ground into fine flour (separately or together). The flour can then be stored in an airtight container for one to three months. The flour is stirred into boiling water and cooked for a short time. The proper amount and consistency of the porridge will depend on the age and condition of the child. Salt should not be added, especially if the child is malnourished.

The exact make-up of the porridge can be varied according to the lentils or cereals available locally.

For example: Dal, carrot and Amaranthus is used with rice or chapati in some parts of Asia, millet and bean porridge in some parts of Africa, rice, beans and liver in South America, and rice lentils and yoghurt in the Middle East.

Traditional ways of preparing cereals can be also encouraged, especially those involving fermentation, which reduces the number of germs present.

Where Vitamin A deficiency occurs (see pages 170, 180), consider giving Vitamin A 200 000 IU every four to six months up to school age, or even up to ages nine or ten in severely affected areas, preferably linked into other CBHC activities.

From one year upwards:
- The child can eat 'from the family pot'.
  Children can generally eat the same food as adults, but they should have their own plate to make sure they get their fair share. By the age of one year children are eating about half the amount per day that their mothers eat.
- Feed four to six times a day.
  Children will not be able to manage on the one or two main meals a day that adults eat.

They have small stomachs and 'like chickens should often be pecking'.

A final point:

> Make sure all health workers and CHWs give identical advice on improving nutrition so as to avoid confusion within the community.

Rule 4. Continue to feed sick children

The belief that food should not be given to sick children is dangerous and many children die as a result. Illness leads to malnutrition and malnutrition to illness. So increase the number of breast-feeds, encourage the child to eat even if not hungry, give soft foods especially if the mouth and throat are sore, give extra fluids if the child has a fever or diarrhoea.

Sick children will have small appetites; they should therefore eat what they wish, as often as they like and in small amounts at a time.

> After an illness there will be plenty of catching up to do. Children will need to eat more than usual and more often than usual, with extra oil added to the food, until they are back on the Road to Health.

Children with diarrhoea should also be fed. Oral rehydration using home-prepared liquid foods such as rice water can be used instead of simple salt-sugar solution (see pages 212–3).

It has been estimated that people living with HIV/AIDS, depending on the state of their illness, need 10 to 15 per cent more calories and at least 50 per cent more protein than uninfected people. We must ensure that infected children eat sufficient amounts so they continue to gain weight and remain on the road to health.

Giving the antibiotic cotrimoxazole daily to all infected children will help to prolong their lives. Ensuring this is available and continuously used should be part of our programme.

Rule 5. Prepare, cook and store food correctly

Mothers or those preparing food should be taught these basic rules:

1. Wash hands thoroughly before preparing or serving food, after any interruption, after cleaning the baby, touching animals or going to the toilet. Finger nails should be kept short.
2. Use clean utensils, containers and surfaces for preparing food.
3. Wash fruit and vegetables using the cleanest water available, peel them if possible, and cook if they are likely to have become contaminated with dirty water or faeces.
4. Cook food thoroughly until steaming hot, and eat within two hours of preparation. However, over-cooked vegetables, especially if in an uncovered container, can lose valuable vitamins.
5. Avoid storing cooked food if possible. If stored food is used it should always be stored in a refrigerator and fully recooked, not simply reheated.
6. Store foodstuffs in safe places, away from chemicals and pesticides and protected from rodents, other animals, and insects, by using closed containers.
7. Avoid contact between cooked food and raw foods, especially poultry and other meat.
8. Avoid feeding infants with a bottle, as bottles and teats are very hard to clean. Use a cup and spoon instead.

Rule 6. Avoid harmful and unnecessary foods

Harmful foods include spoilt or mouldy cereals, beans and groundnuts. Also any food that has been inadequately recooked, or stored in containers that have held pesticides, fuels or chemicals.

The use of unnecessary foods is becoming common in developing countries. This leads to the overweight child who is fed on 'junk foods' such as artificial milk, tinned baby foods, tonics, bottled drinks, including beer and cola, excessive sweets, biscuits, or other fashionable products seen on the latest TV programme or soap.

Money saved can be used to buy nutritious foods to improve the family's diet.

Beware the 'Curse of Malinche' – Malinche was a Mexican who helped the foreign soldier Cortes invade Mexico and conquer the country. The Curse of Malinche is the belief that anything foreign or western is good and must be better than things made in our own country.

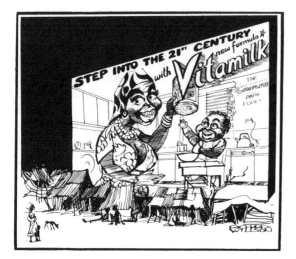

Figure 9.16

The Curse of Malinche makes poor people want to buy the latest drink, food, cigarette, or drug from the nearest 'smart' country. Parents may spend all their savings on fancy foods from abroad. This in turn leads them deeper into poverty.

Mothers need to be taught to use foods from their own communities.

Consider special feeding programmes

Sometimes more serious causes for malnutrition are present in a community meaning that 'The Six Rules' on their own are inadequate.

We need to assess with the community whether this is likely to be a short-term local shortage that the community and project can manage together, or whether this is a more serious problem that requires specialist outside help.

1. Local/short-term food shortages

When is a feeding programme needed?
The community may ask for a feeding programme, either because it is necessary, or sometimes, especially when a project is starting up, because they may hope for free handouts or subsidies.

In CBHC, we should only start a feeding programme if the following conditions exist in the target area:

1. There is evidence of food shortage or severe or worsening malnutrition. Usually we will have become aware of this through many apparently well children failing to gain weight as discovered during clinic weighing or MUAC measurements.
2. The community is able to share responsibility and take action.
   This can be a health committee, or a church, temple, mosque, school or social committee. It can be a single enthusiastic CHW supported by motivated community volunteers.
3. Availability of sufficient food from sources not too distant from the community. We should use the most local and familiar foods that are available.

How is it done?
We can help the community, CHW or committee carry out the following:

1. To select a suitable time and place for feeding. *For example*: Midday or evening in the CHW's house; morning outside the clinic.
2. To collect and prepare suitable food. This must be well balanced and high in energy, protein and micronutrients. A 'super-porridge' may be appropriate.
   Where available at least some food should be supplied by the community itself. Wealthier members can be encouraged to contribute supplies for the programme. Community members should cook the food themselves either in their own homes or as a community activity.
3. To organise cooking stoves and utensils.
4. To gather the children, feed them and keep order.
5. To teach and motivate the parents. This is an excellent time to teach the rules of good nutrition, weigh the children with the parents' help and distribute Vitamin A and worm medicine if needed.

In practice the CHW will usually be the organiser and the motivator. To be successful, she will need effective backup both from the project and from the community.

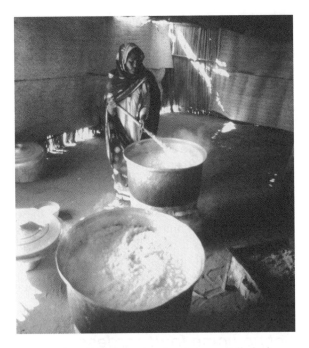

Figure 9.17   Weigh up the situation carefully before embarking on a special feeding programme.

For example: In Jamkhed, India, a feeding programme was needed when villagers first joined the project. Young Farmers' clubs were formed whose members would help to collect the food, gather the children and motivate the community. They were careful always to support the CHW by giving the same advice and teaching as she herself gave. With clubs and CHWs working together the programme achieved quick results and could soon be discontinued.

Some Dos and Do nots:

1. Do run the programme for a short time only. As soon as food supplies improve, discontinue, but follow up vulnerable children.
2. Do include children with moderate malnutrition.
   Choose a cut-off point on the Road to Health chart (see below) and include children below that point. Children should not be included simply because their parents request it or because they come from influential families. Explain entry criteria clearly to the community, otherwise envy or mistrust can easily develop.

Where malnutrition is more widespread and severe, an alternative is to include all children under five at the start.
3. Do follow up each child at home.

> When the feeding programme has been stopped, make sure that each child receives appropriate food at home and continues to gain weight.

4. Do not run the programme for the people. They themselves should do it with our help.
5. Do not give out free supplies unless no food is available and a relief situation applies.
6. Do not start a community feeding programme unless there is a need for it confirmed by someone with expert knowledge on nutrition. It is much easier to start programmes than to stop them, as communities can quickly become dependent.

> We should never give free handouts, supplies or rations through clinics except in famine conditions. Where this is done it creates dependence and in the long term may even worsen nutritional problems.

2. Widespread/longer-term food shortages

If we predict or have been advised by experts that we are entering this situation, we must call on outside experts, be in touch with government agencies and make sure our response involving the community can be as effective as possible.

This is a typical situation when relief and aid agencies will be making a response, often saving lives but sometimes bypassing or disempowering the community.

A good model for us to consider in such a situation is known as CTC – Community-based Therapeutic Care. This has been pioneered by an organisation called Valid International, mainly working in chronic complex emergencies. Adequate resources and training are needed for this to be successful. (See page 191, ref. 8.)

CTC's approach is based on building the capacity of local communities and existing structures to respond as effectively as possible.

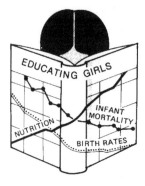

The education of girls is closely associated with a falling infant mortality and birth rate and improved nutrition

Figure 9.18   Improvements in schooling of mothers leads to reduced infant mortality and improved nutrition.

In discussion with the community they define 3 models of care:

a) The need for supplementary feeding: this is the use of additional food when the average weight for height of under-five children is 70–80 per cent of the median, and there is no pitting oedema, or the MUAC is between 11 and 12.5 cm, and the child is alert, well and has an appetite. Guidelines are available that can be adapted and adopted.

b) The need for 'outpatient' therapeutic care. This is needed when the average weight for height of children is less than 70 per cent of the median, or pitting oedema is present, or the MUAC is below 11 cm and the child remains alert, well and has an appetite.

c) The need for inpatient care starts when the child loses its appetite, is unwell with fever, and/or has dehydration.

For a) and b) above the home and the health centre will usually be the best locations to set this up.

Where food shortage is severe, Ready-to-Use Therapeutic Food (RUTF) can be used. RUTF comes in various forms. It is an enriched food, easy to digest and enables children to increase rapidly their intake of energy, protein and micronutrients.

Encourage micro-enterprise

More information on special feeding programmes is given in the Further reading and resources section at the end of the chapter.

Poverty is often the root cause of chronic malnutrition. This means that helping a community to generate its own income can be the most useful service we provide. Ask an expert to help assess this before rushing into it, or cooperate with another NGO that specialises in income generation or micro-enterprise (see page 393).

When starting an income generating programme, make sure that teaching is given about the correct use of extra cash and also about the dangers of extra income when it is not used constructively and for the benefit of the family. Try to encourage women to take a leading part in these initiatives and to control the way the money is spent. This makes it more likely that income will be used for family needs, rather than wasted on alcohol, cigarettes or drugs. Women's clubs or cooperatives can help with this (see pages 31–34).

Set up home food gardens

Often known as kitchen gardens, these can be set up almost anywhere including urban areas where crops can be grown in buckets or old tyres, and placed near the house, or on ledges or roofs.

In many rural areas fewer traditional foods are being grown for family consumption, wild fruit and berries are harder to find and money is often spent on buying less nutritious 'fashionable food'. This makes it valuable to grow a few highly nutritious foods near the home especially for the benefit of children and people living with HIV/AIDS.

This is what we can do:

1. Assess what foods would be most suitable. If protein is in short supply, beans and lentils can be grown. If there is Vitamin A deficiency, green leafy vegetables, and carrots. Pawpaw (papaya) or mango trees can be planted.
2. Choose crops that are easy to grow. They will ideally need a short growing season and a long cropping season, should be familiar to the community, popular with children when cooked correctly, and not prone to disease and pests.
3. Make sure there is sufficient water throughout the growing season. This can be household waste water providing it is not toxic, or rainwater can be collected and stored from roofs.

4. Feed the soil, for example by using compost. If on a slope, protect the soil from being washed away, by stones or fixed contours.
5. Involve children in the project or delegate the care of the garden to children.
6. Consider planting trees that provide nutritious leaves or fruit, especially trees that are, or have been, native in the area.

An example: The San Lucas association in Peru discussed home gardens in village meetings, owing to high rates of malnutrition and because few vegetables were grown locally. They started with a gardening project in four schools, then many families started to set up their own. Now women's groups coordinate these gardens in many nearby villages, childhood nutrition has improved and there are sometimes surpluses that can be sold to increase family income.

Consider mass deworming

Why is deworming useful?

Children, especially those of school age, (i.e. 3–18) may have very high intestinal worm (Helminth) levels. Forty per cent of the world's schoolchildren have intestinal worms and in some areas, such as Zanzibar in East Africa, almost 100 per cent are affected. WHO has set a target that 75 per cent of school-age children in developing countries should be having regular deworming treatment by the year 2010.

Roundworms (*Ascaris*) reduce absorption of food and worsen malnutrition. Hookworm (*Ancylostoma* and *Necator*), whipworm (*Trichuris*) and bilharzia (*Schistosoma*) reduce iron levels and cause anaemia. Two or more of these common Helminths are often found together.

Regular deworming therefore improves nutrition, reduces anaemia, and enables children to have more energy and learn more quickly. Well run programmes are cost effective.

When should we start a programme?

Consider doing this when 25 per cent or more of a sample population of school children has worms. Certainly carry it out when this figure reaches 50 per cent. In practice this means that mass deworming will be useful in most school-age children living in poor rural and urban areas.

Most programmes concentrate on younger age groups, for example: Grades 1 to 4, or children between six and eleven. However, there is increasing evidence that younger children even down to the age of two can benefit.

What drugs should we use?

Two are especially useful – mebendazole 500 mg or albendazole 400 mg given as a single dose. Both are largely free of side effects. Mebendazole is usually the cheaper, but donation programmes can alter this. Seek advice from the DMO about any national programme and what drugs are being used.

Bilharzia has to be treated with a different drug – praziquantel. Measuring sticks are often available that can be used in clinics to calculate quickly the dose needed. Only take part in any control programme in association with the DMO or a regional plan.

How often should these drugs be used?

In order to be effective, mebendazole or albendazole needs to be given every four to six months. Although neither drug is completely effective, by using them this frequently worm levels are kept so low that they cause little harm. Using the drugs less often allows worm populations to build up and iron levels to fall.

How should they be distributed?

This depends on the local situation. If school children are being targeted, the health team can arrange distribution within the school. If school-age children who do not attend school are being included, CHWs or members of the health team can distribute them in the community. The benefits of the programme can be used to persuade families to send their children to school.

Some programmes also distribute other medicines. *For example*: A project in Gujarat, western India, distributes Vitamin A capsules 200 000 IU, and iron tablets (60 mg equivalent Fe) at the same time, making sure that schools use iodised salt for their cooking. Children have become taller, heavier, better able to see in the dark, less anaemic and have felt more active than before the programme started.

What public health improvements should also be carried out?

CBHC should never depend purely on medicine distribution to solve a problem. Our aim is always to improve the health of communities so that outside programmes become less necessary.

We should start a deworming programme only if at the same time we actively consider three other areas:

- Working with the community to provide safe water for drinking and washing (Chapter 16).
- Working with the community to improve sanitation – this may mean promoting latrines (Chapter 16).
- Improving personal and community hygiene (pages 217–8).

Evaluate the programme

This is most simply done by seeing how the nutritional status of children changes over a period of time. The percentage of children under five on the Road to Health, or of those aged one to five years with MUACs of 13.5 cm or more, is compared between the start of the programme and a resurvey two, three or five years later. However, nutritional status varies with seasons and repeat surveys should therefore be done at the same time of year.

All stages of the evaluation should be done in partnership with the community. Results should be explained carefully as changes in child nutrition may not be obvious and the community may not realise that improvements have occurred unless this is clearly presented to them (see also Chapter 18).

Summary

Child deaths in a community can be halved by ensuring that children are adequately nourished. Community health programmes are ideally placed to bring this about. Malnutrition usually indicates lack of energy foods, protein and micronutrients, such as iron, iodine, Vitamin A and zinc. Two extreme forms of malnutrition are marasmus and kwashiorkor.

For each community and family the causes of malnutrition must first be discovered, so the underlying causes can be targeted. A system of health monitoring should be set up, either weighing children or measuring Mid-Upper Arm Circumference. Practical advice can then be offered from house to house, the CHWs taking a leading role. If sufficient food is available, the 'Six Rules of Good Nutrition' may be sufficient, but where causes are deeper rooted further community action may be needed, such as feeding programmes and income generating schemes. Community-based therapeutic care is one model that can be used when malnutrition becomes severe or prolonged such as in chronic complex emergencies. Expert advice always needs to be sought in such situations.

Deworming programmes in school-age children can have positive effects and should be actively considered alongside public health improvements. If malnutrition is a recurrent or continuing problem, consider setting up home food gardens

Regular evaluations should be carried out with the community, by resurveying after two, three or five year periods.

Further reading and resources

1. *Caring for severely malnourished children*, A. Ashworth, A. Burgess, Macmillan, 2003. CD ROM also available. This book is essential reading. Available from: TALC. See Appendix E.
2. *Complementary feeding: Family foods for breast-fed children*, WHO, 2000. Available from: WHO. See Appendix E.
3. *Vitamin A Supplements*, 2nd edn. WHO, 1997. Available from: WHO. See Appendix E.
4. *WHO Global Database on Child Growth and Malnutrition*, M. de Onis and M. Blossner, WHO, 1997. Available from: WHO. See Appendix E.
5. *Healthy Eating*, I. Carter, Tearfund, 2003. Practical advice on making the most of available food. Available from: TALC.

6. *Antiretroviral drugs for treating pregnant women and preventing HIV infection in infants*, WHO, 2004, see www.who.int.
7. *The global strategy for infant and young child feeding*, WHO, 2004.
   Available from: WHO and from www.who.int.
8. *Community-based therapeutic care: a new paradigm for selective feeding in nutritional crises*, S. Collins, Overseas Development Institute, London, 2004.
   Available from: www.odi.org.uk/publications.
9. *Nutrition Matters: People, Food and Famine*, H. Young and S. Jaspars, IT Publications, 1995.
   Extremely useful information on situations of severe food shortage.
   Available from: IT Publications. See Appendix E.
10. *Nutrition For Developing Countries*, F. Savage-King and A. Burgess, Oxford University Press, 1993.
    Still a valuable resource but expensive.
    Available from: TALC. See Appendix E.
11. *How to Grow a Balanced Diet: A handbook for community workers*, A. Burgess, G. Maina, P. Harris and S. Harris, VSO, 1998.
    Available from: TALC. See Appendix E.
12. *The Manual on Nutritional Care And Support Of People Living With HIV/AIDS*, also entitled *Living Well with HIV/AIDS*, UN Food and Agriculture Organisation, 2003.

Also see www.fao.org and www.unaids.org.
For details of vitamin A supplementation see www.who.int/vaccines/en.vitamina.

Slides

The following slide sets are available from TALC. See Appendix E. New sets are continually added.

- Breastfeeding   Bf
- Breastfeeding Problems   BFP
- Charting Growth in Small Children   ChG
- Xerophthalmia (Vitamin A Deficiency)   EyX
- Malnutrition in India   MI
- Malnutrition in an Urban Environment   MUE
- Weaning Foods and Energy   WFE
- Treatment of severely malnourished children TSMC

Accessories

1. TALC Direct Recording Scales Kit contains scale, plastic wall chart, 30 child health charts (available in eight languages). Discounts for five or more kits.
2. Child health charts, weight-for-height charts, etc.
3. Nutrition Growth Monitoring Pack, also available from TALC.

See Further references and guidelines, page 412.

10

Setting up a Childhood Immunisation Programme

In this chapter we shall consider:
1. What we need to know
   - Why childhood immunisation is important
   - Global strategies: EPI and GAVI
   - Details of commonly used immunisations (Table 10.1)
   - Immunisation schedules
   - Equipment needed
   - How to maintain the cold chain
2. What we need to do
   - Assess needs for immunisation in the programme area
   - Discuss plans with the government
   - Set targets
   - Train the team
   - Prepare the community
   - Carry out immunisation in the field
   - Carry out immunisation in the clinic
   - Keep records
   - Evaluate the programme

What we need to know

Why childhood immunisation is important

At the time of writing (2005), measles kills about half a million children a year, most in the poorest communities, and half in Africa. It accounts for almost 10 per cent of under-five deaths worldwide. However, measles has become less frequent over the past few years because of measles immunisation and the disease is no longer endemic in north or South America.

Polio at the time of writing is still present in a few countries of Asia and sub-Saharan Africa but is likely to be eradicated shortly.

Three hundred and fifty million people are chronic carriers of hepatitis B, and over half a million die each year mainly from liver cancer, which arises many years after the infection occurs. Over 2 billion people globally have been infected.

Apart from death, many million more suffer disability, bereavement, and loss of earnings because of diseases preventable by vaccination.

Global strategies: EPI and GAVI

The Expanded Programme on Immunization (EPI) is the global programme started by WHO and UNICEF that implemented and organised worldwide immunisation against several vaccine preventable diseases.

The spotlight has now shifted to the Global Alliance for Vaccines and Immunization (GAVI), a partnership between various bodies, including UN agencies, donors, the pharmaceutical industry and NGOs, which is driving forwards universal immunisation. It aims to improve access, expand the use of vaccines, accelerate research and support national programmes.

Each year more than 130 million children are born, each of which needs to be immunised. Making sure we sustain immunisation programmes needs huge effort both globally but also for us in our own programme area.

Six diseases were originally included in the EPI: diphtheria, pertussis, tetanus (DPT vaccine), measles, polio (OPV) and tuberculosis (BCG vaccine). Hepatitis B (HBV) has recently been added, with the goal that all countries should introduce this by 2007. Yellow fever is being added by some countries in Africa.

Tetanus immunisation, as well as being included in the formulation DPT, is given alone or in combination with adult diphtheria (Td) to pregnant women, women of childbearing age and adolescent girls. This is to prevent neonatal tetanus. (See page 248).

Table 10.1   Details of commonly used immunisations*

Type of vaccine	Who should have it?	How is it given?	How many are needed?	Side effects	Contraindications	Storage	Comments
1. DPT (Triple) against: Diphtheria Pertussis Tetanus	Children from 6 weeks to 5 years	0.5 ml intramuscular into upper outer thigh	3 doses at intervals of 4 weeks or more	Pain, swelling and redness at site of injection. Fever for 24 hours Very occasionally fits	Any child with high fever, seriously ill or who has had severe reaction to previous DPT, especially a fit	Between 2–8°C It is destroyed by freezing	To check if spoiled: shake bottle. If uniformly cloudy, use – if white flecks, discard.
2. OPV** (oral polio vaccine)	Children from birth to 5 years	2 drops by mouth	1 dose at birth, 3 more from 6 weeks at intervals of 4 weeks	Usually none	None	Under 8°C Unharmed by freezing	Continue to use polio vaccine in all countries unless EPI discontinues
3. Measles	Children from 9 months to 5 years or more*	Add diluent to powder and shake. 0.5 ml subcutaneously into left upper arm (or thigh)	1 at 9 months and 2nd at 15 months or more	Fever and sometimes mild rash at 7–10 days	Any child with high fever or seriously ill	Under 8°C. Unharmed by freezing. Any unused reconstituted vaccine should be discarded	2 doses needed for full eradication. Follow national guidelines
4. BCG against Tuberculosis (see also Chapter 14)	Children from birth upwards Upper age limit varies: follow national guidelines	Add diluent to dried vaccine. Give intra-dermally, usually into left upper arm (or forearm, Africa) Below 1 year 0.05 ml Over 1 year 0.1 ml using BCG syringe	One only unless no reaction	0–2 weeks: red, tender nodule 2–4 weeks: small ulcer 4–6 weeks: scar appears and persists	Any child known to have active TB or AIDS, or seriously ill with high fever	Under 8°C. Unharmed by freezing. Any unused, reconstituted vaccine should be discarded. Harmed by light	If no nodule, ulcer or scar develops **repeat**. If nodule appears at once, ulcer is 2 cm or more or glands develop in axilla, report to health centre

Table 10.1   Details of commonly used immunisations* (continued)

Type of vaccine	Who should have it?	How is it given?	How many are needed?	Side effects	Contraindications	Storage	Comments
5. Hepatitis B (HBV)	Children from birth, but linked in with other vaccinations	By intramuscular injection in upper outer thigh	3 doses at interval of 4 weeks or more	Minor pain and swelling, occasionally fever	Any child with high fever or seriously ill	Between 2–8°C. Destroyed by freezing	Follow national guidelines. Countries are increasingly using HBV, often at the same time as DPT
6. Haemophilus influenzae B (Hib)	Children in Africa, some in Asia and elsewhere	By intramuscular injection in upper outer thigh	3 doses at one month intervals, e.g. 6, 10 and 14 weeks	Minor local reaction	Any child with high fever or seriously ill	As instructed by manufacturer	Follow national guidelines, often given at same time as DPT

* Manufacturer's instructions and local EPI guidelines should be followed. There is increasing diversity in the vaccines used.
** Inactivated polio vaccine (IPV) given by injection is increasingly used.

Measles can also be given as MMR (combined mumps, measles, rubella vaccination).

Through GAVI other diseases are being targeted for mass immunisation in areas where they are common. Vaccines already developed or near to use include: meningitis A and C or ACWY, Hib (disease caused by Haemophilus influenzae type B), pneumococcal disease (caused by Streptococcus pneumoniae), an improved cholera and TB vaccine, and immunisation against rotavirus diarrhoea. Japanese encephalitis vaccine is widely used in China, Korea, Thailand and Japan under separate national programmes. Much work is being done to develop effective malaria vaccines.

Immunisation schedules

Although EPI recommends certain schedules for worldwide use there is considerable variation from country to country. There are more than 50 different schedules currently being followed worldwide! Recommendations also change frequently.

> In order to avoid confusion we should generally follow the schedule laid down by the National Ministry of Health or our District Medical Officer. Having decided on one schedule, we should be slow to change to another.

From the practical view it is helpful to consider commonly used schedules and special campaigns.

Commonly used schedules

Our aim should be to immunise all children born into our target population, at the ages recommended by our national or district immunisation plan.

Here is a commonly used schedule, appropriate for most developing countries as recommended by the EPI:

Notes

1. The time interval between successive doses of DPT/OPV is not important, providing it is a minimum of four weeks.
2. Where yellow fever is used, this can be given at nine months, along with measles. Where yellow fever is a high risk, catch-up programmes can be arranged to vaccinate those aged nine months or more.
3. Hib vaccine is being widely used in Africa but less widely in Asia because of varying disease patterns.
4. Some programmes in highly malarious areas give iron supplements and antimalarials between two and nine months of age at EPI visits.
5. Vaccines that combine DPT with either hepatitis B or Haemophilus influenzae B (Hib) are likely to become more widely available.

Special campaigns

Sometimes normal immunisation programmes need extra campaigns to make them fully effective.

Here are some important examples:

- **Polio**
  At the time of writing this is still found in South Asia and Africa. To speed up eradication two strategies are useful. National or Subnational (i.e. involving part of a country) Immunisation Days. Where NIDs or SNIDs are held we can help to make these known and encourage families to attend. Where pockets of polio remain we can help take part in 'mopping up campaigns'. Visits are made to homes where children are known not to have completed immunisations. In CBHC we are very well placed to know which these families are and to visit them ourselves. Polio immunisation must

Table 10.2   Commonly used schedule for immunisations

First visit	Birth (or as soon after birth as possible)	BCG OPV1 (HBV1)
Second visit	6 weeks	DPT1 OPV 2 (Hib 1) (HBV 2)
Third visit	10 weeks	DPT 2 OPV 3 (Hib 2) (HBV 3)
Fourth visit	14 weeks	DPT 3 OPV 4 (Hib 3)
Fifth visit	9–12 months	Measles Vitamin A (200 000 IU)

be continued worldwide until such time as WHO confirms the disease is fully eradicated.

- **Measles**

  Measles cannot be fully eradicated until 98 per cent of children are immunised, otherwise outbreaks can still occur. Reaching this target level is extremely difficult, but building a two-dose schedule into a national programme is a useful strategy. Instead, or in addition, mass campaigns such as NIDs or SNIDs can be arranged to revaccinate all children between 1 and 19 years regardless of when and whether they were immunised before. Similar to NIDs and SNIDs are supplementary immunisation activities (SIAs) held every three or four years where every child from 9 months to 14 years of age is immunised over a one- to two-week period.

  An alternative to setting aside particular days is to target high-risk areas for special approaches such as poor urban communities, or any district where measles immunisation rates are below 80 per cent.

  In CBHC we should know both the immunisation coverage of our target area and the number of cases of measles occurring. We can use this information to discuss plans with the DMO and work alongside district and national programmes.

- **Hepatitis B**

  Most cases in Asia are transmitted at the time of birth. In Africa the majority during the second or third year of life. However, the first dose is ideally given within 24 hours of birth, meaning that a midwife or other health care worker should usually be responsible for giving this or making sure it is given. If this is not possible, it can be given at 6 weeks.

It is estimated that official immunisation rates are often over-recorded by us much as 20 per cent. If we keep our programme figures, e.g. from household surveys, these are likely to be more accurate than official figures

Equipment needed

In considering the equipment needed we must remember our two main priorities: to maximise coverage and to promote safety.

Our success will depend mainly on good organisation and especially in having the right equipment, vaccines and supplies at the right place, e.g. base, clinic or field, at the right time.

We will need the following:

1. **Needles and syringes**

   How we choose these has become a very important question. Because so many needles and syringes are reused without proper sterilising, it is estimated that one third of all injections (the majority not immunisations) are unsafe: one third of hepatitis B cases in developing countries is caused by unsafe injections, as are 42 per cent of hepatitis C infections, and 2 per cent of new HIV infections. This totals over 20 million cases of these three diseases. Many health workers also develop hepatitis B and occasionally HIV through needlestick injuries.

   For example: one recent study estimated that each year unsafe injections (from all causes) lead to an estimated 1.3 million early deaths.

   There are three types of syringe we can use:

   a) Autodestruct syringes, with needles (e.g. Auto-disable (AD) devices).

      These are used once only, after which the plunger jams. They must be burnt after use. They are the best type to use, but are currently more expensive than alternatives in most countries.

   b) Disposable plastic syringes and stainless steel needles.

      These are designed to be used once only, but are frequently and incorrectly reused. They have to be burnt at high temperature to be destroyed, so in practice are often dumped and then picked up and used by others. There is a high risk of needlestick injuries.

   c) Sterilisable (reusable) glass or plastic syringes with stainless steel needles. They can be reused many times but have to be taken apart, cleaned and steam-sterilised for 20 minutes at 121–126 °C, i.e. in an autoclave or pressure cooker. They are cheap but sterilisation is often done inadequately (or not at all). If this system is used, temperature spot indicators must be attached to the items being sterilised or

Best infection control practices for injections

These best practices are based on evidence and the advice of experts.

1. Use sterile injection equipment

- Use a sterile syringe and needle for each injection and to reconstitute each unit of vaccine.[a]
- Ideally, use a new, single-use syringe and needle. Discard a needle or syringe if the package has been punctured, torn, or damaged.[b]
- If single-use syringes and needles are not available, use equipment designed for steam sterilization. Sterilize equipment according to WHO recommendations and document the quality of the sterilization process using time, steam, temperature (TST) spot indicators.[b]

2. Prevent contamination of injection equipment and medication

- Prepare each injection in a clean designated area, where contamination from blood or body-fluid is unlikely.
- Use single-dose vials rather than multi-dose vials.[c] If multi-dose vials must be used, always pierce the septum with a sterile needle.[a] Avoid leaving a needle in place in the stopper of the vial.[c]
- Select pop-open ampoules rather than ampoules that need to be opened by using a metal file. If an ampoule that requires a metal file is used, protect fingers with a clean barrier (e.g. small gauze pad) when opening the ampoule.[c]
- Inspect for and discard medications with visible contamination or cracks, leaks.[b] Follow product specific recommendations for use, storage and handling.[b] Discard a needle that has touched any non-sterile surface.[b]

3. Prevent needle-stick injuries to the provider

- Anticipate and take measures to prevent sudden movement of patient during and after injection.[c]
- Avoid recapping of needles and other hand manipulations of needles. If recapping is necessary, use a single-handed scoop technique.[a]

- Collect used syringes and needles at the point of use in an enclosed sharps container that is puncture-proof and leak-proof and that is sealed before it is completely full.[c]

4. Prevent access to used needles

- Seal sharps containers for transport to a secure area in preparation for disposal. After closing and sealing sharps containers, do not open, empty, reuse, or sell them.[c]
- Manage sharps waste in an efficient, safe and environment-friendly way to protect people from exposure to used injection equipment.[c]

5. All devices

- Whenever possible, use devices that have been designed to prevent needle-stick injury that have been shown to be effective for patients and providers. Auto-disable (AD) syringes are increasingly available.
- Hand hygiene and skin integrity of provider. Perform hand hygiene (i.e. wash or disinfect hands, e.g. with alcohol) before preparing injection material and giving injections. The need for hand hygiene between each injection will vary depending on the setting and whether there was contact with soil, blood or body fluids.
- Gloves. Gloves are not needed for injections. Single-use gloves may be indicated if excessive bleeding is anticipated.
- Swabbing vial tops or ampoules. Swabbing of clean vials tops or ampoules with an antiseptic or disinfectant is unnecessary.
- Skin preparation of patient before injection. Wash skin that is visibly soiled or dirty. Swabbing of the clean skin before giving an injection is unnecessary. If swabbing with an antiseptic is selected for use, use a clean, single-use swab. Do not use cotton balls stored wet in a multi-use container.

a Category I: Strongly recommended and strongly supported by well-designed experimental or epidemiological studies.
b Category III: recommended on the basis of expert consensus and theoretical rationale.
c Category II: recommended on the basis of theoretical rationale and suggestive, descriptive evidence.

Adapted from WHO Bulletin, 2003, 81, p. 492

Figure 10.1   Best infection control practices for injections.

their covers, to ensure sterilisation has been adequate.

There is also a high risk of needlestick injuries when reusable needles and syringes are being used.

In deciding which type of syringe to use we will be partly guided by what is available and partly by the costs of each. Where possible we should use AD devices.

If we don't use AD devices we should select the following sizes of needles and syringes:

needles:

• 10 mm, 26 gauge for intradermal (used for BCG, usually with a one-dose BCG syringe)
• 30 mm, 22 gauge for intramuscular and sub-cutaneous injections (used for all other EPI immunisations)
• 18 gauge for mixing or reconstituting.

syringes:

• 0.05 or 0.1 ml for BCG
• 0.5, 1 ml or 2 ml for other injections
• 5 or 10 ml for adding diluent.

Auto-disables are manufactured in appropriate sizes and combinations.

2. **Vials**

These come either as multidose vials usually containing 20, 10, 6 or 2 doses, but commonly 10. These can be used for both liquid vaccine and those that need to be reconstituted, such as BCG and measles.

Single dose vials can be standard design or prefilled auto-disable devices, suitable for hepatitis B, DPT, and TT.

Advantages of multidose: usually cheaper, take less space in fridges and in cold chain containers, and provide a smaller volume of medical waste. Often used when larger numbers are being immunised.

Advantage of single dose vials: can be used when only a few children are likely to need immunisation, leading to less vaccine wastage. They are also safer and the prefilled auto-disable makes it safer to dispose of as it can't be reused or cause injury. GAVI is promoting and financing AD devices.

3. **Safety boxes (also called safety or sharps containers)**

These should be used for all autodestruct or disposable needles and syringes. They need to be made of tough material and not cardboard as otherwise disposable needles can pierce through them. Place supplies in them immediately after giving the injection without recapping, in order to avoid needlestick injuries. After the immunisation session this box should be destroyed by burning. Special incinerator boxes that self-ignite after a simple manoeuvre are becoming available in some areas. Alternatively, special incinerators can be built (see Further reading and resources).

WHO/UNICEF has recently introduced the idea of 'bundling'. A 'bundle' comprises good quality vaccines, AD syringes and safety boxes. Ideally these three components should always be considered together.

4. **Other field supplies needed:**
   • A tray for placing syringes ready for use.
   • Forceps for fixing needles on to syringes, if using reusable needles.
   • Spirit for cleaning.
   • File for opening ampoules.
   • Cold box (or cup with ice) in which to place vaccines currently being used.
   • Bowl and disinfectant if reusable syringes and needles used, otherwise a safety box.
   • Rubbish bag or bin.
   • Equipment for washing hands: alcohol gel or wipes for more frequent cleaning of hands.
   • Supply of clean water.
   • Adrenalin (Epinephrine) and an antihista-mine for emergency use.
5. **A vaccine carrier** with ice packs.
6. **A kit bag** in which to pack all supplies.
7. **Records and registers.**
8. **A supply of vaccines.**
9. **Paracetamol** and other simple medicines.
10. **A transportable table.**

How to maintain the cold chain

The cold chain refers to the set of cold containers in which vaccines are stored and transported, from the moment of manufacture to the time of injection. If the cold chain is broken, a vaccine may become useless. However, some vaccines are more sensiive to heat than others.

> Unless vaccines are kept at the right temperature, they lose their effectiveness. **Millions of doses are spoilt and lives lost because vaccines have been allowed to warm up, or (with some vaccines) to freeze.**

We can help to maintain the cold chain by taking careful precautions at each link:

1. **The source**
   Identify a reliable source as near as possible to the point of manufacture or import. Only use sources known to be kept cold. If supplies are obtained from the District Medical Officer, from a government hospital or private pharmacy, we should ensure that the fridge is working when we collect supplies.
   Where possible use EPI/GAVI approved sources.

2. **Source to base**
   On collection, we should place supplies immediately in a vaccine carrier, usually with ice packs, but freezing the vaccine must be avoided.

On returning to base, we place them immediately in the refrigerator. If the vehicle breaks down, the vaccine carrier is placed in the shade, outside the jeep, while repairs are being made.

3. **Base**
   Supplies should be kept in a refrigerator.

   - Place supplies in the back of the main part of the fridge. The door compartment gets too warm, and the cold box gets too cold, especially for DPT and tetanus.
   - Do not put food or drink in the fridge.
   - Place any vaccine brought back from the field in a separate section, or in front of other supplies, where it can be used first.
   - Vaccines that are expired should be thrown away as should those that have warmed up.
   - Keep a thermometer with the vaccines so that the temperature can be readily checked. Keep a twice-daily chart. It is good practice to use vaccine vial monitors (VVMs) on all vaccine supplies (see page 200).
   - Maintain the fridge in good working order.
   - If the fridge works on electricity, set up an alternative store in case of power cuts, keeping a good supply of ice in the fridge in case this happens.

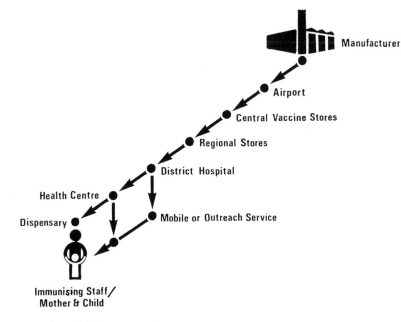

Figure 10.2   Maintaining the cold chain is vital.

- Defrost the fridge regularly and while doing so place the vaccines with ice in the vaccine carrier, or in a second fridge.
- Do not open the fridge unnecessarily; check the rubber door seal regularly; seal the electric plug into the socket with tape to avoid accidental disconnection.
- Ensure the vaccines do not freeze.

Heat stability of vaccines

1. **The most heat stable**
   Usually stable for up to 30 days at or below 37 degrees C
   Hepatitis B, tetanus toxoid, diphtheria/tetanus
   Use vaccine vial monitor (VVM) 30
2. **Moderately stable**
   Usually up to 14 days at or below 37 degrees C
   DPT vaccines
   Use VMM 14
3. **Unstable**
   Keep below 8 degrees C but can be frozen
   Oral polio, unreconstituted measles and BCG
   (Adapted from *Bulletin* of WHO, February 2004, page 103, Box 1)

---

4. **Base to field**
   Place vaccines within a box in the vaccine carrier, usually with an ice pack.
5. **Field**
   Keep the vaccine carrier in the shade with the lid tightly closed. Take out supplies as they are needed, keeping the multidose vial or supply of single dose vials or AD devices currently being used in a table cold box or bowl filled with ice. Discard any unused, reconstituted vaccine at the end of the session.

Vaccine Vial Monitors (VVMs) are increasingly being used. These are markers made of heat-sensitive material placed on the outside of vaccine vials. They respond to heat over a period of time and change colour when a vaccine is no longer safe to use because of warming. VVMs therefore tell us if the cold chain has been broken at any stage.

VVMs usually consist of a square within a circle. Providing the square is lighter than the circle, the vaccine is safe to use. If it matches the circle or becomes darker we should throw the vaccine away. Read instructions carefully.

We should also dispose of any vaccine if it has passed its expiry date, regardless of what the VVM shows.

What we need to do

Assess needs for immunisation in the programme area

Before starting a programme we will need to discover:

1. Past immunisation coverage in the area we are covering. We can find this out from the community survey; if we are using a family folder, the immunisation status of each child is recorded on the front of the folder.
2. Programmes currently being carried out by other organisations, both government and voluntary. Some areas will already have effective programmes. In others there may be good plans on paper but little being done in practice. Sometimes there is a difference between the coverage claimed by the government and the immunisations that have actually been given. In many areas, effective programmes have been set up in the past, but have been allowed to lapse since.

Discuss plans with the government

We should make contact with the District Medical Officer or person responsible for implementing the EPI in our project area. As well as building trust and friendship, we will need to find out:

- Schedules being used nationally or locally.
- Any immunisations, including hepatitis B and Hib, used in addition to the EPI's original six target vaccines.
- Where to obtain vaccines and details of the cold chain.
- Records needed by the government and how our own records can be used with minimum change and duplication.

- Ways of working together so we can reach the community most effectively.
- Details of any National Immunisation Days (NIDs, or SNIDs) that we can make known and provide services for, and in the case of measles, supplementary immunisation activities (SIAs), (see pages 195–6).

Set targets

An example might be to aim for 90 per cent of all children under five in our project area to be fully immunised within three to five years, or we may aim to increase uptake of measles immunisation from say 50 per cent to 80 per cent within three years. To accomplish this we will need to set yearly targets, appropriate for the area, and enter these in our logframe (see page 106).

At this stage we can also work out the total number of children needing immunisations and hence the number of injections we will need to give each year. These figures can be obtained from the family folder or other records. In most developing countries the number of children needing to start immunisations each year will be approximately 3 per cent of the total population.

Reaching targets may not be difficult where people are educated or where parents have been made aware through radio and television. In poor, backward areas or scattered communities it may be a major challenge.

> Often those who need vaccines the most want them the least. We will need to target extra time and energy to these individuals and communities.

Train the team

1. **The team will need to be motivated.**
   Encourage all those involved in the programme to help set targets and contribute to planning. Let them enjoy the results of successful programmes and make suggestions to help improve coverage. The more team and community members feel this is their programme, the stronger will be their motivation. Any supervisor appointed must be fully involved in the giving of immunisations.

2. **The team will need to be informed.**
   All team members will need to know:
   - why each immunisation is needed.
   - how each immunisation is given.
   - how a clinic station and how an outreach session are organised. This will include knowing how to:
     - prepare all the equipment, in plenty of time and using a checklist;
     - maintain the cold chain; use cold boxes and refrigerators correctly;
     - give injections safely and effectively especially if using informally trained staff;
     - dispose of needles and syringes using any safety box;
     - avoid needlestick injuries;
     - clean and sterilise supplies unless using disposable syringes or AD devices
     - incinerate used supplies safely and thoroughly.
   - which children should not be given immunisaitons:
     - any child who is seriously ill or with a high fever;

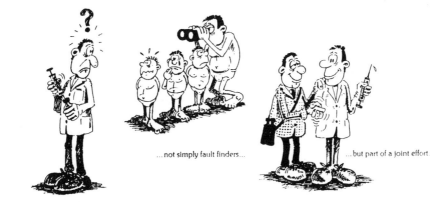

...not simply fault finders...   ...but part of a joint effort.

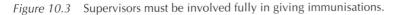

Figure 10.3   Supervisors must be involved fully in giving immunisations.

- any child who has previously had a serious reaction to a vaccine or is known to be allergic to the vaccine;
- any child whose family refuses permission after careful explanation;
- children with symptomatic HIV infection should not be given BCG or yellow fever. Otherwise HIV positive children can be given all immunisations;
- children with active TB should not be given BCG.

Prepare the community

Although most communities are now familiar with immunisation programmes and willingly join in, there are still many remote areas or family groups who are resistant and suspicious. It is also easy for a programme to become unpopular or for a wrong idea to take hold. To increase immunisation coverage we often have to work hard to gain, or regain, the community's cooperation. The immunisation should be carried out in full partnership with the community.

Health committee members or CHWs can help to plan and organise any field vaccination session. They can help to raise awareness amongst parents – and amongst older family members who may oppose the programme.

It is common to see eager health workers forcing immunisations on unwilling people. Health workers will first need to spend time and patience in raising community awareness. Only when parents are ready should the programme be started.

No family should be forced to have immunisations against their will but we should try hard to encourage their cooperation.

> Perhaps the most important, and most difficult, part of any programme is creating awareness. Parents, especially in remote communities, may find it strange that we refuse to give penicillin injections when their children have colds, but that we plan to give a whole series of injections when their children seem completely healthy.

In raising awareness for any CBHC activity there are two distinct stages:

1. **Answering fears and objections.**
   Each individual and each community will have its own beliefs, and suspicions, about immunisation. Here are some common examples of what people may be thinking:

> - We don't understand why our children need these injections.
> - The diseases you talk about don't occur in our area.
> - Your centre is too far away for us to reach.
> - A child in our village died shortly after an injection and we don't want you to come back.
> - I've heard that these injections are a secret form of family planning.
> - We can't afford to lose half a day's wages each time we have to bring our children.
> - We always have to wait such a long time at the clinic and there's not enough shade to sit in.
> - The nurse shouted at us last time we came.
> - We are afraid of making the spirits angry.
> - We have heard that needles spread AIDS.

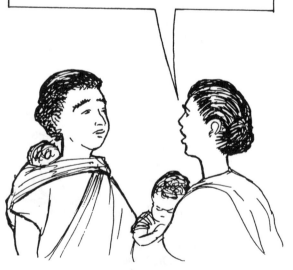

Figure 10.4   Motivation is the key to high immunisation coverage.

2. **Giving appropriate teaching.**
   After discovering common objections, we can now give appropriate teaching. In doing this we will use a variety of methods, places and people.
   Useful methods include: drama, puppetry, question and answer, flash cards, billboards, radio. *Suitable places include*: individual homes, the clinic, a convenient meeting place in the community, the CHW's home or verandah, a temple, church, mosque or school.
   Appropriate people to give teaching are: CHWs, health committee members, mothers who have completed immunisations, members of women's groups, youth and adolescent groups, young farmers' clubs, priests, teachers and older children.

> Community members themselves are often more effective than health workers in motivating parents for immunisation.

Here are examples of methods that have proved successful:

1. **Special immunisation days**
   NIDs, SNIDs and SIAs are described above on page 195 and we should promote these and join in with them where possible.
   We can also arrange an annual 'Pulse Strategy'. Each year at a convenient time the health team working with community leaders arranges, well in advance and with careful publicity, three successive immunisation days at monthly intervals. Some programmes that have had poor results with weekly or monthly visits have found this very successful, achieving almost 100 per cent coverage.
2. **'High-uptake' families get special recognition**
   Some programmes give special status to mothers whose children have completed their immunisations. They may be given a flag to fly from their home, a badge to wear on their clothes, a reduction in fees at the clinic or hospital, or bonus points in the next baby competition.
3. **House-to-house preparation**
   For example: One successful programme taught each household about immunisations at the time of the first community survey, giving

a time and place the following week where immunisations could be obtained. Many villages in that project reported 80 per cent of their under-fives completing immunisations within one year of the project starting.
4. **Using religious leaders to promote immunisation**
   For example: UNICEF reminds us there is hardly any community without a place of worship, even though many have no school or health facility. A two-year collaboration between UNICEF and Christian and Muslim leaders in Sierra Leone increased coverage of children under one year of age from 6 per cent to 75 per cent.

Carry out immunisation in the field

Where should this be done?

> Any community programme must be at a place that is convenient for the mother and the child. The best site is within the community itself.

When should this be carried out?

At a time of day that is easy for the family. Depending on the community, this may be an evening, a midday break from the fields, or a full day planned well ahead.

At a time of year convenient for the community. In rural communities it should not be during harvest, sowing or other busy times in the fields. It should not be just before major festivals when mothers are busy, or just after them when the community is recovering.

Who should carry this out?

A team of three is ideal for most immunisation sessions: two can manage small groups, four or five may be needed for larger ones.

The ideal team leader is a nurse, medical assistant or experienced health worker. The leader or another qualified person can give the injections and deal with other problems or illnesses that may need attention.

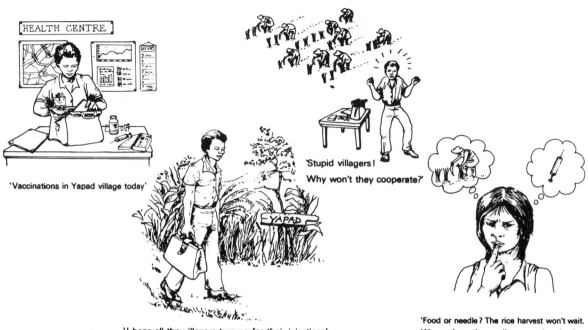

'Vaccinations in Yapad village today'

'I hope all the villagers turn up for their injections'

'Stupid villagers! Why won't they cooperate?'

'Food or needle? The rice harvest won't wait. We can have the needle some other time'

Figure 10.5   Immunisation sessions should be convenient for the community.

Other team members can be multipurpose health workers, trainees and students, community health workers and members of a village health committee.

Motivated community members can make the best workers of all. They can organise the mothers and children, keep records, and give polio drops.

Generally, immunisations should be given only by trained and accredited health workers, otherwise in case of accidents or side effects there may be legal problems especially if community members become angry or suspicious.

How should this be carried out?

This will be a joint venture with the community, who each year should take increasing responsibility for setting up the programme.

Before the programme:

1. The community must know in plenty of time:
   • when and where the session will be held.
   • what equipment it should provide (tables, chairs, a room, etc.)
   • what helpers will be needed.
   • its responsibility in telling and gathering the children and informing parents.
2. The team must have prepared its supplies (see pages 196–8).

At the time of the programme:
1. The team should set up its equipment before parents arrive (see Figure 10.6).
2. All team members should know their exact function.
3. Parents and children should wait in an orderly way out of the sun and rain, coming forwards one at a time.
4. Health teaching should be given to waiting mothers and other family members. This is also a good chance for weighing children – 'Weights can be done during waits'.

After the programme:
1. Supplies are carefully gathered up, including all syringes and needles.
2. The time and place of the next immunisation session is fixed. Community members are encouraged to make this known.

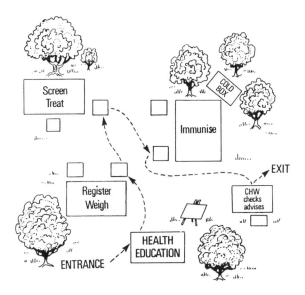

Figure 10.6   Plan for an outside immunisation session, making good use of available shade.

3. CHWs have supplies of paracetamol and are ready to visit and advise any parent worried about side effects.

Carry out immunisation in the clinic

Most of the details just described also apply to clinic sessions.

Many parents are unwilling to come for immunisations alone, but may be willing if a visit to the clinic is needed for other reasons.

> All clinics should have all immunisations available on all occasions and offer them to all children who are eligible.

Many health centres will also arrange weekly or monthly immunisation days or have regular mother and child health clinics where immunisations are given.

Here are some ways of increasing clinic immunisation uptake:

1. Waiting times are kept as short as possible. Children who only require immunisations go direct to the nurse, bypassing the doctor or other health worker seeing patients (see page 147). A separate immunisation room or corner can be set up.
2. Immunisations are given free.
3. Health workers immunise all children who come to the clinic, unless there is a strong reason against doing it.
4. Health workers send for unimmunised family members. The health worker can check the record cards of other children in the family (*for example*: through the family folder system or their diary) and ask the parent to bring any child still eligible. Today if convenient, next time if not.
5. Teaching is given on immunisations. This can be given both to waiting groups of parents and children, and to each individual parent when seen by the health worker.
6. No eligible child leaves hospital or clinic without being offered immunisation.
7. The CHW or TBA gives first OPV (see page 195).
8. No mother is scolded or made to look foolish.

> Treating mothers with dignity and respect improves immunisation coverage.

Remember: the better our injection technique, the more efficiently we immunise and the more friendly our attitude, the more likely it is that parents will bring their children for further immunisations.

Keep records

The following records can be kept:
1. The child's own self-retained health card (Growth Chart). Immunisations are recorded as they are given.
2. The immunisation register.
   Here all children under five are recorded family by family. All eligible children are written beforehand in the register, space being left under each family for new members to be added as they are born.
   The register is filled at the time of immunisation, the correct entry quickly being found if each child has his code number written on his self-retained card.

Twelve suggestions for giving immunisations to children

1. Where possible, children awaiting immunisations do not watch other children being injected.

2. Where possible, the injection is prepared without the child seeing it.

3. The smallest needle possible is used: 26 gauge for intradermal, 22 for IM or SC. It is neither blunt nor barbed.

4. The parent is asked about serious reactions. If the child has ever collapsed or been severely ill after a previous injection the doctor is consulted.

5. The skin is cleaned with soap and water if visibly dirty. Otherwise, cleaning, e.g. with spirit, is not necessary.

6. Explanations are given to the mother. Before her child is injected, she is told what the immunisation is for, what side effects she might expect and when to bring the child back. She is given two or three paracetamol tablets in case of fever or pain and told the correct dose to give.

7. The mother is shown how to hold her child in a comfortable position.

8. Injections are given in the correct part of the body. This should be in the upper outer thigh, but not the bottom, for intramuscular injections, or the upper outer arm for subcutaneous and intradermal injections. The reason (reducing the risk of nerve damage) may need to be explained.

9. In the case of reusable syringes, the needle and syringe are placed immediately into a bowl with chlorine solution with no recapping.

10. In the case of autodestruct and disposables, needle and syringe are placed directly into the safety or sharps container, with no recapping.

11. Procedures to be followed in case of severe reactions are known by all.
Adrenalin is ready and all team members know how to use it.

12. Parent and child wait for 15 minutes after the immunisation.

Treating mothers with dignity and respect improves immunisation coverage.

Figure 10.7   Twelve suggestions for giving immunisations to children.

When this system is used, the exact immunisation status of any child can be seen at a glance. Every six or twelve months the immunisation statistics can be copied into the Master Register. Some projects may prefer to use a tally sheet at the time the immunisations are given, or record a simple list of names to be added to the register later. Where family folder inserts cards are used, immunisation status can be regularly updated for each child directly from the register.

If the project is computerised, we can complete any Due List or computer-generated form and return this to base for data entry the same evening or the following day.

3. A proforma for the District Medical Officer. Immunisation details should be sent on time and recorded according to the DMO's design. These details can be copied down from the register or tally sheet.

Alternatively, and to save time, standard national forms used for recording immunisations are used alone, sent to the DMO or immunisation officer, with copies being kept by the project. GAVI has recommended reporting systems.

Evaluate the programme

This is done with the community, and results are explained to all community members.

1. **Make yearly totals.**
Each year we can calculate the total numbers of each injection given, first, second, third, fourth, etc. for each community.
From this we can calculate the percentage of children under five who have completed each immunisation, the percentage who have partially completed and the percentage of children who remain unimmunised.

2. **By occasional questionnaires.**
If coverage is poor we can design a questionnaire to find out why parents are not bringing their children.

3. **By regular assessment of target disease incidence.**
Every two or three years we can work out whether the target diseases are becoming less common (see page 342).

Summary

The lives of millions more children could be saved each year if immunisation against preventable diseases was universally carried out. With effective community partnership and good planning this is within reach of all health programmes.

Equipment needs to be prepared, vaccines obtained and a cold chain maintained. The project needs to decide whether to use autodestruct, disposable or non-disposable syringes and needles, along with a policy on how to destroy any non reusable items. Where available and affordable, single prefilled auto-disable devices should be used. Care needs to be taken to avoid neeedlestick injuries and to ensure that any reusable needles and syringes are adequately sterilised. Schedules need to be calculated according to local and national guidelines. Immunisations should be given by teams of health workers who have been carefully trained, to communities whose awareness has been raised.

Immunisations should be offered at places and at times that are convenient to parents and children. Such sessions are best carried out in the community itself and in the neighbouring clinic. Waiting times must be kept to the minimum and any child attending the clinic should be offered immunisation, unless seriously ill. The project should cooperate with and promote any national immunisation day

Accurate records should be kept and regular returns sent in to the District Medical Officer. Yearly evaluations of coverage should be made.

Further reading and resources

1. *Immunization in Practice: a practical guide for health staff*, WHO, 2004.
   This is an excellent manual for health workers, giving detailed and practical advice. Also available as a CD ROM.
   Available from: WHO. See Appendix E.

2. Expanded Programme on Immunisation (EPI) publishes *EPI Update*, and WHO's Global Programme for Vaccines and Immunizations publishes *Vaccine and Immunization News*.
   Both are extremely useful and obtainable from WHO, see Appendix E. This office will also provide information about autodestruct syringes, safety boxes, incinerators and VMMs. See also www.vaccinealliance.org.

3. *How to Look After a Refrigerator*, AHRTAG, 1992.
   Available from: Healthlink. See Appendix A.

4. *State of the World's Children*, UNICEF, Oxford University Press, 2006.
   A new edition of this is published each year.
   Available from TALC. See Appendix E.

5. *V and B Catalogue*, Department of Vaccines and other Biologicals, WHO, 2003, with regular planned updates.
   This contains a very wide range of resources and is worth ordering.
   Available from: WHO. See Appendix E.

6. *Management of wastes from immunization campaign activities: practical guidelines*, WHO, 2004.
   A complete guide on this important topic.
   Available from: WHO. See Appendix E.

7. Applied Sustainable Technologies Group.
   For information on incinerators and other useful technologies, contact ASTG, De Montfort University, Gateway, Leicester LE1 9BH, UK.

8. Useful information on vaccines is available from www.vaccines.org.

9. Websites on vaccination safety.
   There are a number of these in different languages. Accredited sites can be seen at www.who.int/immunization_safety/safety_quality.

Slides

The following slide sets are obtainable from TALC. See Appendix A.
- Cold Chain – Target Diseases CoTD
- Cold Chain   CoV
A variety of slides is available from the V and B Catalogue from WHO.

Video, CD Roms and Software

A variety is available from the V and B Catalogue.

See Further references and guidelines on page 413.

11

Dealing with Childhood Illnesses: Diarrhoea, Pneumonia and Malaria

Community Based Health Care (CBHC) is ideally suited to prevent and treat most of the illnesses that seriously affect children. Before looking at three of the most important we need to understand the health needs of under-five children and how they are being met.

Diseases that kill children

At the time of writing (2005) about 11 million children die before the age of five years. About six million of these die from infectious diseases that can be prevented and treated: these include two million from diarrhoea, just over two million from pneumonia, one million from malaria and nearly half a million from measles. Malnutrition contributes to many, and poverty underlies all of them.

In Africa, child mortality rates are about 150 deaths per 1000 live births, almost eight times the rates in Europe. In several African countries there has been no improvement over the past 50 years and some countries that started to make gains have fallen back.

The Millennium Development Goals and the rights of the child

It is helpful to look at the health needs of children in the context of the Millennium Development Goals and from a human rights angle.

Millennium Development Goal 4 is to reduce child mortality and Goal 6 is to combat HIV/AIDS, malaria and other diseases (see page 12).

Article 24 of the Convention on the Rights of the Child states that it is a child's right to enjoy the highest attainable standards of health and to have access to health services.

The Integrated Management of Childhood Illness (IMCI)

We need to understand an important worldwide strategy now being carried out in virtually all developing countries. (See page 233, ref. 1.)

This is the Integrated Management of Childhood Illness introduced by WHO in 1998. This programme looks at the commonest causes of death and disability in children, recognises they are often linked, and seeks to prevent and cure these by an integrated or horizontal approach (see pages 3, 4). When well managed, IMCI is proving effective at reducing under-five death rates and improving the health and well-being of children.

IMCI has three related aims. We should understand these and adopt them if our programme is in an area where IMCI is operating. These are:

1. Improving the case management skills of health workers through training, using locally adapted guidelines.
2. Improving the health systems we set up or are involved with, including making sure that essential drugs are always available.
3. Training families and communities to prevent illness where possible and to know how and when to seek medical help.

As IMCI programmes are introduced into each country, pilot projects are set up from which locally adapted guidelines are written. Programmes are then scaled up. The success of IMCI depends to a large extent on how effectively health workers are trained to recognise the signs of serious illnesses, the correct ways of treating them, and when to refer seriously ill children.

Recent evaluations in many countries show that, where IMCI programmes are working well, children become healthier and fewer die. IMCI is becoming one important way of attempting to reach the fourth and sixth Millennium

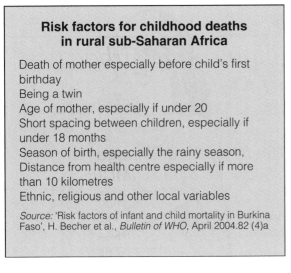

Risk factors for childhood deaths in rural sub-Saharan Africa

Death of mother especially before child's first birthday

Being a twin

Age of mother, especially if under 20

Short spacing between children, especially if under 18 months

Season of birth, especially the rainy season,

Distance from health centre especially if more than 10 kilometres

Ethnic, religious and other local variables

Source: 'Risk factors of infant and child mortality in Burkina Faso', H. Becher et al., *Bulletin of WHO*, April 2004.82 (4)a

Figure 11.1

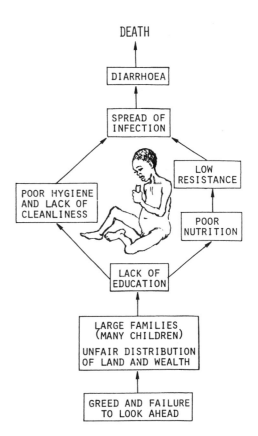

Figure 11.2   The chain of causes leading to death from diarrhoea.

Development Goals. However, in the poorest communities setting up IMCI programmes is difficult. This throws us back to our main responsibility: to help set up the most effective CBHC programmes possible, with a strong emphasis on both the prevention of illness and the empowerment of communities. Figure 11.1 shows some of the risk factors we can help to reduce through a community based approach.

Linked with IMCI are programmes to reduce death rates amongst adolescents – currently about one million per year. We need to be aware of these programmes and where possible to work with any local initiatives that are being set up.

DIARRHOEA AND DEHYDRATION

In this section we shall consider:
1. What we need to know
   - Why treating diarrhoea is important
   - Understand different forms of diarrhoea
   - The meaning of ORS and ORT
   - Understand the dangers of diarrhoea
2. What we need to do
   - Set aims and targets
   - Choose suitable approaches with the community

- Prepare ORS appropriately
- Feed ORS correctly
- Teach the use of ORS to all family members
- Use other ways to treat diarrhoea
- Explain how diarrhoea can be prevented
- Evaluate the programme

What we need to know

Why treating diarrhoea is important

Diarrhoea kills at least two million children per year, making it the commonest cause of death in children under five, after pneumonia. If we set up really effective programmes, nine out of ten of these deaths can be prevented.

Diarrhoea has several serious effects. It weakens children so they become more likely to become seriously ill from other infectious diseases. It causes them to lose weight and undermines their nutrition, especially important if they have HIV/AIDS or TB. It can cause death from dehydration – the main reason children die from diarrhoea.

Understand different forms of diarrhoea

WHO defines diarrhoea as: the passage of loose or watery stools at least three times in a 24-hour period.

Blood in the stool indicates possible dysentery, not always accompanied by diarrhoea as defined above.

There are different types of diarrhoea and WHO's IMCI approach (see page 233, ref. 1) suggests these categories:

* Acute watery diarrhoea – lasting 14 days or less, usually starting suddenly and normally caused by infections.
* Persistent or chronic diarrhoea – lasting more than 14 days and often present because of other factors such as malnutrition or AIDS.
* Dysentery – diarrhoea with blood, with or without fever.

Many different germs cause diarrhoea. In developing countries more than half are caused by rotaviral infections. In practice, all forms of diarrhoea are treated with Oral Rehydration Solution (ORS). In addition, for persistent diarrhoea, we should try to find a cause, e.g. amoeba or *Giardia* and treat this. For dysentery we should usually use antibiotics.

The meaning of ORS and ORT

ORT stands for Oral Rehydration Therapy. This is a treatment for dehydration where Oral Rehydration Salts (ORS) – either packeted or home prepared – are mixed with water and given to those with diarrhoea.

This special solution, which contains added sugar and salt, is life saving. The child needs the fluid and the salt to replace that lost in diarrhoea.

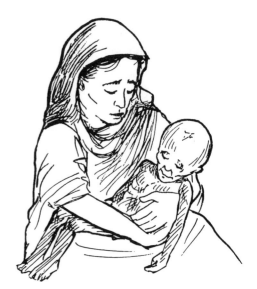

This child is dying from dehydration. The nearest clinic is closed. The mother does not know how to make a rehydration drink.

Figure 11.3

Added sugar helps water and salts to be absorbed from the stomach and also gives energy.

The use of salt-sugar solution in treating diarrhoea has been described as one of the greatest medical discoveries of the twentieth century. Nearly all cases of dehydration could be prevented and nearly two million lives saved per year if parents worldwide knew how to make it and give it. Probably one million lives are already being saved by those who do know.

> It has been calculated that on average it takes a health worker about 30 minutes per community member to teach the effective use of ORS. This may seem a long time, but in terms of saving lives is there any more effective way of spending half an hour?

Understand the dangers of diarrhoea

1. **Diarrhoea itself is dangerous, causing death by dehydration.**
   In addition:
   * It leads to malnutrition if prolonged.

- It is highly infectious, rapidly spreading in communities, especially where there is poverty and overcrowding.

2. **The wrong treatment of diarrhoea can be dangerous.**

   Many doctors and health workers still believe that diarrhoea should be treated by medicines and injections. They may give intravenous glucose when the patient is able to drink by mouth. Some know little about ORS, and many more will not use it because it brings less profit than antibiotics or injections. One reason why medicine continues to be used is because it appears to cure diarrhoea. Usually however diarrhoea is self-limiting and would have stopped anyway.

   Medicines for diarrhoea may be dangerous in themselves, but the greatest danger is through the delay they may cause. Instead of starting home-based ORS at once, parents will delay treatment while they waste valuable hours seeking the wrong remedy from a clinic or pharmacy.

   ---

3. **The incorrect use of ORS may be dangerous.**

   Although ORS potentially saves more lives worldwide than any other treatment, it does have occasional dangers.

   - Too much salt can be given, which occasionally causes convulsions. For this reason ORS needs careful measurement and the solution must always be tasted before it is given.
   - Too little ORS may be given so failing to treat dehydration rapidly enough.
   - It may be fed too fast or impatiently, causing vomiting or refusal in the child.
   - The water used to dissolve the salts may be contaminated with germs. Ideally the water should be boiled and if this is not possible the cleanest possible source must be used.

4. **Serious types of diarrhoea may be present.**

   Dysentery caused by shigella and some other organisms usually needs antibiotics. Diarrhoea may be persistent (lasting more than 14 days) needing diagnosis and further treatment. Serious epidemic forms of diarrhoea may be present, including cholera and typhoid, needing a coordinated community approach.

Regardless of cause, some children may need intravenous treatment and referral to hospital. (But even in hospital feeding ORS by naso-gastric tube is often possible.)

Health workers need to train parents to be alert to danger signs (see Table 11.1, page 214).

What we need to do

Set aims and targets

Our ultimate aims are these:

1. To make sure that every family member in our project area knows how to make and use ORS.
2. To make sure that every child with diarrhoea does actually receive ORS.

In an area where ORS is little used, our targets could be for 50 per cent of parents to understand and use ORS after one year, 90 per cent after two years. In areas where ORS is known about but little used, our target will be to increase the proportion of families who use this at the first sign of diarrhoea.

For example: a recent study of 225 mothers in Garwhal, North India, showed only 18 per cent recognised an ORS packet or knew how to use it, and only 6 per cent knew how to prepare and administer it. After face to face education, 86 per cent knew how to use ORS packets and 80 per cent how to prepare home-made solutions.

However, the real test is whether mothers translate this knowledge into practice and are actually using it six months later. This was not checked.

Also see Logical Framework on pages 103–5.

Choose suitable approaches with the community

There are many different ways of preparing ORS. Before starting a programme we must work out carefully with the community which method is most suitable. We will make our task harder if we start using one method at the beginning, then change to another later.

We can follow these guidelines:

1. **Decide which overall method is most suitable:**
   - Consult with the people
     Discover which containers and measurers are commonly used at home. Find out if ORS packets are available locally. Discover what liquid foods are fed to children. Ask for the community's suggestions.
   - Follow national guidelines
     Many countries now have national programmes. Find out about these and follow them where possible.
     Even if there is no national programme, there may still be a method in use in our district or project area that we can discover by consulting with the DMO and any other programmes working nearby.

2. **Decide whether to use packeted or home-made ORS.**

> Unless packets are cheap, easy to obtain and always available, families should learn how to prepare their own ORS at home. They can still use packets when available, but their children will not die when supplies of the packets run out.

Home-made ORS can either be a salt-sugar solution or traditional liquid food such as rice water, soups, gruels, fruit juices, dilute tea, potato water, carrot juice or coconut milk.

Liquid foods have various advantages: they are easily available, children are familiar with them, they reduce the stool volume if some salt is added, and they provide food as well as fluid.

3. **Decide on containers in which to make up the solution.**
   Containers used should be known by everyone, be available in the homes and be always the same size. They should also be carefully washed out with clean water before use.
   Here are some examples:
   - Beer bottles holding 1 litre or soft drink bottles holding 0.75 litre
   - Medium sized glasses or cups holding 0.25 litre
   - In south Asia a 'Lota' usually holding 0.5 litre.

4. **Decide on measuring devices for the salt-sugar.** Again these must be widely known, easily available and of standard size. In addition, they must be simple to use so that mistakes are not made in the amounts measured out. Here are some examples:
   - A 5 ml teaspoon
   - A human fistful of sugar and a thumb-and-two-fingers pinch of salt. Although less accurate, this remains an important method in poor communities.
   - A TALC or similar measuring device, either bought or home-made.
   - A bottle top.

Prepare ORS appropriately

Having decided what is most appropriate in terms of container, measurers, packets or home-made preparations, we now prepare the solution.

Here are some examples of how ORS can be prepared:

1. **Home-made sugar-salt solution**
   - To make a one litre solution (as currently recommended by WHO):
     Add eight level (5 ml) teaspoons of sugar (previously 6 were recommended and some programmes still use this) plus one level teaspoon of salt to one litre of clean water. Mix carefully and feed.
   - To make a half-litre solution:
     Either halve the above amounts or, if teaspoons are not available, add one fistful (four-finger scoop) of sugar plus one pinch (thumb and two fingers) of salt to half a litre of clean water.
     To each of the above we can squeeze in lime, lemon or orange if available to give taste and provide potassium.

2. **Home prepared liquid foods.** Do not use in children under six months.
   To make one litre of rice water:
   - Grind any sort of ground rice into powder.
   - Take two to three large level tablespoons of the above powder (total 50–80 g) and pour on one litre of water.
   - Add two pinches of salt.
   - Boil and stir for five to seven minutes.
   - Cool and feed.

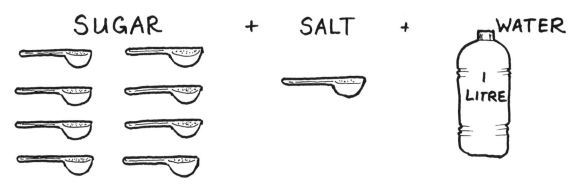

Figure 11.4 Home-prepared ORS kit.

Ground dried wheat, sorghum, millet, maize, or potato can be prepared in similar ways. Coconut juice can be given with two pinches of salt added per litre. Do not add any potassium. Weak tea can be used to which are added salt and sugar in the same amounts as in preparing salt-sugar solution.

3. **Packeted ORS.**
The new standard WHO recommended packet should contain the following measured in mmol/litre: (note change from original ORS packet)
Sodium 75
Chloride 65
Glucose, anhydrous 75
Potassium 20
Citrate 10
Total osmolarity 245
If not available locally, ORS can be ordered from other suppliers (see Appendix A).
We should make sure that any packets used or recommended contain the substances in the correct proportions, are not overpriced, and have instructions in a language that is easily understood by the local people. Those with only written instructions will be unsafe for use by illiterate members of the community. Pictorial instructions are often useful.

Feed ORS correctly

ORS should be given to the child by the mother or other family member. We should first demonstrate this and then make sure the mother does it herself.

How to prepare it

1. Prepare the solution (as described earlier) by mixing and stirring.
2. Taste it.
   It should taste less salty than tears. If it is saltier, it may be harmful to the child.
3. Feed it as detailed in 'How to feed it'.

When to give it

Start giving it at the same time as the diarrhoea starts. Continue giving it until both the diarrhoea stops and a normal amount of urine is being produced.

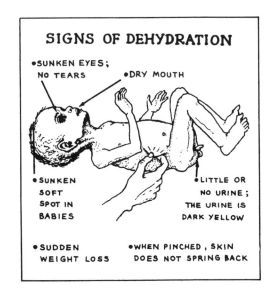

Figure 11.5 Signs of dehydration.

Table 11.1   How to assess dehydration

ACTION		PLAN A	PLAN B	PLAN C
1. LOOK AT:	CONDITION	Well, alert	*Restless, irritable*	*Lethargic or unconscious; floppy*
	EYES	Normal	Sunken	Very sunken and dry
	TEARS	Present	Absent	Absent
	MOUTH and TONGUE	Moist	Dry	Very dry
	THIRST	Drinks normally Not thirsty	*Thirsty, drinks eagerly*	*Drinks poorly or not able to drink*
2. FEEL:	SKIN PINCH	Goes back quickly	*Goes back slowly*	*Goes back very slowly*
3. DECIDE:		Patient has NO SIGNS OF DEHYDRATION	If patient has 2 or more signs, including at least 1 *sign*, there is SOME DEHYDRATION	If patient has 2 or more signs, including at least 1 *sign* there is SEVERE DEHYDRATION

Adapted from Section 3 of *The Management and Prevention of Diarrhoea: practical guidelines*, 3rd Edition. Geneva; WHO, 1993. Now go to Table 11.2.

How to feed it

• Feed young children from a spoon, giving one teaspoon every 1–2 minutes. Give older children frequent sips from a cup.
• If the child vomits, wait 5–10 minutes, then try again more slowly. ORS often helps to reduce the feeling of nausea.
• Breastfed children should continue to be breastfed.
• As soon as possible start giving soft foods that are easy to digest in small amounts, e.g. bananas and cereals. As soon as the child has recovered from diarrhoea, give extra food, with a small amount of added vegetable oil.

How much to feed

1. Assess the level of dehydration according to Table 11.1.
2. Feed the amounts as detailed in Table 11.2.

A simple rule for those not seriously dehydrated is to give children one glass after every stool, adults two glasses.

Teach the use of ORS to all family members

Our aim is for every community member to know about ORS; for the use of ORS to enter the folklore of the community.

We will need to make sure that every member of every family:

• Knows how to make it.
• Knows how to use it.
• Believes in it so that when diarrhoea occurs ORS is given at once and with confidence.

Here are some ways of encouraging the community to use it:

1. **Understand local beliefs about diarrhoea.**
   Communities are often reluctant to use ORS. We must discover local beliefs about diar-

Table 11.2   How to treat dehydration

PLAN A	PLAN B	PLAN C
Diarrhoea with **no** dehydration	Diarrhoea with **some** dehydration	Diarrhoea with **severe** dehydration
After each loose stool	*First 4 hours: catch-up phase* Give these amounts within the 4-hour period:	*Refer the child* for intravenous treatment or feeding through a nasogastric tube without delay, continuing to give ORS if possible
Children under 2 years: 50–100 ml Children 2–10 years: 100–200 ml Children 10 years+: As much as wanted	Children under 4 months or less than 5 kg: 200–400 ml Children 4–11 months or 5–8 kg: 400–600 ml Children 1–2 years or 8–11 kg: 600–800 ml Children 2–4 years or 11–16 kg: 800–1200 ml Children 5–14 years or 16–30 kg: 1200–2000 ml Simplified version of PLAN B 1. Double amounts of ORS given in Plan A after each stool for first 4 hours. 2. After 4 hours, reassess dehydration. 3. If not present, use Plan A. If still present, use Plan B. 4. If the child is deteriorating, use Plan C.	

Adapted from *The Management and Prevention of Diarrhoea: practical guidelines*, 3rd Edition. Geneva: WHO, 1993.

rhoea and why people are suspicious of using ORS.

For example (1): In parts of Africa and South Asia many people believe that giving fluid makes diarrhoea last longer; therefore children with diarrhoea are not given fluids. This is quite logical when people believe that diarrhoea rather than dehydration kills the child. Explain to parents that children die, not from the diarrhoea itself but because they dry out. Show them an orange dried out in the sun or a leaky gourd that only keeps holding water if it is continually filled up.

Explain also that giving fluid does not necessarily stop the diarrhoea. Mothers know this anyway. In fact, ORS may seem to make diarrhoea worse and children will often pass a stool shortly after receiving ORS. Explain to mothers that this may happen. (This is less likely to happen with a liquid food (page 212). *For example (2)*: People with easy access to practitioners and pharmacies often believe that the only effective treatment for diarrhoea is a medicine, injection or intravenous drip given by doctors; that home-made remedies are useless. These wrong ideas have to be discussed with the community until they are made aware of the situation. Unless objections are faced up to, people will listen politely, then go away and ignore our advice.

2. **Demonstrate the use of ORS in clinics.**
Whenever a child comes to the clinic with diarrhoea, a health worker should show the mother how to make and how to feed ORS.

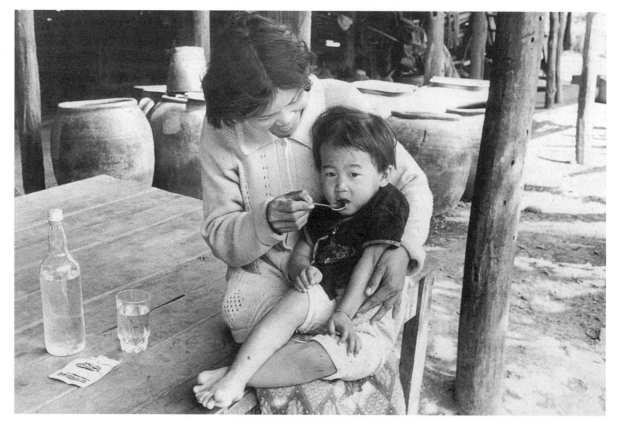

Figure 11.6   A mother in Thailand feeding ORS by glass and spoon.

Then the mother herself gives it to her own child.

> Clinics can have special ORS or rehydration corners where equipment needed for making ORS is always available and ready for use.

3. **Demonstrate the use of ORS in homes.**
   This is usually the task of the CHW, who should continue until family members are confident about using it.
   Make sure that CHWs themselves use ORS in their own families.
4. **Help community leaders to know about ORS,** to use it themselves and to encourage its use in the community. Teachers, religious leaders and shopkeepers must all be aware of its value.
5. **Teach children and pre-school children.**
   Older siblings can give it to younger ones. Teaching on ORS should be a central part of school health programmes.

Pre-school children can be taught in crèches and balwadis.
6. **Encourage the community to tune in to radio and TV programmes about ORS.**

Use other ways to treat diarrhoea

Although using ORS is much the most important thing to do, we should also know:

1. **When to use antibiotics.** As mentioned above these are usually recommended for:
   • Dysentery, i.e. blood with diarrhoea, e.g. as caused by shigella.
   • Cholera and typhoid.
   • Amoebiasis and giardiasis, which a lab usually needs to confirm.
2. **National guidelines on which antibiotic to use and the correct dose.**
   Discover what these are and use them.

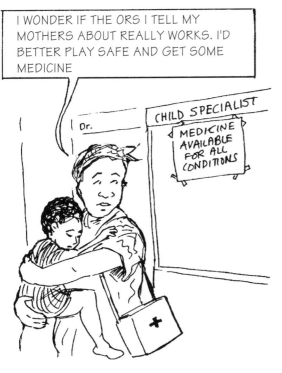

I WONDER IF THE ORS I TELL MY MOTHERS ABOUT REALLY WORKS. I'D BETTER PLAY SAFE AND GET SOME MEDICINE

Figure 11.7   Test of a successful ORT programme: does the CHW trust oral rehydration alone when her *own* child is at risk?

3. **About the use of zinc supplements,** which are known to reduce death rates from both acute diarrhoea and dysentery – 10 mg daily of elemental zinc for infants and 20 mg for children over one year of age are often recommended and are likely to become more widely available.
4. **When to refer.** Follow IMCI guidelines and see tables 11.1 and 11.2. If referral is not possible consider using a naso-gastric tube to give oral rehydration solution, if health team members are trained and correct equipment is available in the health centre.

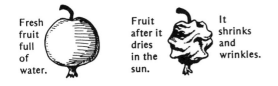

Fresh fruit full of water.

Fruit after it dries in the sun.

It shrinks and wrinkles.

Figure 11.8   If the child with diarrhoea is not given water, he will dry like a fruit in the sun.

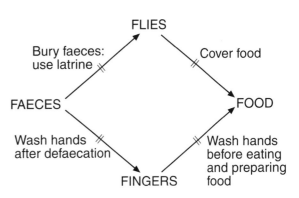

Figure 11.9   Diarrhoea prevention: breaking the '4F cycle'.

Explain how diarrhoea can be prevented

Teaching on how to prevent diarrhoea must always go alongside our teaching on how to treat it.

This is a list of key tasks:

- **Promote breastfeeding** up to two years and encourage no mixed feeding until six months (see page 180). (Where HIV/AIDS is common we need to modify this to help prevent mother to child transmission – see pages 182–3.)
- **Teach good personal hygiene** especially hand-washing (see Figure 11.9). The CHW should promote hygiene. Regular hand-washing with soap has been shown to halve the rate of diarrhoea, even if the water is not clean. Those giving and preparing food, infants and children (with help from older family members) all need to wash their hands. Families that start using soap and water often gradually stop doing this, so we must continually reinforce this teaching.
- **Use the cleanest water available** for drinking and preparing food. If possible improve a community water source (see page 307). Where this is not possible, use other methods. *For example*: Masai children in east Africa have been trained to place plastic water bottles in full sun for at least five hours on the roof of their huts, where heat kills the germs. Diarrhoea rates have fallen as a result. This is known as the Sodis system, see page 310.

- **Promote the use of latrines** and the burial of children's faeces, which are usually highly infectious (see pages 312–3).
- **Design or use fly traps.**
- **Set up school teaching programmes** on the importance of hygiene and sanitation. Use Child-to-Child approaches (see page 406). Make teaching specific, e.g. 'always wash both hands with soap after using the latrine'.
Also see WHO's 5 key strategies below.

WHO's 5 key strategies for preparing and consuming food:
1. Keep hands and cooking surfaces clean
2. Separate raw and cooked food
3. Cook food thoroughly
4. Keep food stored at safe temperatures
5. Use safe water

For more information see www.who.int/foodsafety.

Evaluate the programme

After an agreed period of time the programme should be evaluated to see if targets are being met. We can discover:

1. **Whether family members are using ORS in practice.**
   Supervisors can find this out informally by keeping alert, enquiring from community members and CHWs, doing spot checks.
   We can find out more formally by preparing a questionnaire for use on a sample of homes. We would ask:
   - How, When and Why ORS is used.
   - How families have treated actual cases of diarrhoea in the past three or six months.
2. **Whether deaths from diarrhoea are decreasing.**
   We could use our own project statistics to calculate this by comparing community surveys carried out before and after ORS was introduced, providing our sample is large and our methods are accurate. Alternatively, we could total the various causes of under-five deaths from CHW's record books.
   If deaths from diarrhoea have become less common, other factors may be responsible, such as improved nutrition (see also Chapter 18).

Summary

Diarrhoea and dehydration cause two million, largely unnecessary, deaths each year. By the simple use of home-based ORS most of these deaths could be prevented.

In preparing a programme with the community, decide which forms of ORS are most appropriate for the area, and which containers and measuring devices most suitable. Any method used must be acceptable to the community and follow national guidelines.

All community members should learn how to make and prepare ORS and be able to feed it to those with diarrhoea. Repeated and imaginative teaching methods are needed to raise community awareness and change incorrect beliefs. Unnecessary medicines should always be avoided, but zinc supplements help in diarrhoea and antibiotics are useful in dysentery. As well as treating dehydration, we must teach methods to prevent diarrhoea. Usually these will include developing cleaner water sources, improving sanitation and careful handwashing of both adults and children.

The programme should be evaluated after an agreed length of time, to make sure ORS is actually being used in practice.

ACUTE RESPIRATORY INFECTION (ARI)

In this section we shall consider:
1. What is acute respiratory infection?
2. What is the importance of ARI?
3. What are the causes of ARI?
4. How can ARI be prevented?
5. How can ARI be recognised and treated?
6. What is the role of the CHW in ARI?

What is acute respiratory infection (ARI)?

Acute Respiratory Infections (ARIs) include those illnesses where there is cough, sore throat and runny nose with or without an increase in respiration rate or fever. Most are not serious and require only care at home, including extra fluids, good nutrition and ensuring that symptoms do not become worse. On average, an African child suffers six to ten episodes of ARI per year.

Although most cases of ARI need no drug treatment and soon improve, there is always the risk that ARI can turn into pneumonia, often very quickly and with little warning.

Pneumonia is an infection of the lungs that can rapidly cause the death of children (and adults), especially those who are weakened by other conditions such as measles, diarrhoea, AIDS and malaria, or who are malnourished.

The two most important symptoms of pneumonia are easy to recognise. First, a fast respiratory rate – over 50 breaths per minute in children aged two to eleven months, over 40 in children between one and five years of age. Second, lower chest wall indrawing. In addition there may be cough, fever, and blue lips and, when very serious, stridor, drowsiness and coma. (Children under two months have variable breathing rates – two successive counts of 60 or more suggests pneumonia or severe ARI.)

What is the importance of ARI?

ARI, mainly in the form of pneumonia, kills about two million children under five per year. Up to 40 per cent of children seen in health clinics are suffering from some form of ARI.

About one quarter of all cases of pneumonia in under fives will lead to death in a few days if not treated. This makes quick recognition and immediate treatment the two keys for a successful programme.

> Nearly all cases of ARI can be prevented and treated at community level without the need for a doctor.

What are the causes of ARI?

Most cases of pneumonia in developing countries are caused by bacteria, in Africa, four out of five. Most of the rest are caused by viruses.

Nearly one quarter of all fatal cases follow measles or TB. An increasing number is associated with AIDS.

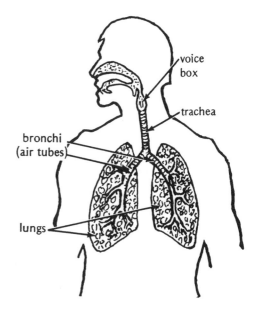

Figure 11.10   The respiratory system.

Some conditions increase the likelihood of getting ARI and make recovery more difficult. These include malnutrition, Vitamin A deficiency, anaemia and household smoke – both from open fireplaces and from cigarette smoking.

> Deaths from ARI occur mainly in poor, remote, backward or crowded conditions. Fatal childhood pneumonia is largely a disease of poverty.

Some of the factors that can lead to pneumonia were recorded in a health workshop held in Bangladesh. They are shown in the 'spider chart' (see Figure 11.11). We can make a similar chart for our own area.

How can ARI be prevented?

Much can be done including:
1. **Correcting malnutrition** (see Chapter 9). Make sure that all children climb on to the Road to Health section of the growth chart as soon as possible. They should get more nutritious food after any illness. Children who are malnourished can be given Vitamin A and zinc supplements and those who are anaemic, iron supplements.
2. **Immunisation.**

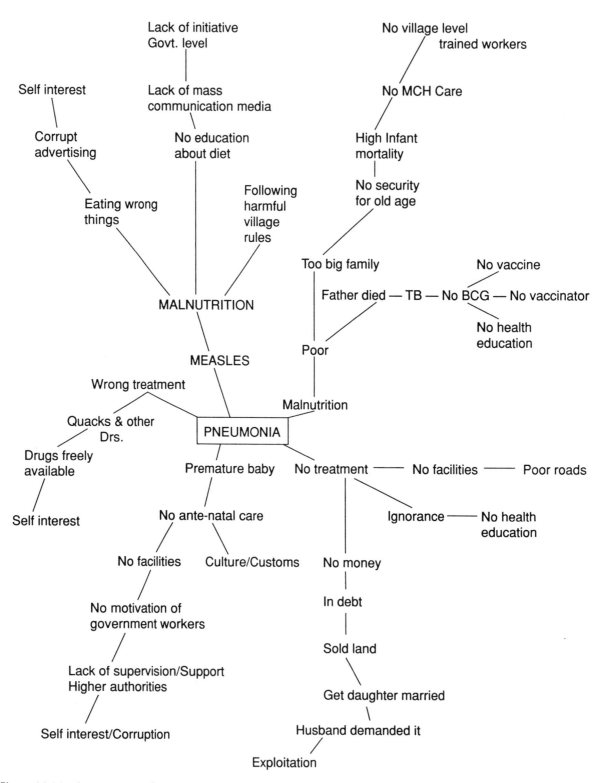

Figure 11.11   Some causes of pneumonia (from a workshop held in Bangladesh).

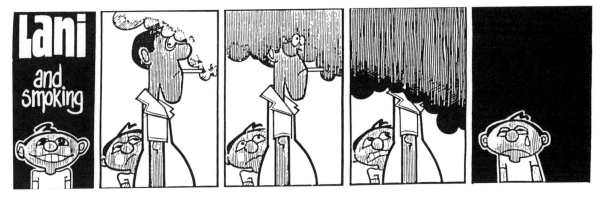

Figure 11.12   Smoking not only kills smokers, but affects children and others who breathe in the smoke.

Check that all children are fully immunised against DPT, polio, TB, measles and where possible Hib. Measles, Hib and Pertussis (P) immunisations are especially important in preventing pneumonia.

3. **Reducing household smoke.**

   If cooking is done inside with no ventilation, the community can be encouraged to install chimneys or build outside cookhouses. Charcoal is less polluting than wood smoke (see Chapter 16, pages 320–21).

   Tobacco smoking must be discouraged. We can explain that smoke causes serious lung (and eye) disease in children and that one household member who smokes puts children at risk through passive smoking.

How can ARI be recognised and treated?

Assess severity

Plan A: Simple cough or cold: no pneumonia.
Simple cough and cold, with or without fever, breathing rate less than 50 per minute in infants aged two to eleven months, less than 40 in children over one year old.

Give supportive treatment only (see 'supportive treatment and feeding' page 222). Antibiotics are not needed. Check regularly to make sure child does not deteriorate. If it does, follow Plan B.

Plan B: Non-severe pneumonia.
Cough or cold with breathing rate more than 50 per minute in infants between two and eleven

months, more than 40 in children over one year old, but no lower chest wall indrawing.

Give supportive treatment (see 'supportive treatment and feeding') plus antibiotics (see 'supplying antibiotics' page 223). Treat at home. Watch for any deterioration, which may be sudden. If deterioration occurs, follow Plan C.

Plan C: Severe pneumonia.
Child seriously ill with breathing rates faster than 50 per minute in infants two to eleven months, more than 40 per minute in children over one year old. Indrawing of ribs plus either vomiting or blue lips or stridor (noisy breathing) or drowsiness or coma.

Give antibiotics (by injection if possible) and refer at once, accompanying mother and child, or arranging escort.

> The treatment of ARI depends on recognition of key symptoms, having antibiotics always available in the community and treating cases without delay.

Type of antibiotic to be used

The choice will depend on cost, availability and which antibiotic is recommended in our country or district. Possible choices would be as follows:

1. Amoxycillin three times daily or ampicillin four times daily for five to seven days in correct dose for age or weight. Suitable for all children except those allergic to penicillin. For those too young to swallow pills, the tablet can be crushed and the capsule opened,

added to milk or other suitable liquid and fed at correct dose. Recent research suggests that taking amoxycillin for just 3 rather than 5 days is just as effective in non-severe pneumonia (but not severe pneumonia) providing no doses are missed. (Ref. see Pakistan, page 414.)

2. Sulfamethoxazole and trimethoprim (SMT/TMP, cotrimoxazole) for five to seven days in correct dose for age or weight. Suitable for all children over six weeks of age except those who are allergic to sulfa drugs.

3. Benzyl penicillin injection once daily for five to seven days in correct dose for weight or age. This can be used in clinics for children who are seriously ill or unable to take medicine by mouth.

   Recent research shows that oral amoxycillin is as effective as injectable penicillin even in severe pneumonia, providing the child can swallow it. (Ref. see Addo-yobo, page 414.)

When using injectable penicillin, ask the parent if the child has ever had any reaction or rash following a previous injection or medicine. If they have, do not give it. An alternative for seriously ill children is to give chloramphenicol by mouth, if injections of penicillin cannot be given.

Remember:

> Antibiotics should not be used for ordinary coughs and colds.

Supportive treatment and feeding

Teach mothers to carry out the following in all cases of ARI:

1. Ensure plenty of fluids.
2. Reduce fever by removing extra clothes and giving paracetamol, but not aspirin, if necessary.
3. Give frequent energy rich drinks, such as fruit juices, soups, etc. Children being breastfed should continue, even if their noses seem blocked.
4. Continue giving extra foods until children are back on the Road to Health and have regained their original weight.
5. Reduce indoor smoke pollution.

What is the role of the CHW in ARI?

CHWs have a key role in the treatment of ARI. They are usually available and can therefore start treatment early, before the disease has become too serious.

For example: In the BRAC programme in Bangladesh (a large, established NGO) community health volunteers, mainly poor middle-aged women, mostly with just five years of schooling, underwent three days of intensive training in the recognition and treatment of children with ARI. Each was assigned 100 to120 households. These volunteers identified children with pneumonia and treated them at household level, referring severe cases. They proved to be almost as accurate, and more cost effective, than physicians, in both identifying and treating ARI, provided they were carefully trained and managed.

> Most of the two million deaths caused by ARI in the world today could be prevented if each community had an effective, well trained CHW or other primary health worker living in the community, with a supply of antibiotics.

The CHW will have the following roles:

Teaching

She will teach her community:
- How to prevent ARI
- The dangers of ARI
- The warning signs of ARI.

She will demonstrate to parents and older siblings that fast breathing rates spell danger and that the child must be brought to her at once.

It is not necessary for the CHW or parent to be able to read a watch, or to count to 50. With practice nearly everyone can learn to recognise fast breathing by careful observation alone.

The CHW will make sure that all community members understand the two golden rules, which are:

1. Children with simple coughs and colds need no medicines.

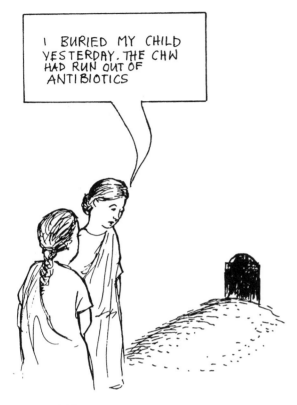

Figure 11.13

2. Children with fast breathing rates are brought for treatment at once.

Supplying antibiotics

The CHW will ideally keep a supply of antibiotics. If so, this supply must never run out.

> Only when community members know that the CHW always has the correct medicines available will they trust her to care for serious illnesses.

If the community perceives that the CHW cannot be relied upon, children will continue to be taken on long and delaying journeys to distant health centres and doctors. Often these journeys will be unnecessary because the child will not need antibiotics. Sometimes, however, they will be too late and the child will be dying on arrival.

The CHW will use the correct antibiotic at the correct dose for the correct length of time, taking care that the parent knows how it should be used, and that the course is finished. She will record details in her book.

Referring

The CHW will refer seriously ill children. First, she will recognise a child who needs to be referred. Second, she starts the child on antibiotics at once. Third, she sends or accompanies the child and its parent to the nearest reliable referral centre without delay.

Follow-up

The CHW will follow up all children with ARI until they have completely recovered, have regained their weight and are back on the Road to Health.

Any child who has a persistent cough for more than three weeks she will refer to the clinic or doctor to check for TB, or another cause of illness.

Identifying risks

She will try to identify any preventable risk factors in the home. She will encourage immunisations and breastfeeding and discourage smoking.

In addition

1. Regular handwashing with soap, of both children and carers, has been shown to reduce greatly the likelihood of children getting ARI.
2. Give zinc supplements if available (see page 217).
3. The use of long-term cotrimoxazole in children who are HIV positive prolongs their lives. In many programmes the CHW will be the most appropriate person, either singly or as part of a home care team, to make sure such children receive regular supplies and take them daily.

Summary

Acute respiratory infection (ARI), usually in the form of pneumonia, kills two million children per year. Nearly all these deaths can be prevented at community level, if simple guidelines are followed. These indicate which children need antibiotics and suggest ways in which they are immediately available when needed.

The CHW plays a key role in this process. She teaches the community how to prevent ARI, working with them in reducing the risk factors. She keeps and uses antibiotics according to simple guidelines. She knows when and how to refer children who are seriously ill.

MALARIA

In this section we shall consider:
1. Why malaria control is important.
2. Ways of preventing malaria.
3. How to set up a community control programme.
4. How to treat malaria.

Why malaria control is important

Over two billion people in over 100 countries (40 per cent of the world population) live in areas where malaria is present.

Most malarial deaths occur in children under five years of age. At least one million children die from malaria each year, that is 3000 African children per day, about one every 30 seconds. Where malaria is endemic (present all the year round) children are at greatest risk between the ages of six months (when immunity inherited from mother fades) and about five years (when their own immunity is increasing). Malaria slows economic development in sub-Saharan Africa by more than one per cent per year. Some experts predict that, unless drastic measures are taken, malaria will double in some of the most affected countries over the next 20 years. Hopefully, by then an effective cheap vaccine will be widely available

In many countries malaria is becoming more common at the present time. In Niger alone, out of a population of ten million, there are 850 000 cases of malaria notified each year, equally distributed between adults and children.

Research from the University of Oxford (2005) suggests the number of cases of malaria worldwide is about twice that of previous official estimates. (See Snow, 'Malaria Risk', *Nature*, 2005:437.)

Attempts at malaria control appeared to work during the 1970s but are now failing for various reasons, partly due to the phasing out of the use of DDT to control mosquitoes, and of the malaria parasite's resistance to chloroquine and other commonly used forms of malaria treatment. It is also a result of more widespread poverty, an increase in human migration due to war and famine, and the opening up of frontier regions to development as in the Amazon region of Brazil.

The situation has become so serious that a new worldwide initiative known as Roll Back Malaria was started in 1998 with the aim of halving the number of malaria deaths by the year 2010. RBM is run by four agencies working together, WHO, UNICEF, The World Bank and the United Nations Development Programme. RBM consists of regional and national strategies that can help to reduce malaria through governments, health workers and communities working together in partnership. (See ref. 2, page 233.)

In addition to RBM, there is a variety of experimental control programmes, use of new drugs and drug combinations and other approaches being used at local or country level. The control and treatment of malaria is frequently changing. We need to know about the major programmes going on in our country and work with them as far as possible. But we should also be ready to try new approaches relevant to our community providing they are based on good evidence and are likely to be sustainable.

> Within a national malaria programme, community based health care can greatly reduce the incidence of malaria within a target population.

In this section of the chapter we shall look first at ways of preventing malaria. Only then can we understand the most effective ways of developing a community control programme.

Ways of preventing malaria

Malaria is caused by an infected female anopheles mosquito injecting Plasmodium into the human bloodstream. Non-infected mosquitoes that feed on people with malaria become infected themselves and so the cycle continues.

Map 1. Global distribution of malaria transmission risk, WHO, 2003

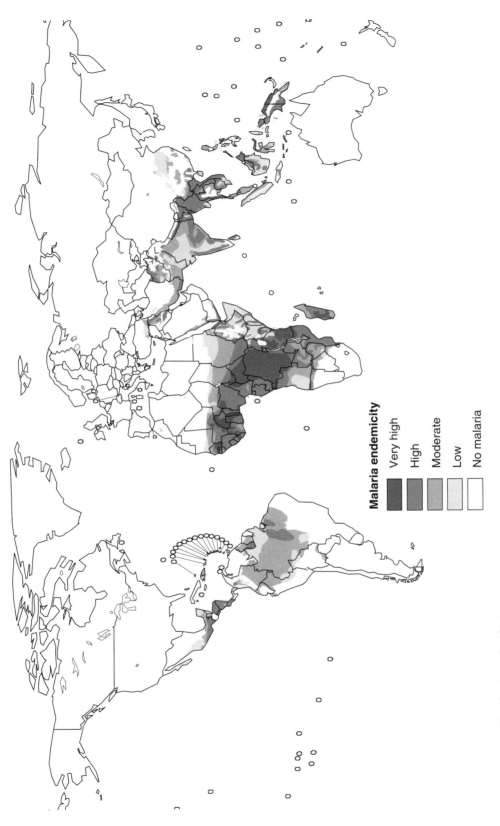

Figure 11.14   Distribution of malaria.

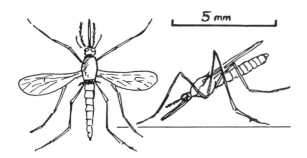

Figure 11.15   An *Anopheles* mosquito.

There are three important ways we can use to help break this cycle and make malaria less common:

A. Reduce mosquito breeding sites

Mosquitoes can breed in very small amounts of water, such as water-filled wheel ruts and hoof prints. All sources of standing water need to be identified and dealt with. Here are examples of

measures that will also help to reduce the number of *Aedes* mosquitoes, which cause dengue fever:

Ways to reduce breeding mosquitoes
1. Remove or fill areas near houses where mosquitoes breed, such as holes, ditches, the tops of bamboo canes, old cans and tyres.
2. Drain areas where water collects, such as near boreholes or around standpipes.
3. Build soakage pits to remove household waste.
4. Cover wells and drains.
5. Plan any new building or development programmes with care so that new breeding sites are not created.
6. Clear away vegetation from the banks of streams so that water flows more quickly.
7. Introduce larva-eating fish, e.g. guppy, into areas where mosquitoes breed, such as rice paddies and small reservoirs.
8. Add polystyrene beads to pit latrines and septic tanks.
9. Pour petroleum oil onto the surface of small amounts of standing water that cannot easily be drained.

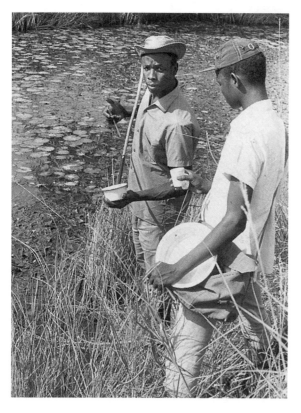

Figure 11.16   Health workers in Africa surveying a mosquito breeding site.

B. Kill adult mosquitoes

Spraying insecticides was the main form of malaria control until the 1970s. Now it is just one aspect of control programmes.

1. For *personal* protection spray pyrethroid insecticides into rooms before going to bed.
2. For *community* protection work alongside any teams that spray residual (persistent) insecticides on the walls of houses. DDT is effective for this and its careful use is approved by RBM, though at the time of writing there is no agreement to reintroduce this on a wide scale. Health committee members can accompany any spraying team to give confidence to the local community and explain the reason it is being done.

C. Prevent mosquitoes from biting people

This is becoming an increasingly important part of malaria control.

1. Use bed-nets. These work most effectively when impregnated with an insecticide, originally permethrin, which gave protection from six to twelve months. This is being gradually replaced by the use of other insecticides, using processes that make the net effective for up to four years. These 'long-lasting insecticide treated nets' (LLITNs) are being manufactured in Africa and becoming increasingly available. Others, known as permanets, which contain deltamethrin, last for a year or more and can withstand several washings. Wherever treated nets are widely used malaria becomes less common and fewer children die from it. Even mosquito nets that are not treated with insecticide give some protection.
2. Hang insecticide-treated netting in windows and curtains in doorways if the house design is appropriate. This reduces malaria but is less effective than using treated nets. Where permethrin is used, curtains and bed-nets can be soaked at the same time.
3. Apply insect repellent (e.g. containing DEET) or burn mosquito coils. These are useful for personal protection of those especially at risk, or for use in the evening before climbing under mosquito nets. Many poorer families cannot afford these.
4. Screen windows and doors to prevent mosquitoes entering the house, and keep doors and windows closed from an hour before sunset until well after sunrise.

How to set up a community control programme

For the most effective malaria control, each country (or district) selects a variety of measures that are most appropriate for its circumstances.

For example (1): Indonesia has had success using a combination of case finding and treatment, indoor spraying with insecticide, use of larvicidal fish, tree-planting in marshy areas and the use of bed-nets.

For example (2): Parts of Tanzania have been experimenting with the widespread use of bed-nets through robust health promotion and social marketing.

For example (3): In Pakistan, sponging of cattle (on which mosquitoes feed and rest) with deltamethrin insecticide has proved effective.

For example (4): Vietnam has been very successful distributing bed-nets to all households with biannual retreatment, training staff in health posts to diagnose malaria using microscopes, and making it possible for early diagnosis and treatment. There is a regular supply of drugs, and a programme of community involvement and health education.

Central to all programme stages is active partnership between project, community and national programmes. We can follow these steps:

Step 1. Meet with the District Medical Officer

At an early stage we need to meet with the DMO or other official responsible for any RBM or IMCI programme.

The reason for this meeting is to learn about national control programmes, discover any district or local strategies and discuss ways in which the project can tie in with any government plans. It is very important that everyone works together.

Step 2. Assess the local malarial situation

We can find answers to questions such as:
- How common is malaria?
- Which ages are most affected?
- What percentage of infants and children aged one to four years die from malaria?
- Is malaria seasonal or irregular (epidemic), or present the whole year round (endemic)?
- Where/what are the main malaria breeding sites?
- Is there widespread resistance to chloroquine, sulfadoxine-pyrimethamine (SP, Fansidar) or other commonly used drugs?
- Are there local beliefs and practices that affect treatment?
- Where and how do community members currently receive treatment?
- Do community members buy treatment and self-treat at home?

- Is malaria either overtreated or undertreated?
- Are mosquito nets easily available and used? Are they treated with insecticide?

Step 3. Assess the resources of the community

- How much community understanding is there?
- How much community commitment to action is present?
- What control measures are already being carried out?
- Does the community have resources to buy mosquito nets or use more effective drug treatments?

This information – on the local malarial situation and resources of the community – can be discovered from:

- The community through a survey or discussion with community leaders and CHWs. As we do this we can also create awareness about how malaria control can be improved.
- The DMO or malaria control experts, such as those working in assocation with Roll Back Malaria or the latest district or national initiative.
- Records or health offices in the nearest hospital or primary health centre.
- Our own personal observation.

Knowing answers to these questions will help us select control strategies that are both effective against malaria and acceptable to the community.

> The key to community-based malaria control is to select a combination of control measures that are most appropriate for our particular community. Depending on one form of control alone will be insufficient.

Step 4. Plan with community and government

During these sessions we can match up the most effective control strategies with their acceptability to the community. We can help to liaise between community and government.

We can then draw up an action plan for each control measure to be adopted.

Step 5. Empower the CHW and health committee

We may first wish to carry out a pilot project. This will be important before we introduce any community-wide programme, such as the use of treated bed-nets.

In carrying out a malaria programme:

- The CHW will have a key role in the care and treatment of individuals with malaria, backed up by the health team. She will have a reliable supply of the nationally recommended drug for treatment and know how to use it. Sometimes a volunteer will work specifically in a malaria control programme
  For example: In Uganda a man named Steven is one of a number of peasant farmers trained as volunteers and working in a government programme called home based management. He keeps antimalarials and is available continually for anyone who needs treatment in his village. Mothers in this community no longer have to walk miles to the nearest health centre.
- Health committee members or any specially trained malaria group will be largely involved in community wide prevention. *For example*: They can mobilise the community to clear malarial breeding sites, or plant trees in marshy areas to help drainage. They can work with the health team and development experts to set up fish-breeding ponds near health centres from which larva-eating fish can be distributed. They can liaise with the government spraying team.

Step 6. Include mothers and care-givers in malaria control

In areas where malaria is common and family members are familiar with symptoms, they are in fact the main providers of antimalarial treatment. *For example*: in several African countries, including Nigeria and Mali, mothers have been shown to manage almost three quarters of their children's cases of malaria with home-based treatment. (See page 414, ref. Deressa.)

Where malaria is common we need to ensure that correct treatment is available at least within

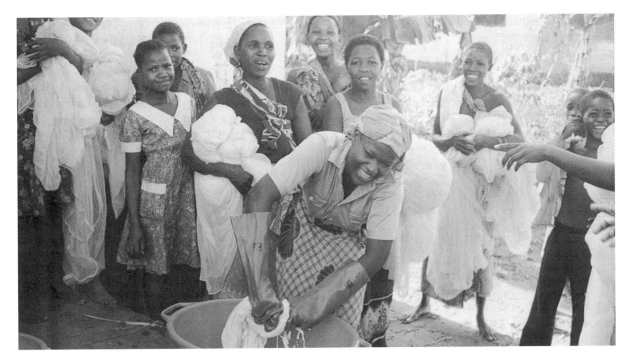

Figure 11.17 Villagers in Tanzania bring their bed-nets for soaking in permethrin.

24 hours of symptoms starting and preferably earlier. Home-based care is one obvious answer.

In practice CHWs can train mothers, other family members and care-givers how to recognise and treat malaria.

Family members will do this most safely if they are included in the health programme and obtain supplies from the programme or other trusted suppliers, rather than from unregulated private practitioners.

Step 7. Organise a community bed-net programme

This is an effective way of reducing malaria, and helps to save the lives of children. Long-lasting insecticide treated nets (LLITNs) are becoming increasingly used in malaria control.

We should start a programme only if the following apply:

1. Malaria is a serious problem in the community, and is a common cause for children dying. Contact the district medical officer, local referral hospital or Roll Back Malaria offfice to get an estimate of how common malaria is and details of any seasonal variations. Follow any guidelines that have been drawn up regarding the use of impregnated bed-nets.
2. The community is fully involved and willing to cooperate.
3. Careful training has been given to health committee members or others involved in management.
4. Bed-nets and permethrin, or LLITNs are available at a price most people can afford. Encourage people to obtain nets if they are free, or to seek out reduced priced nets available through social marketing or subsidised sources. If these are not available, the community and programme can advocate for nets to be available at affordable prices.
5. The programme will be sustainable after any initial subsidy or donation is no longer available.
6. A pilot programme is run first, to see if the idea works in practice, and to discover and solve problems.

If LLITNs are not available we can soak nets as follows:

1. Fix a day when members of all community households will come to soak their nets.
2. Prepare the site – preferably in the open air: wash used nets before treatment and dry them: have long rubber gloves and bowls available.
3. Make up the solution by calculating the amount of solution, mixing and storing it in clean drums or tubs.
   Different substances are used – permethrin is the most common. Different nets are used, which absorb different amounts of solution. Follow instructions carefully and calculate the amount of solution needed according to the type of insecticide, type and size of net and total number likely to be soaked.
4. Dip the nets. Soak thoroughly, then wring out over the container. Nets should be dry and clean before soaking.
5. Dry the nets either by hanging, or better still laying flat on the bed. A plastic bag will be needed to take the wet net home.
6. Clear up and clean up. Unused solution should be kept.

> No permethrin should be disposed of near lakes, river or water, as it can kill fish and invertebrates.

Advantages of using treated nets:

- They help to kill mosquitoes, so reducing their numbers.
- Nets that have holes or are not correctly tucked in still give good protection (but nets should still be mended and tucked in).
- Those using bed-nets are also protected from other insects, sleep better and have fewer skin infections.
- Children are more likely to survive, and pregnant mothers less likely to become seriously ill or to have miscarriages.

How to treat malaria

The problem

Malaria is dangerous and can kill rapidly. It also mimics many other diseases, making diagnosis difficult. The malaria parasite is developing resistance to chloroquine and other commonly used and relatively cheap types of malaria treatment. New and effective treatments are becoming available but they are more expensive. Without subsidy most people or countries can't afford them.

WHO recommends that, once resistance to a malaria drug reaches 25 per cent, the country should change to another more effective treatment. In sub-Saharan Africa chloroquine is no longer effective. Many countries have changed to sulfadoxine/pyrimethamine (SP) but this too is fast losing its effectiveness.

When affordable or strongly subsidised, artemisinin combined therapy (ACT) is the best treatment to use for sub-Saharan Africa, usually in the form of co-artemether (Coartem). It appears safe and effective.

At the same time, many of the most vulnerable people live too far from any clinic. *For example*: in a recent survey of mothers in Uganda, 44 per cent said the nearest health centre is too far from their homes.

Pregnant women and children under five are at greatest risk and these find it even harder to reach treatment centres.

To overcome these problems we need:

- **CHWs** – carefully trained to recognise, treat and refer; always available and with a reliable supply of medicines. In remote seriously affected areas, mothers can be trained to recognise malaria and hold supplies to treat it.
- **Health centres** where severe cases can be referred and treated without delay. This is important because without accurate diagnosis malaria can be overtreated, especially where effective home treatments are available. Serious diseases can be missed when it is assumed that every case of fever is malaria and is treated as such.
- **Mothers and care-givers.** See step 6 above.
- **An effective referral system.** This involves a protocol to follow, (see Figure 11.18 as an example), access to care within the community, reliable transport and a dependable referral centre. See Chapter 8, pages 164–5 for other actions we can take when referral is not possible.

Integrated Management of Childhood Illness (IMCI) categories of referral

Urgent referral
Any child who exhibits one of the general danger signs under IMCI including:
- convulsions
- inability to drink
- vomiting everything
- unconsciousness or lethargy
- specific combinations of signs and symptoms that identify severe illness

Non-urgent referral
The child coughs for more than 30 days or has a fever for more than 7 days.

Other referrals
Referral of 'other problems' not identified by the IMCI classification, but still in need of specialized management – for example, trauma, osteomyelitis of long duration, etc.

Source, WHO Bulletin, 2003, 81 (7), p. 523.

Figure 11.18   Integrated Management of Childhood Illness (IMCI) categories of referral, not specific to malaria.

Recognising malaria

Here are some suggested guidelines we can adapt or adopt:

1. Be familiar with the pattern of malaria in the project area, how commonly it occurs, which time of year it is usually found, (usually commonest during and just after the rainy season/s), the symptoms most commonly seen, and other diseases that frequently mimic it. (Remember both malaria and other illnesses may be present.)
2. Recognise cases of malaria.

A. Mild malaria
Fever above 37.5 °C when seen by health worker or in past three days, plus one or more of the following: headache, shivering, sweating, vomiting, cough or diarrhoea.

At the same time ask for and observe other symptoms to see if there is another obvious cause of the illness, such as ARI or measles, especially where malaria is relatively uncommon. Typhoid fever, dengue fever and acute bilharzia can also mimic malaria.

To discover if there is a temperature use a clinical thermometer, a new crystal thermometer (see Appendix A) or estimate with the back of the hand. Studies show that many mothers can estimate fever in their child with sufficient accuracy, but may find it hard to understand – or afford – a thermometer.

B. Severe malaria
Any of or all the symptoms in 'A' will be present plus, in addition, one or more of the following: very high fever (39 °C or above) drowsiness, coma, rapid deep breathing, convulsions, very pale mucous membranes, yellow whites of eyes, cold clammy skin with weak pulse.

Many of these severe cases will be in children under five. In areas where malaria is common, treatment should usually be based on symptoms and not depend on blood slide examinations, which are often not available, often cause delay and may be inaccurate.

Treating malaria

If mild malaria is suspected:
- Give paracetamol if the fever is high.
- As fever reduces give the first-line treatment as used in the national malaria programme, at the correct dose for age and weight. These are commonly: sulfadoxine/pyrimethamine (SP) – given in a single dose; chlorproguanil/dapsone(Lapdap) – given daily for three days; or artemisinin combined therapy (ACT) usually co-artemether (co-artem) – given every 12 hours for three days.
- Give children a sweet drink.
- Observe for one hour and repeat medicine if first dose is vomited.
- Teach the mother to observe the child carefully, to continue the course of treatment and to report any worsening of symptoms immediately.

If severe malaria is suspected:
- Inject or treat with the drug recommended by national programme.

  In addition: rectal artemether has been shown to work as well as intravenous quinine to treat severe or cerebral malaria, and this can be used in the health centre or even by a well trained CHW.

- Refer immediately to the health centre or hospital with a referral note and accompanying the patient if possible, but start treatment first.

In the case of pregnant women:

- Those in their first pregnancy are especially prone to malaria. It can be dangerous for mother and child.
- Make sure women are treated promptly, take their full course of medicine and are reassured that the medicine will not harm either them or their child – rather, it may save their lives.
- Provide them with iron and folic acid tablets.
- Consider giving intermittent preventive treatment (IPT), e.g. sulfadoxine/pyrimethamine (SP). WHO recommends IPT should be given to women in their first and second pregnancies in areas with high rates of malaria. This should be started from the second trimester and given at monthly intervals.
  IPT can be provided at the antenatal clinic or by a trained CHW or TBA. The mother should in addition be sleeping under an insecticide treated net.

In the case of children:

Two additional methods that may reduce childhood malaria are as follows:

1. **Intermittent preventive or presumptive treatment (IPT)**
   For example (1): In one Tanzanian project, children received their third dose of DPT polio immunisation with the first of three daily doses of amodiaquine. After 60 days children who took this treatment had fewer malaria fevers than those who did not.
   For example (2): In another programme in Tanzania, sulfadoxine/pyrimethamine (SP) was given as a single dose at two, three and nine months, at the same time as the EPI immunisations. This reduced childhood malarial attacks by nearly two thirds and also halved severe malarial anaemia.
2. **Regular deworming medicine to reduce roundworm infection**
   We may already be giving mebendazole or albendazole to children every four or six months. Studies suggest that there is some-

times a link between severe malaria and high levels of roundworm.
For example: in Togo, West Africa, a campaign has been launched to reach one million under-five children with measles and polio vaccine, mosquito nets and deworming tablets. (WHO/UNICEF Press Release 96, 2004.)

Evaluate the programme

Evaluation will be done in part by visiting malaria control experts, under the RBM programme.

Community based evaluation can show how effective our programme is proving. It can help to tell us the following:

- Is the community satisfied with the malaria programme?
- Has the amount of standing water in the community been reduced?
- Does the community perceive any change in the number of mosquitoes or the number of mosquito bites?
- Is the number of patients with suspected malaria attending the CHW or health post declining?
- Are the number and percentage of children dying from malaria decreasing?

Summary

Malaria is one of the three main causes of death in children and is found in over 100 countries. It is best prevented by destroying breeding sites, killing adult mosquitoes and preventing mosquitoes from biting. Community-wide control measures use a variety of methods suitable for each particular situation. Project, community and government must work in close partnership. The use of insecticide-treated bed-nets, especially those that are long lasting are a vital part of control.

CHWs and health clinics need to work in unison to develop effective ways of recognising and treating malaria, especially amongst children under five and pregnant women. Mild cases can be treated by CHWs in the community, or by mothers at home; severe cases must be recognised promptly, treated and referred without delay. We should follow national programme guidelines, or those from the IMCI or RBM, ideally using drugs currently recommended in the country we are working in.

Further reading and resources

The most useful information on topics in this chapter are found on the following websites
1. www.who.int/child-adolescent-health. This and other linked sites give information on the Integrated Management of Childhood Illness.
2. www.rbm.who.int. This is the website of Roll Back Malaria
3. www.healthlink.org.uk/pubs.html. This website has back copies of a large number of publications on diarrhoea and acute respiratory infection in addition to regional newsletters on these topics.
4. www.rehydrate.org is a valuable website on the treatment of childhood diarrhoea, including the use of oral rehydration solution.

In addition the following books are useful:
1. *Malaria Vector Control*, J. Nagera and M. Zaim, WHO, 2001.
   A useful book on insecticides.
   Available from: WHO. See Appendix E.
2. *Child Health: A Manual for Medical and Health Workers in Health Centres and Hospitals*, 2nd edn, P. Stanfield (ed.) AMREF, 1999.
   Full details on child health, simply written and relevant for all health programmes.
   Available from: TALC. See Appendix E.
3. *Management of Severe Malaria: a practical handbook*, 2nd edn, WHO, 2000,
4. *Malaria: A Handbook for Health Workers*, Malaria Consortium, Macmillan, 2006.
   Available from Macmillan. See Appendix E.

See Further references and guidelines, pages 413–4.

12

Setting up a Maternal Health Programme

This chapter will include details on antenatal care, delivery care and postnatal care.

1. What we need to know
   - Why maternity care is important
   - Why mothers and newborn babies die
   - What can be done to reduce the deaths of mothers and newborns?
2. What we need to do
   - Prepare the community
   - Set aims and targets
   - Train traditional birth attendants
   - Set up antenatal care
   - Set up delivery (or intrapartum) care
   - Set up postnatal care
   - Keep records
   - Evaluate the programme

What we need to know

Why maternity care is important

The first reason is to prevent the huge number of unnecessary deaths of mothers during pregnancy and childbirth, and long-term complications afterwards. One woman dies each minute in developing countries during childbirth.

Three of the Millennium Development Goals are concerned with what we discuss in this chapter. Goal 4 is to reduce child mortality, Goal 5 is to improve maternal health, and Goal 6 is to combat HIV/AIDS malaria and other diseases (see pages 11–12).

Half a million mothers die each year from causes related to pregnancy, most of which could be prevented. Ninety-nine per cent of these deaths occur in developing countries.

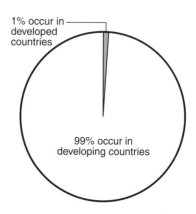

1% occur in developed countries

99% occur in developing countries

Figure 12.1   Maternal deaths

In sub-Saharan Africa, one woman in twelve dies from pregnancy-related causes. A mother in the poorest parts of Asia or Africa is nearly 200 times more likely to die during the births of her children than a mother in many developed countries. Many millions more worldwide suffer from long-term complications, including one million from fistulae causing leakage of urine or faeces from the birth canal, which makes them virtual outcasts.

The second reason is to prevent the unnecessary death of babies at the time of birth, and disability afterwards. Each year there are about one million stillbirths and one million more dying in the first few days, caused largely by the same underlying causes that kill mothers. In addition, one million children per year are left motherless and such children are three to ten times more likely to die within two years than children living with both parents.

More than half of women in Africa and south Asia give birth at home without a skilled attendant. This means that in CBHC we can play a very important role in working at community level to increase the understanding of families, and to use low-tech community based solutions. At the same time we will be wanting to build the capacity of the health care system to bring in more effective long-term solutions.

There is a variety of international initiatives and organisations of which we should be aware (we live in an age when new plans, strategies and initiatives are being set up all the time, frequently changing, merging or being superseded). The first was the Safe Motherhood Initiative in the 1990s, still active. The Making Pregnancy Safer Initiative is a WHO-led programme and is currently the body that forms worldwide strategies, guides countries in their national programmes and is probably the most important group for us to know about in CBHC. We should also be aware of the Integrated Management of Pregnancy and Childbirth (IMPAC), (an equivalent of IMCI) and the Partnership for Maternal, Newborn and Child Health.

However, in CBHC we should always look beyond health activities alone.

For example: In urban areas of east Africa it has been shown that the level of education of the household head relates directly to maternal death rates. So by linking with programmes that help to improve both male and female education, we can save the lives of mothers and newborns.

Why mothers and newborn babies die

Mothers die from a variety of causes:
1. **Haemorrhage** (25 per cent) usually during birth or shortly afterwards. This usually requires treatment within two hours at a health facility, but misoprostol used in the home can save many of these lives (see below).
2. **Infection or sepsis** (15 per cent) usually from unsterile procedures during delivery or from prolonged labour. Antibiotics are necessary.
3. **Unsafe abortion** (13 per cent) usually because of unclean instruments and unhygienic conditions. When abortion is illegal, women are reluctant to seek help.
4. **Eclampsia** (12 per cent) caused by high blood pressure, which leads to fits and, unless carefully treated, to death. This can often be recognised by good quality antenatal care. Magnesium sulphate injections, possible to give at home, can save many lives.
5. **Obstructed labour** (8 per cent) where the womb bursts or the mother dies from exhaus-

tion. This needs early operative delivery and advocacy against the use of oxytocin from untrained practitioners, which makes the problem worse. (See page 252, refs 4 and 5.)

In addition, 20 per cent of deaths occur from diseases that are made worse during pregnancy and delivery, including malaria and TB. Areas with a high level of HIV/AIDS have higher maternal mortality rates. Mothers suffering from anaemia are more likely to die from any of these causes; malaria and iron deficiency are the commonest causes of anaemia in tropical Africa.

Adolescent mothers are twice as likely to die from childbirth as women in their twenties.

Even small increases in average birth weight, e.g. 100 g, greatly reduce neonatal mortality so good nutrition and supplements for underweight and malnourished mothers are important.

Newborn babies die for various reasons:
1. Maternal malnutrition and illness during pregnancy leading to low birthweight babies; twins increase the risk.
2. Complications during delivery including maternal haemorrhage, infection, eclampsia and obstructed labour.
3. Inadequate care and nutrition after birth.

We know that poverty is closely linked with higher maternal and perinatal mortality. The reasons are complex but include the following:
1. Appropriate health care is not available.

> Facilities for the poor are not usually present either when they are needed or where they are needed.

There may be plenty of doctors working in private clinics and larger towns, but their services have very little effect on the overall death rates of mothers and babies. They are largely out of reach of the poor majority because they are too distant and too expensive.
2. Health care that is available is not used. One study from a developing country has shown that 98 per cent of rural women and 85 per cent of urban women failed to use locally available maternity services. There are several possible reasons:

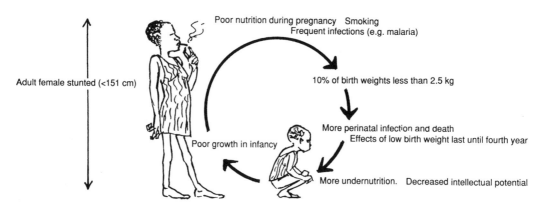

Figure 12.2   Effects of poverty on mothers and infants.

- Pregnancy is considered a natural process that does not require the presence of doctors and clinics.
- Traditional birth attendants and local remedies usually exist, and are preferred.
- Women are busy, with jobs in home, field or factory considered a greater priority than spending half a day visiting a clinic.
- Customs may not allow women to travel when pregnant, nor to see a male doctor.
- Clinics are disliked often because they are too far, too crowded, too frightening and too expensive. Also the quality of care is often perceived to be poor because the staff do not treat the women with kindness and courtesy.
- Transport is inadequate.

> The secret of preventing deaths during pregnancy and delivery is to set up effective community based health care, backed up by quick referral to reliable delivery units.

What can be done to reduce the deaths of mothers and newborns?

We know from evidence that the following activities will help:

1. **Train and deploy skilled birth attendants.**
   Skilled attendants are defined as people with midwifery skills (for example, midwives, doctors and nurses) who have been trained in the skills needed to manage normal deliveries and to diagnose or treat complications due to childbirth.
   SBAs are higher level workers than TBAs, though there is some overlap. The wider use of SBAs is ideal in practice but many of the neediest communities will rely on the use of TBAs for many years to come (see below). The training of SBAs goes beyond the scope of this book.

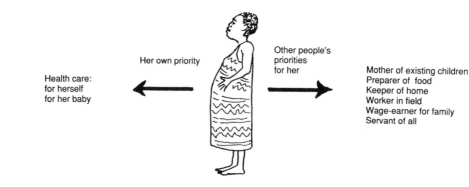

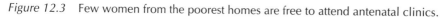

Figure 12.3   Few women from the poorest homes are free to attend antenatal clinics.

2. **Increase access to good quality services.**
   This is perhaps the biggest challenge of all in the neediest communities where death rates are highest. It calls for careful preplanning to make sure that the quickest referral systems possible are in place. This needs to be discussed with the community, who may come up with creative ideas.

3. **Encourage pregnant women to develop a birth plan.**
   We should help pregnant women draw up a plan and to discuss it at home with the decision makers such as husband, mother-in-law, and brother. Together they will need to decide where the birth is to take place, what transport to use either for an emergency, or for a planned referral before delivery so as to be nearer a health centre if this is advised. They will need to set aside costs for transport and other expenses. When pregnant women and their families are able to decide these matters in advance it reduces delays and uncertainty at times at or near delivery, which can be life saving.

4. **Develop the skills and understanding of women, families and the community** through health promotion and education.
   This makes it more likely that women will seek out good quality services both for antenatal care and for delivery. Encouraging and giving guidance on *health seeking behaviour* is at the heart of what our CBHC programme is all about.

5. **Make sure that maternity services are linked in with other aspects of primary care programmes.**
   These linkages should include IMCI, control of sexually transmitted illness, family planning, immunisation, and programmes directed towards people living with HIV/AIDS.

> It should be obvious from the first part of this chapter that effective community based programmes can significantly reduce deaths of mothers and newborns. This will depend on excellent training and good management, helped by the use of new drugs and technologies that are appropriate at community level.

For example: a study in rural India showed a 62 per cent reduction in neonatal mortality through a community based approach that included training of TBAs and local women to treat sick newborn infants at home.

What we need to do

Prepare the community

> Because care of the mother during pregnancy is not usually a felt need in poor communities, we must help the community understand that the good health of mothers and babies will benefit the whole family, including the husband.

The key to bringing this about will be raising awareness of health issues connected with childbirth, and the actions that families and communities can take.

Some of this will occur before starting the programme. We will discuss ideas and draw up plans with community leaders and representatives.

Awareness will also grow after the programme begins. As traditional birth attendants (or CHWs) are trained and mother and baby clinics are set up, mothers will start using them and come to understand their value.

Set aims and targets

Our overall aim will be to reduce the number of maternal and perinatal deaths in the target population. (A maternal death is a death from a pregnancy-related cause either during the pregnancy or within 42 days of the end of the pregnancy; perinatal deaths comprise stillbirths and deaths of the newborn within seven days of delivery.)

Our targets will be to establish:

1. **Antenatal care (care during pregnancy).**
   To increase the number of women receiving at least four check-ups during pregnancy (this is the official WHO target).

2. **Delivery care (or intrapartum care).**
   To increase the number of deliveries being attended by a skilled attendant or a trained traditional birth attendant or CHW.

To make sure that whoever attends the delivery uses a sterile delivery kit.

3. **Referral services.**

   To do all things within our power to set up speedy referral to health centres that can provide essential obstetric care (EOC), see page 249.

4. **Postnatal care.**

   To increase the number of women having at least two checks in the clinic or community for care and advice.

Specific targets for each of the above must be realistic for the populations we are serving. An example might be for 50 per cent of mothers to receive four or more antenatal appointments within three years, 80 per cent within five years. We should add these into our logframe (page 101).

Train traditional birth attendants

Most communities have TBAs, and some CHWs will serve as TBAs. With careful training and upgrading they can become effective primary health midwives, assisting most births in the mothers' homes. They can also carry out some antenatal and postnatal care. However, TBAs are often not sufficiently trained to carry out some of the antenatal activities we know can be most effective, such as giving tetanus immunisation. Unless carefully trained, they may not be able to recognise anaemia or distribute the antimalarials that are recommended in areas where malaria is common.

TBAs can have a major role in areas where HIV/AIDS is common in sharing information, arranging Voluntary Counselling and Testing (VCT), and helping to supervise the use of anti-retrovirals for mothers and infants where the mother is HIV positive.

As more skilled attendants are trained and functioning near or in communities, the role of the TBA may gradually change from being the main front-line worker to carrying out more of a support role in the community. Probably only very few TBAs will have the skills and background to enable them to be trained as SBAs.

However, we must realise that in the poorest and most traditional communities TBAs are likely to have a key front-line role for many years to come.

For example: In Yemen, the lowest income country in the Arabian peninsula, where the maternal mortality rate is estimated at 850/100 000 births, virtually all home deliveries are attended by TBAs whose skill upgrading is a high priority.

What are the characteristics of TBAs?

1. They live in or near the community and are usually available when needed.
2. They are usually older women, often of low social status, though in many communities highly respected.
3. Their skills are traditional, learnt from other TBAs – often their mothers or mothers-in-law.
4. Until trained they carry out little antenatal care and have poor understanding of hygiene.
5. They assist at births by advice (often strongly expressed), and through various interventions, some of which may not be appropriate.
6. They are usually rewarded by gifts or small cash payments.
7. Another important point to be aware of is that TBAs are often reluctant to transfer women when there are problems in labour because of their fear of criticism. This will be an important area on which to focus our training.

What should be the function of trained TBAs?

In an ideal situation, they will assist and work alongside skilled attendants. However, in many situations they will continue to be the only people with training who attend the delivery or can give antenatal and postnatal care.

In practice they will carry out or assist in:

1. Antenatal examinations (see page 242).
2. Deliveries in order to:
   a) encourage and instruct the mother;
   b) monitor the progress of labour;
   c) recognise danger signs early and refer quickly;
   d) assist the delivery of the baby;
   e) assist the delivery of the placenta and check it is complete;
   f) cut the cord using a sterile blade, and tie with a clean cord tie;

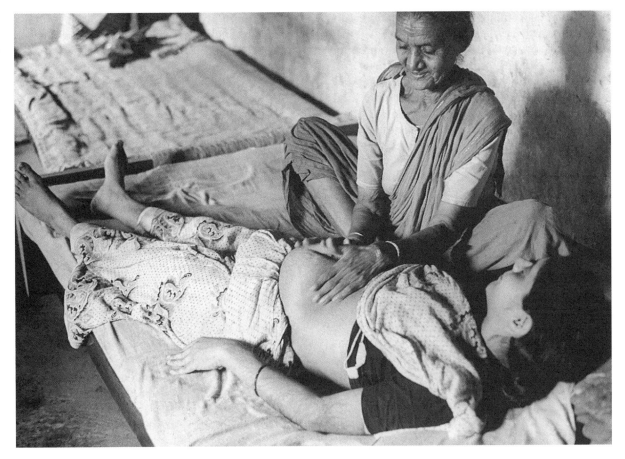

Figure 12.4   Traditional birth attendants still continue to have a vital role in poor communities.

g) care for the newborn by:
   - drying, keeping warm and giving any necessary first aid;
   - putting to the mother's breast to suck colostrum;
   - simple resuscitation measures;
   - working with other health team members to ensure the child has its first polio immunisation within 24 hours or as soon after as possible and ideally its BCG vaccination. In practice this will often be difficult to do at home. (Latest guidelines from IMPAC are now suggesting to delay the first hepatitis B immunisation until 6 weeks.)

h) when appropriately trained, offer HIV prevention services and help with antiretroviral prophylaxis for HIV positive mothers and their infants.

i) care for the mother by:
   - making sure she is comfortable;
   - making sure the bleeding is controlled.

In carrying out these activities she will use the sterile delivery kit and ensure she has:
a) clean hands – washed with soap and water after taking off all rings;
b) clean cutting and tying of the umbilical cord;
c) clean surfaces – she will place clean cloths under the mother and baby.

3. Carry out postnatal care (see page 250).

We should encourage village health committees and women's groups to work with and support the work of TBAs.

For example: In one area of Nepal, trained female facilitators work with a village development committee to help with problems through pregnancy, delivery and the newborn period. This is based on improving what is known as essential newborn care: hygiene of mother and child, simple home-based resuscitation of the newborn, keeping the child warm, early breastfeeding and strengthening the bond between mother and baby. This carefully planned programme is being assessed to see how far it will reduce maternal and newborn deaths and illness. (See page 415, second Osrin ref.)

What should TBAs be taught?

Teaching should cover all the listed functions as well as basic delivery techniques.

Training manuals are available in many countries and should be adapted and used.

How should TBAs be trained?

The trainer can be a nurse, midwife, skilled attendant or any female member of the health team with practical experience in delivering babies. Doctors can be called in to teach selected lessons.

In practice TBAs will often be taught by the same person who teaches the CHWs.

The timing of training should be coordinated with the rest of the community health programme. Normally a CHW training programme is a higher priority than the training of TBAs.

The location should be the nearest place to the community that has sufficient deliveries to make teaching worthwhile. Often this will be a health centre or small hospital. Alternatively, basic teaching can be given in the community and extra practical sessions can be arranged. Community-based visits must always be part of any training programme.

If training is done in hospitals by nurses or doctors, we need to make sure that TBAs do not start trying to adopt complicated methods or expect to use special equipment unsuitable for a delivery at home.

Remember that the purpose of training TBAs is to enable them to deliver babies as safely as possible in their communities using the simplest equipment.

The duration of training might total 30 days. This can either be given in a single 30-day term, in several separate blocks, or one day per week over a period of time. An alternative is to give seven days together, followed by a weekly training day, until the course is complete. Many TBAs will find it hard to leave their communities for more than a few days at a time.

TBAs should be given thorough examinations, especially in practical procedures and methods of referral and only then should they be 'accredited' by the project. They will also need continuing development of their skills.

Ways of ensuring successful TBA programmes

Although many TBA programmes are working well and reducing mother and child deaths, others have not been so successful. As a result many countries are putting more effort into training skilled attendants (see above).

But because TBAs continue to have an essential role in most poor communities we need to make sure they are trained and used as effectively as possible. Here are some pointers taken from a variety of projects, which may help to make programmes more effective:

- **Appropriate women must be chosen.** As maternity services gradually improve we will need health workers with more education and training than in the past. There is a conflict here because TBAs are deeply embedded in their communities and their roles and skills are often passed down in families. Outsiders should be reluctant to interfere with this and get involved in selection. However, where younger TBAs are available for training, it gives us a greater opportunity to develop their skills more effectively.
  For example: in Bangladesh the government officially ended TBA training in 1998 and switched to training skilled birth attendants. But most SBAs still come from the lower skill bracket and are typically aged between 21 and 45 with appropriate levels of education.
- **The services of trained TBAs must be wanted.** The people themselves should request the use

of TBAs and be happy with their further training, often by being helped to realise that mothers (and newborns) die unnecessarily. We can help this process by creating awareness of the TBA's value and how the community will benefit.

- **Relationship with the community should be defined.**
  If a CHW is being selected whose functions will include working as a TBA, make sure the community selects an appropriate person, fully understands their function (usually quite different from the community's understanding of what they think the TBA should do) and agrees about methods of payment or reward.

- **Appropriate training must be arranged.**
  This needs to be kept simple and practical with short, interactive training sessions. Many TBAs are illiterate especially when first selected.

- **Support and affirmation from project staff is necessary.**
  TBAs must be fully accepted by the health team, treated with dignity and respect and included in wider health activities if they wish to be and have the time.

- **Regular and reliable supervision is essential.**
  A trained midwife (ideally the TBA's trainer) or person of equivalent ability will need to make regular visits, ideally every month and at least every three months, to the TBA in her community. This should be mainly to give training, support and encouragement. Where this is not possible, TBAs may be willing to travel to the health facility and collect supplies of delivery kits and at the same time to have a training update.

- **Regular update is required.**
  Programmes that start with enthusiasm often run down, skills are lost and the community loses interest. We must ensure that the knowledge and skills of TBAs are regularly updated, especially as many will only carry out a few deliveries and rarely see complications.

- **Literacy training is an advantage.**
  Becoming literate empowers TBAs, CHWs (and mothers) to be more effective carers. However, many TBAs will find literacy training difficult because of their age.

How should delivery kits be organised?

Why is a kit necessary?
Infection of the mother's birth canal and infection of the baby's umbilicus are common causes of death or illness. The main purpose of the sterile delivery kit is to make these infections less likely.

What should a delivery kit contain?
- Soap and a nail brush or nail sticks.
- Gloves.
- Antiseptic solution and cotton wool.
- A small metal or plastic bowl.
- Two clean sheets or towels – one to place under the mother, another on which to place the delivery kit.
- A sterile razor blade for cutting the cord.
- Cord ties (three sterile pieces of cotton).
- Clean gauze to cover the stump.
- String to wrap around the cord dressing.
- A simple set of instructions.

How should kits be used and replaced?
There are various ways this can be done. Here are some examples:

1. The TBA is given a separate prepacked kit for each delivery.
   This works well where the TBA/CHW does only a small number of deliveries, e.g. fewer than 20 per year. In some areas UNICEF or other agencies provide these kits.

2. The TBA is equipped with a delivery box containing reusable items, including delivery kits.
   This system is only likely to work for those TBAs, CHWs or other health workers who have been thoroughly trained, carry out at least 20 deliveries per year, and are carefully supervised.
   Experienced TBAs can make up their own kits, cleaning reusable items, and obtaining expendable and sterile items from the health centre or project stores. Less experienced TBAs can collect prepacked delivery kits from the project. The delivery box might contain the following:

   - Fetal stethoscope.
   - Fundal height measurer.

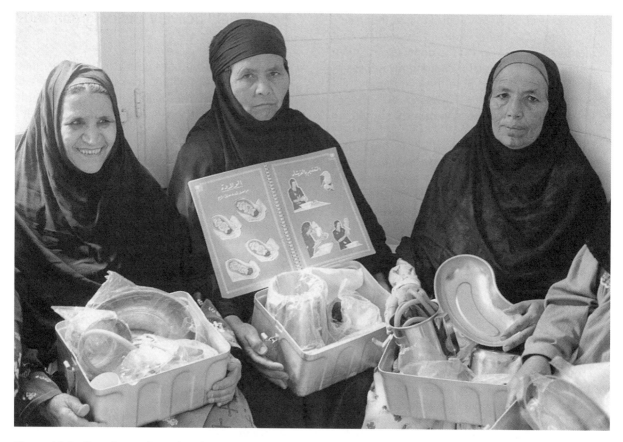

Figure 12.5   Egyptian traditional midwives with their new delivery kits.

- Tubular scales for weighing the newborn or a mid-upper arm circumference (MUAC) measurer.
- Bowls for swabbing perineum; antiseptic.
- Forceps and scissors.
- Clean cloth or towel for the newborn.
- Nail file.
- Gentian violet, paracetamol, ergometrine.
- Full course of antibiotics.
- 15 cm pot for boiling supplies.
- Gloves.
- One or more prepacked delivery kits.
- Stationery and record cards.

TBAs can also help the mother prepare her own similar kit, making sure the ties, gauze and blade are sterile.

3. The mother is given a simple delivery kit. This is useful where relatives do the delivery, where there is no TBA or where the home is remote. The mother collects or buys a kit from the clinic at not later than 36 weeks, being instructed what to do with it.

4. Kits are sold in the market or other retail outlets. This method has been used successfully in parts of rural Bangladesh, and in some other countries.

Set up antenatal care

In this section we shall look at:
- The purpose of antenatal care
- Clinic or community?
- Selecting a Home-based Record Card
- Seeing patients in the clinic
- Caring for those with At-Risk Factors (ARFs)
- Preventing neonatal tetanus

The purpose of antenatal care

Recent figures show that over the past ten years the number of women receiving antenatal care in Asia and Latin America has increased, but in most countries of sub-Saharan Africa there has been little change.

WHO recommends women should ideally have at least four antenatal visits. Here are some important reasons:

- Health promotion: for advice on nutrition and health care: counselling on danger signs in the pregnancy, preparing for a safe delivery and caring for the newborn.
- Assessment by health worker: history, examination and screening tests to discover early warning signs that alert us to extra care or action needed, including referral for delivery.
- Prevention: to give nutritional advice and supplements, manage complications, prevent malaria with intermittent preventive treatment (IPT), and insecticide treated bed-nets, and to give tetanus toxoid injections.
- To develop a birth plan (see page 237).
- Treatment: to treat anaemia, sexually transmitted illness and other serious conditions.
  Where HIV is common, encouragement of women to come forward for voluntary counselling and testing (VCT) and to start on anti-retroviral therapy when needed to lower the risk of mother to child transmission. Each year over half a million infants become infected with HIV from their mothers.

Clinic or community?

This depends on the closeness of the clinic, the presence of any skilled attendant and the training of the TBA. Ideally, pregnant women should attend the clinic monthly from the fifth month, and more often in the last three months, if At-Risk Factors (ARFs) are present (see page 246). Well trained TBAs can carry out some of these checks in the community. She would refer to the clinic any women with ARFs.

Most clinics will see mothers at any time when they are open, which may be daily, weekly or monthly in the case of remote areas or mobile clinics. Clinics serving larger populations may run separate antenatal clinics on certain days.

Selecting a Home-based Record Card (HRC)

We will need to choose or design an HRC according to these guidelines:

- It should be easy to use, able to record key information accurately, and be in an appropriate language and style. WHO has designed a prototype record that can be adapted. It details previous pregnancies on one side (Figure 12.6) and the present pregnancy on the other (Figure 12.7).
- Ideally it should have ways of highlighting at-risk patients.
- It should be the right size and shape so mothers can carry it conveniently and bring it for all examinations – by TBA, skilled attendant, in clinic, health centre or hospital. Ideally it should be kept in a plastic envelope.
- A duplicate card can be kept in the family folder for clinic records (or key details can be copied into a register).
- If much of the care will be done by illiterate TBAs, we can design cards using symbols instead of writing. An example is given in Figure 12.8.

Please note: it is essential that any HRC used is adapted so it is appropriate for our community. Some governments have introduced adapted HRCs, and these will often be the cards we should use.

Seeing patients in the clinic

The simplest way of doing this is to link the examination of the pregnant woman with the sequence on the record card. However, our purpose is to give high quality care not just complete a form. As each stage is reached the clinic worker passes on health information or advice, for example on the best foods to eat and any supplements needed.

1. At first attendance, the registrar fills in name, number and address of patient.
2. At first attendance, the health worker (HW) does the following:
   - Completes age, height and previous history.

Name _____

Address _____

_____

Date of first visit _____

Age	18-35	below 17	above 35
Height		more than 145 cm	less than 145 cm

Previous history

Number of deliveries	1	2	3	4	0	5 or more
Abortions	no					yes
Oedema	no					yes
Fits	no					yes
Stillbirths	no					yes
Abnormal deliveries	no					yes
Excess vaginal bleeding after delivery	no					yes
Labour lasting more than 24 hours	no					yes
Low birth weight (less than 2500 g)	no					yes
Death of child during first week	no					yes

Other health problems:

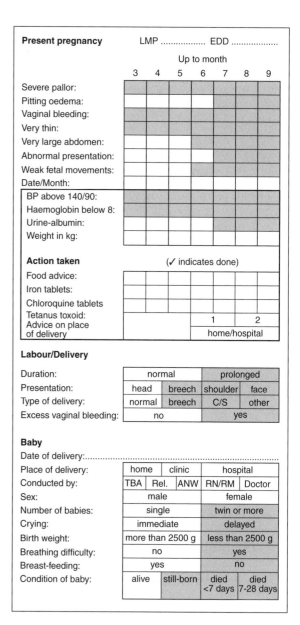

Figure 12.6 The WHO prototype home-based maternal record: Mother's health record (Side 1). Adapted from Chapter 1 of *Home-based Maternal Records: guidelines for development, adaptation and evaluation*, Geneva: WHO, 1993.

Figure 12.7 The WHO prototype home-based maternal record: present pregnancy (Side 2). Adapted from Chapter 1 of *Home-based Maternal Records: guidelines for development, adaptation and evaluation*, Geneva: WHO, 1993.

- Completes relevant parts of section on present pregnancy – date of Last Menstrual Period (LMP), Expected Date of Delivery (EDD).

3. At first and all other attendances the HW:
- Weighs the patient.

- Takes blood pressure.
- Checks urine for sugar and protein.
- Arranges blood tests. These may include haemoglobin (Hb) if there is a way to measure it, and a malaria slide, VCT where HIV/AIDS is common or concerns are

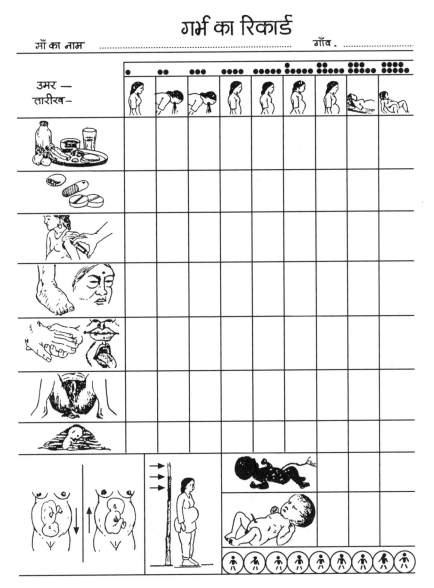

Figure 12.8   Pictorial home-based maternal record from Chandigarh, India. Adapted from *Home-based Maternal Records: guidelines for development, adaptation and evaluation*, Geneva: WHO, 1993.

raised, and tests for other relevant problems or locally important illnesses. Treatment for intestinal worms, e.g. albendazole 400 mg, has been used successfully in one programme (unsafe in first trimester).

• Records details on HRC. This will include placing a tick, if any conditions are present, in the shaded boxes that represent at-risk factors.

4. Skilled attendant, e.g. nurse, midwife, or other trained health worker:
   • examines patient for any other pregnancy-related problems, and other illnesses, including sexually transmitted illness.
   • completes further entries on HRC including Action taken box.
   • gives teaching and reassurance on: correct feeding and nutrition (page 179); how to

keep healthy during pregnancy; preparing for the delivery; the need for regular check-ups; future needs for family planning (Chapter 13) and the importance of breast-feeding (page 180).

- arranges Tetanus Toxoid if due, gives iron and folic acid and any other medicines needed.
- gives a delivery kit if this is project policy.
- follows WHO's recommendation, where there is a high level of malaria, of using inter-mittent preventive treatment (IPT), most commonly sulfadoxine/pyrimethamine (SP) as single doses at not less than monthly intervals starting in the second trimester of the first and second pregnancies. See also page 232.
- counsels the mother if she is HIV positive about the use of antiretroviral therapy both for herself and the newborn. Options for breastfeeding or the use of infant formula are also discussed with her. Ideally infant formula is available if the HIV positive mother opts to use it. We need to make sure this is done sensitively so as not to infer to other clients that those using formula are likely to be HIV positive.

For time-saving and convenience at all attendances ensure that:

1. Pregnant women are able to sit down at each clinic station and that waiting is kept to a minimum.
2. Weights, blood pressure, urine and blood tests, are taken before the woman sees the health worker or trained attendant.
3. Packets of iron and folic acid tablets, prefer-ably as a combined preparation, are pre-counted and handed out by the health worker, not the dispenser.
4. Charges are kept as low as possible so that the poor can easily afford the services.
5. Health teaching is given to waiting patients.
6. Preparations are ready for unexpected deliveries.

For further details on clinics see Chapter 8.

Caring for those with At-Risk Factors (ARFs)

What is the importance of ARFs?

Most health problems are found in a small minority of pregnant women. We can usually predict which women are more likely to have problems by our observations at antenatal checks. Features known to be connected with difficulties at the time of birth are known as ARFs.

This can be a useful approach from the view-point of identifying at-risk individuals in our community and targeting extra care for them. *But, in practice, as many problems at the time of birth will occur in the majority with no ARFs as in the minority with obvious ARFs, because so many problems are not easy to predict.* This means we need to be vigilant in the care of our whole maternal population especially near or at the time of delivery.

This is one main reason why policies have shifted towards the training of skilled attendants in preference to that of risk screening and TBA training. However, the ARF approach is still valuable in the poorest communities where skilled attendants are likely to be beyond reach for many years.

> By targeting our care towards those with ARFs we will bring quicker benefits. In addition, we will save the time of patients and health workers and reduce expenses of the project.

How do we discover important ARFs in our project area?

Some ARFs are found everywhere, others may be specific to our target population. We can discover important ARFs in two ways:

1. Before starting the project by learning from the experience of doctors and midwives working in nearby hospitals and health projects. We can also question local TBAs.
2. After the project starts by gathering our own information.

We should try to include in this category only those pregnancies that are most at risk. This means that, as a guide, we need to define the 20 per cent of pregnancies most at risk and target care towards them.

WHO's list of At-Risk Factors

The following factors have generally been found to increase a woman's risk of developing serious complications during delivery, which may put her or her child at serious risk. ARFs are shaded in the prototype record cards in Figures 12.6 and 12.7.

- She weighs 38 kg or less before pregnancy.
- She weighs 42 kg or less at the eighth month of pregnancy.
- She gains less than 1 kg a month after the fifth month of pregnancy.
- She is less than 145 cm tall.
- She is less than 18 or more than 30 years of age when she has her first pregnancy.
- She has a history of abortion or stillbirth during a previous pregnancy.
- Her previous child died within one month of birth.
- Her previous delivery was by Caesarean section.
- She has given birth to 4 or more children previously.
- She has swollen legs during pregnancy.
- There is a possibility she may have twins.
- She has high blood pressure.
- In addition, known or probable HIV infection is an ARF.

How do we care for those with ARFs?

This group of women needs the following extra care over and above routine antenatal care already described:

1. Regular checks in the clinic, preferably once per month and more often in the last few weeks. This should include examination by a skilled attendant, e.g. a doctor, nurse or midwife.
2. Regular visits in the community by the TBA or CHW, who will keep a list in her book of all those known to have ARFs.
3. Early referral to a hospital or health centre for supervised delivery where there is a high risk of complications during delivery, e.g. there has been a previous ruptured uterus or there is a Caesarean section scar.

For example (1): Some countries, including Cuba, Ethiopia and Nicaragua, have been setting up a network of maternity waiting homes, located near hospitals. Here, women with ARFs from remote areas are referred a month before the delivery is due. As labour starts they are easily transferred to the nearby hospital.

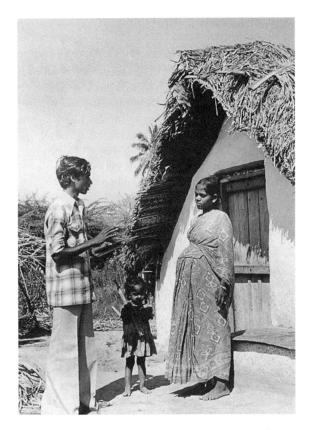

Figure 12.9   CHW advises a mother on antenatal care.

For example (2): Malaysia has set up community birth centres attached to health clinics. Here mothers with ARFs wait in units with four to six beds, which are staffed by experienced midwives with doctors available. Most deliveries occur in the centre, but those with serious complications can be transferred to a nearby hospital.

> We must do everything possible to reduce complications during delivery by the following methods:
> - Refer early any patient with At-Risk Factors.
> - Set up the quickest transport system possible for immediate referral, to use when serious complications develop.
> - Ensure the referral centre sees patients without delay.
>
> Quick referral is the most effective way of reducing mother and child deaths at the time of delivery.

Prevent neonatal tetanus

What is neonatal tetanus (NNT)?

This is a disease that kills nearly half a million babies each year, though this number is falling.

All forms of tetanus cause muscles to contract so that breathing becomes impossible. Germs enter the body through wounds and in newborn babies through the umbilical cord. Traditional dressings often contain tetanus germs.

Infected babies go through these stages:

- They are healthy at birth.
- At 3–5 days after birth they stop sucking and close their mouths.
- At 5–8 days they go stiff, have fits and die.

Preventing NNT by tetanus toxoid injections

1. **The best time to do it:**
   Antenatal checks offer the best opportunity. However:

> Many mothers at greatest risk will not come to antenatal clinics. This means that Community Health Programmes should offer tetanus immunisations to girls and young women of childbearing age at every possible opportunity.

Such opportunities will include:
- During childhood – as part of DPT;
- During school years – as TT, or combined Tetanus and adult Diptheria (Td);
- Whenever a woman of childbearing age attends any clinic or hospital for any reason;
- During national or district immunisation days.

2. **The number of injections needed:**
   Follow any official national and regional guidelines. If not available or in doubt we can follow this schedule:
   - During the first pregnancy two injections of 0.5 ml intramuscular into the upper outer arm, at least one month apart, the first any time after the third month of pregnancy, the second at least four weeks before the EDD;
   - A booster dose during each further pregnancy up to a total of five injections;
   - If records prove three previous doses of DPT, TT or Td have been given earlier, give one single dose of TT or Td during pregnancies, up to a total of two TT or Td injections.

3. **Possible side effects.**
   There may be pain, firm swelling and redness for up to three days. This is not serious and needs no treatment. Later injections tend to give a greater reaction than earlier ones.

4. **Storage of TT and Td.**
   As for DPT (see pages 198–200).

5. **Recording of TT.**
   This should be done:
   - On the Home-based Record Card (HRC) and any duplicate if a family folder system is used, (see page 86).
   - In a clinic register or, if the project is computerised, on a Due List or computer-generated record for later data entry onto the computer.
   - Possibly onto a separate Tetanus Immunisation Card.
   - Onto the new baby's Growth Card when this is prepared.

Preventing NNT by other measures

- By clean practices during delivery.
- By cutting the umbilical cord with a sterile blade or razor.
- By placing a dry, sterile dressing on the stump, or by applying chlorhexidine 5% solution.
- By making sure that no traditional dressing, dung or ash is put on the stump.

These measures alone, even in the absence of TT injections, can be very effective.

For example: In Rwanda, NNT has been almost eliminated. This has occurred through the twin approach of high TT coverage and more hygienic delivery practices, including care of the umbilical stump.

Set up delivery (or intrapartum) care

Birth is the most dangerous time of life both for mother and child. The purpose of good delivery care is to make birth as safe as possible for both.

WHO recommends a skilled attendant should be present at every birth who can:

- provide continuing good quality care that is hygienic, safe and sympathetic.

- recognise and manage complications, and carry out life-saving measures for mother and baby.
- refer promptly and safely where necessary and without delay. This involves preplanning quick methods of referral, and making sure each pregnant women has a birth plan.

> An essential part of any maternity programme is an emergency referral system, which both TBAs and CHWs know how to operate with the minimum of delay.

There is no way skilled attendants can be present at birth in many of the poorest communities. Although this should be our eventual aim as we help to build capacity, we need to ensure that TBAs, CHWs, women's groups and village health committees work together to ensure the best possible care is available with the resources we have.

Where should the birth take place?

1. In the mother's home.
   This can be appropriate providing conditions are clean and a sterile delivery kit is used. It is the only place most mothers in the world's poorest countries are able to afford.
2. In a TBA delivery unit.
   In some areas and programmes TBAs conduct deliveries in their own home or informal units rather than that of the woman. We need to make sure any such site has been checked in advance and we have worked with the TBAs in making conditions as clean and appropriate as possible.
3. In the health centre or hospital.
   Mothers with At-Risk Factors should be referred in advance for a hospital or health centre delivery. Those developing problems before or during birth should be referred as emergencies.

A referral centre should ideally be able to provide essential obstetric care (EOC) (see Figure 12.10).

Who should assist at the birth?

Deliveries where possible should be carried out by skilled attendants. If this is not possible, trained TBAs or CHWs can carry out home deliveries. Skilled attendants are a good choice for health centres, but doctors should only be involved in the management of difficult births or complications.

In some communities, mothers, mothers-in-law or relatives do deliveries. Where possible, TBAs should be trained to replace them. In these situations any person likely to attend the delivery should be given training by the project. The mother should previously have been given a sterile delivery kit, with an explanation about how it should be used. She should also have drawn up a birth plan.

How should the delivery be carried out?

With skill and compassion. In homes with good hygiene using a sterile delivery kit. In health centres with skilled attendants, hygienic conditions, adequate equipment and where appropriate the use of a partograph to identify problems in labour.

There is evidence that better results are obtained where a woman has the continuous support throughout her labour of an attendant whom she trusts.

> **WHO's list for essential obstetric care**
>
> The list includes:
> Facilities for surgery and anaesthesia
> Use of intravenous oxytocin
> Medical treatment for disorders related to delivery
> e.g. shock and sepsis
> Safe blood transfusions
> Safe manual procedures
> Monitoring of labour
> Management of problem pregnancies
> Manual vacuum aspiration
> Special care for neonates.
>
> (We should also include the use of misoprostol and magnesium sulphate, available in the community, see page 250.)

Figure 12.10

Some life-saving activities are easy to carry out even at local level. *For example*: the use of injectable magnesium sulphate halves the rates of mothers dying from eclampsia; the use of miso-prostol greatly reduces deaths from postpartum haemorrhage. However, the use of these needs to be carried out in the context of local training and following careful protocols. We should ask a specialist to help guide us in their use at community level. (See below and Further reading and resources.)

All deliveries, especially in regions where HIV is frequent, must be carried out using gloves. Training must be given to all staff involved in deliveries about minimising their risk of becoming infected with HIV.

How should the delivery be recorded?

By the person carrying it out filling in details on the Home-based Record Card under the sections 'Labour/Delivery' and 'Baby'.

On the Family Folder Insert Card, Register or other system used by the project.

Set up postnatal care

For postpartum (postnatal) care, WHO recommends integrated care that includes the following:

- Identification and management of problems both in the mother and in the newborn.
- Counselling, information and services for family planning.
- Health promotion for mother and newborn, including immunisation, nutrition, advice on breastfeeding and safer sex.

Many women die after birth because of infection or blood loss. Blood loss is the commonest cause of maternal death, nine out of ten within four hours of delivery. Many children die after birth because of poor feeding practices, infection, ignorance, neglect and neonatal tetanus (NNT) – also from hypothermia as a result of poor practice, including bathing newborn babies and failing to wrap them up in warm enough coverings. (A thermospot temperature indicator is now available from TALC.)

In many traditional societies, the mother is prevented by custom from leaving her home or community for several days or weeks. For this and other reasons postnatal care usually takes place in the home and by the TBA, CHW or equivalent health worker.

A suggested plan for community postnatal care:

1. **Immediately after the birth the TBA checks the mother and child as part of delivery duties.** She makes sure the uterus remains well contracted and there is no excessive blood loss. She ensures the newborn is breathing well and is comfortable and warm, by being placed next to the mother and with wrapping when not sharing her body heat. She encourages the mother to put the child to the breast within an hour. She discourages the use of early bathing.

   TBAs can also be equipped to provide one new life-saving action. Misoprostol stimulates uterine contractions, prevents death from postpartum haemorrhage (PPH), is safe to use and can be given by trained TBAs and other providers in the home. It is being used in various ways:

   For example: In Tanzania, TBAs are using 1000 micrograms rectally to treat PPH; in the Gambia, women are given 600 mcg to prevent haemorrhage; and in Indonesia, women themselves are given misoprostol to self-administer as soon as the baby delivers.

   The person carrying out the delivery should leave only when she is sure there are no danger signs in mother and baby. She should refer at once if she is concerned, and especially if vaginal bleeding continues.

2. **Within the first 24 hours the TBA sees the newborn:**
   - She checks for obvious abnormalities such as breathing problems, swelling of the stomach, deformity or jaundice.
   - She weighs the baby or measures the mid-upper arm circumference (MUAC).
   - She records details of the birth, on the Home-based Record Card if she is able, or a specially designed chart for illiterate TBAs. Alternatively in her record book or diary.
   - She gives the first polio drops (OPV Zero), and gives or arranges BCG. (See page 286.)

The TBA sees the mother.
- She checks for any fever or continuing blood loss.
- She checks for any feeding problems.
- She discusses any other concerns.

3. **During the next two weeks the TBA visits daily for a few days,** then gradually less often if mother and baby remain well. This may not always be possible where TBAs have a large workload.

During this time she pays special attention to fever and any vaginal loss in the mother, feeding problems, any sign of NNT or other infection in the baby and any other concern of the mother. She discusses family planning and, where relevant, safer sex practices. She advises how other immunisations can be given (see page 195).

If the mother is HIV positive, she can give guidance on using infant formula or help to ensure exclusive breastfeeding, i.e. whichever method the mother has opted for. If mothers or partners are concerned that they might be HIV positive, the TBA can explain when and where VCT is available.

If the community has both a TBA and a CHW, now is the time for the TBA to hand over care for the mother and child to the CHW.

Make sure that the TBA, CHW or other person who attended the delivery passes full details to the relevant project health worker. This ensures that health care for mother and newborn can be properly integrated into the programme.

Keep records

The following records can be kept:
1. **Home-based Record Card (HRC)** (see Figures 12.6 and 12.7).

This is the definitive card on which full details of the pregnancy are recorded. It is used not only during the pregnancy to help patient care, but also as the source of maternity statistics. Mothers should keep the HRC and make sure that any health worker who sees her checks it and enters notes on it – from the first antenatal visit to the last postnatal one. A duplicate or summary can be kept in the family folder.

2. **Record card with symbols** (see Figure 12.8).

This is for use by illiterate CHWs or TBAs. It needs to be purpose-designed for each country and district.

Symbols are used to represent both the factors the TBA needs to check, and any ARFs that are present.

This card is kept by the mother. It may be used in addition to the Home-based Record Card (HRC).

3. **The master register or project computer.**

Details from HRCs, or duplicates kept in the family folder, or from registers or tallies can be entered monthly, or every three to six months.

Evaluate the programme

After an agreed time we will need to evaluate the project to see whether targets are being met.

Here are some useful annual percentages to measure:

1. **Antenatal coverage.**

The percentage of pregnant women who have attended for four or more antenatal checks either in the clinic or with the TBA. All women who have given birth (whether live or still) over a one-year period are eligible (see page 342).

2. **Nutritional status of the newborn.**

The percentage of newborn babies weighing more than 2500 g or having MUACs of 8.7 cm or more.

3. **Supervised deliveries.**

The percentage of births attended by a skilled attendant or by a trained TBA or CHW. The percentage of deliveries where a sterile delivery kit was used.

4. **Maternal tetanus coverage.**

The percentage of women who have had three or more tetanus immunisations (in total throughout her life).

5. **Maternal mortality rates and perinatal mortality** (see pages 237, 343).

We can compare rates at the start of the project with those after three or four years. Only large-scale projects will obtain valid statistics.

The figures needed for these measurements are obtained from HRCs or tallies or via the master register, or project computer.

The results of any evaluation should be shared with the community as a basis for joint planning.

Summary

Many millions of mothers and babies die each year from causes related to childbirth. Nearly all such deaths can be prevented through setting up effective, community-based maternity care backed up by a good referral centre.

The most ideal primary health workers are TBAs and CHWs. They will work in cooperation with clinics to provide antenatal care, delivery and post-natal care. However, deliveries should be carried out by skilled attendants where possible, otherwise by carefully trained TBAS or CHWs.

An important tool to coordinate the care of pregnant women is the Home-based Record Card (HRC). This also identifies those with At-Risk Factors (ARFs) so they can be targeted for extra care. Information from these cards is fed through to the project headquarters and entered on the database for regular evaluations.

Further reading and resources

1. *A Book for Midwives: Care for pregnancy, birth and women's health*, S. Klein, S. Miller and F. Thomson, Hesperian Foundation, 2004.
   A new edition of this outstanding book on all aspects of maternity care. Available from the Hesperian Foundation. See Appendix E.
2. *Primary Mother Care and Population*, M. King, Spiegl Press, Stamford, 2003.
   This can also be downloaded from www.leeds.ac.uk/demographic_ entrapment/.
3. *Home-based Maternal Records*, WHO, 1994.
   An excellent manual to help guide not only recording systems but the coordination and content of maternity programmes.
   Available from: WHO. See Appendix E.

4. *Making Pregnancy Safer* is at www.who.int/ making_pregnancy_safer and see below.
5. The Safe Motherhood Initiative and Partnership for Safe Motherhood and Newborn Health is at www.safemotherhood.org.
6. *Basic Newborn Resuscitation: A Practical Guide*, WHO, 1997.
   Available from: WHO. See Appendix E.
7. *Managing Maternal and Child Health Programmes: A Practical Guide*, WHO, 1997.
   Mainly aimed at the District level but with helpful ideas to improve management in larger programmes.
   Available from: WHO. See Appendix E.
8. *Mother-Baby Package: Implementing Safe Motherhood in Developing Countries*, WHO, 1996.
   Describes ways of implementing 18 simple interventions to reduce mother and child deaths.
   Available from: WHO. See Appendix E.
9. *Training Manual for TBAs*, G. Gordon, Macmillan, 1990.
   A useful and comprehensive guide, but has not been updated.
   Available from: TALC. See Appendix E.
10. *Where Women Have No Doctor: A health guide for women*, A. Burns, R. Lovich, J. Maxwell and K. Shapiro, Macmillan, 1997.
    A comprehensive guide to women's health problems and how to prevent and treat them.
    Available from: TALC. See Appendix E.
11. Basic Delivery Kit Guide, PATH, 2001: a guide for organisations wanting to develop locally based delivery kits.
    Available from PATH, 4 Nickerson Street, Seattle, WA 98109-1699 USA, Website: www.path.org; email: apallat@path.org.
    PATH gives a step-by-step guide to organisations wanting to make up their own delivery kits relevant to the country and community.
    The Making Pregnancy Safer website is also found at www.who.int/reproductive-health/mpr and the information is available on CD for those who do not have good internet access.

Slides

A number of useful slide sets are available from TALC. See Appendix E.

See Further references and guidelines, pages 414–5.

<h1 style="text-align: center;">13</h1>

Setting up a Family Planning Programme

In this chapter we shall consider:

1. What we need to know
   - Why is family planning important?
   - What are the common objections to family planning?
   - What methods can be used?
   - Dual protection – against unwanted pregnancy and against infection

2. What we need to do
   - Decide whether to develop a programme
   - Set aims and targets
   - Prepare the community
   - Ensure supplies
   - Organise a family planning clinic
   - Arrange community-based distribution of supplies
   - A summary of FP stages
   - Include facilities for controlling sexually transmitted infection
   - Evaluate the programme

What we need to know

Why is family planning important?

Family planning is important to reduce world population growth

Many areas of the world are already grossly overcrowded. Currently the world population is about 6500 million, rising by over 70 million each year. Reducing or stabilising population levels through family planning will continue to be a top priority.

Currently only about half the eligible couples worldwide use any form of family planning. Although progress has been made over the past 20 years, this figure is challenging and disturbing. An estimated 105 million married women in the developing world face an unmet need for contraception.

However, recent figures indicate that the average number of children born to families in developing countries has fallen over the past ten years largely because of the success of family planning. In areas with high death rates from HIV/AIDS the number of children born who survive into adult life is also falling. (See page 270, ref. 7.)

> In India alone, 13 million people are added to the population each year meaning that 127 000 new primary schools are needed annually simply to educate the extra children.

When a population is either too large or increasing too fast the following problems are likely to get worse:

1. **Poverty:** there is less money, less food and less space for the poor. The rich remain largely

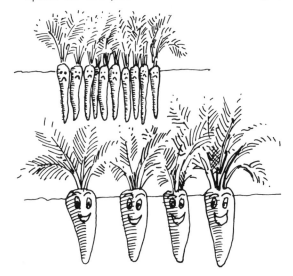

Figure 13.1 Well-spaced children, like well-spaced carrots, grow better.

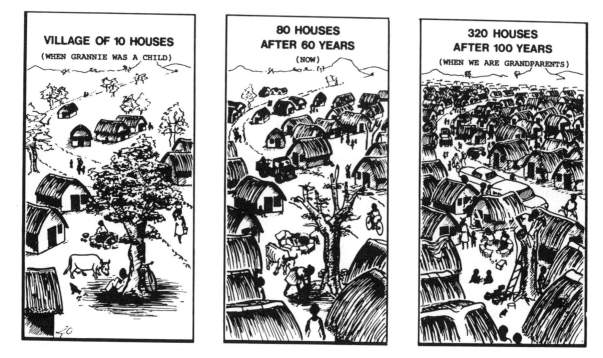

Figure 13.2   Expanding villages.

unaffected. We must remember that the resources of the family have to be shared amongst all the children and often amongst other dependent relatives.

2. **Disease:** overcrowding increases the spread of infection. Existing hospitals and clinics cannot cope with additional patients.
3. **Urbanisation:** cities grow in size rapidly. Overcrowding, lack of sanitation, water pollution and shortage, drug abuse and prostitution become more widespread. AIDS spreads more rapidly. In South America it is estimated that 20 million children live on the streets.
4. **Social breakdown:** overcrowding triggers off a chain reaction: exploitation, injustice, riots and war within countries and between countries.

Family planning is important for each family

Poor families have only limited space, money, food and resources. The more children that are born to them the more likely these children will become seriously ill or die.

Spacing between children is just as important as the total number of children born.

Child spacing leads to healthier mothers:
1. They have fewer children to look after at once, so have more time and energy.
2. They have an opportunity between pregnancies to regain strength and build up their iron stores.

Child spacing leads to healthier children:
1. They have more milk, more food, more love and more attention from their parents.
2. By the time the next child is born, the next youngest has passed the most dangerous age for malnutrition.
3. Healthier children do better in school and so become stronger, better educated adults. They in turn will be able to provide more successfully for their children.

In addition recent research tells us that a short interval between pregnancies makes it more likely that the next child will be born prematurely and that neonatal death is more likely.

Kofi Annan, director general of the United Nations said in Bangkok in 2002:

The Millennium Development Goals, particularly the eradication of extreme poverty and hunger, cannot be achieved until questions of population and reproductive health are squarely addressed. And that means stronger efforts to promote women's rights, and greater investment in education and health including reproductive health and family planning. (See www.unfpa.org.)

The third Millennium Development Goal is to achieve gender equality and to empower women (see page 12).

Important results of this goal lead to women having greater control over their own fertility, and having an equal share with their partner in deciding family size. It also affirms their power to protect themselves against sexually transmitted illness, by negotiating safe sex.

Family planning is important as part of reproductive health

WHO has adopted a strategy on reproductive health that includes antenatal, delivery and post-partum care, high-quality services for family planning, eliminating unsafe abortion, and combating sexually transmitted infections, including HIV.

This has come about because 20 per cent of the burden of illness amongst women in their childbearing years is directly related to sex and reproduction.

For example: the link between family planning and maternal health has been shown in Sayaboury in the Lao People's Democratic Republic. Family planning increased from 12 per cent to 67 per cent over a six-year period and, where contraceptive use is high, maternal deaths have fallen dramatically. (WHO *Bulletin*, 2006; 84: 132–8.)

What are the common objections to family planning?

National objections

Some governments disapprove of family planning (FP) either because they perceive themselves as

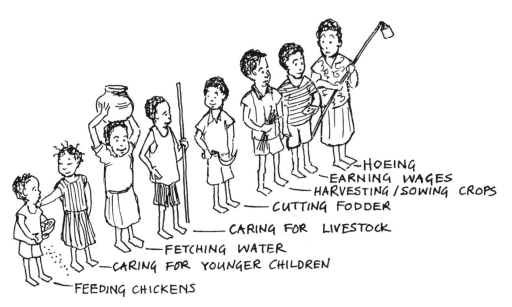

Figure 13.3   The poor person's question: 'How can I afford *not* to have a large family?'

having relatively low populations, or for political or religious reasons. AIDS and other emerging infections will slow or even reverse the rate of population growth in the most affected parts of the world, e.g. sub-Saharan Africa and eventually possibly in south and south-east Asia.

Family objections

Help from children is needed to:
- assist on the farm and in the home;
- earn money;
- look after and provide for older parents and relatives;
- give the family status in the community, and
- carry on the family name, farm or business.

In many cultures boys are valued more than girls, meaning families will increase in size until at least two or three healthy boys are growing up.

Despite these objections, recent data from the World Fertility Survey shows that half of all mothers questioned did not wish to have another baby. This makes the availability of contraceptive services ever more important.

Personal objections

> **Common or moral objections to family planning**
> - What will people think?
> - What happens if my children die?
> - Will my method be reversible?
> - Will I lose my manhood or womanhood?
> - What will happen to my periods?
> - Will my sex life be affected?
> - Will there be side effects?
> - Will my husband be suspicious?
> - Will my partner agree to use FP methods?
> - Will the government force me to use FP?
> - Will it be difficult to get good advice and obtain regular supplies?

Each country, community and couple will have its own questions and objections. Sometimes several minor fears, combined with a reluctance to discuss FP, may prevent a couple seeking advice. We will need to discover and meet these objections.

For example: In Bangladesh, family planning workers have discovered people's real objections by setting up 'focus groups'. These comprise eight to ten people of similar background, with a facilitator who encourages the people to share their ideas and fears. Objections are discovered and ways of overcoming them are suggested by the community.

What methods can be used?
Reasons why birth rates fall

1. As a result of reducing poverty and increasing education.
   This in turn increases the age of marriage and delays the age when couples start having children. Because children are more likely to survive, there is less need to have such large families. Because family income increases, fewer children are needed to carry out household tasks, bring in extra money or act as financial security for old age.

> This means that in the long term tackling poverty helps to reduce population growth.

2. Through increased use of family planning methods.
   Although there are new methods available, few of these are being used, even though the use of family planning has become far more widespread.

HIV/AIDS as mentioned above is reducing the number of children who survive. This is especially true in communities where ways of reducing mother to child transmission are not being used and where antiretroviral therapy is not yet available or too expensive.

> The ideal we are working towards is a massive reduction in deaths caused by HIV/AIDS, twinned with voluntary birth planning and accessible contraceptive services.

Main contraceptive methods

1. **Permanent methods** include vasectomy in the male and tubectomy (tubal ligation) in the female. These are used when no more children are wanted.

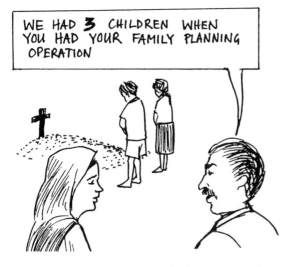

WE HAD **3** CHILDREN WHEN YOU HAD YOUR FAMILY PLANNING OPERATION

Figure 13.4   Permanent FP methods are appropriate only if the couple has **at least 3 healthy children** likely to survive into adult life.

Couples will only accept these methods if there is a high chance that all their existing children will survive to adulthood, and where little stigma is attached to having these procedures carried out.

Many experts argue that too much emphasis is given to these methods, especially for the reasons highlighted in Figure 13.4. We should encourage these methods only in areas with relatively low child mortality and/or in the few areas where a reversal service is easily available.

2. **Long-acting methods** include Norplant or Jadelle (the name for the improved Norplant 2), and copper-coated IUDs in the female. These are used when couples have had children but are not yet ready to use a permanent method. Also when couples wish to delay having children for a number of years. We should be giving more emphasis to these methods.

3. **Temporary or short-acting methods** include all other forms of FP methods. They are used:
   • to delay starting a family;
   • for child spacing;
   • to prevent any further children if the parents are not willing or ready to use a permanent or longer-acting method.

In addition, condoms reduce the spread of sexually transmitted infections, including hepatitis B and HIV/AIDS

Table 13.1 gives a summary of family planning methods.

We need to aim for methods that are as effective and acceptable as possible. *Effectiveness* refers to methods that are as reliable and dependable as possible, with low failure rates. *Examples include*: long-acting contraceptive injections, the latest designs of IUD and Jadelle.

Acceptability refers to methods that are relatively easy to use, free from serious and worrying side effects, and socially acceptable.

For example: Any method that stops or reduces periods may not be accepted by some women. Some Cambodian women believe it darkens their skin, making them less attractive; south Asian women are more concerned that their husbands may consider them unfaithful.

In addition there is value in women using methods where they have control over their own fertility, such as the contraceptive pill or female condom.

Dual protection – against unwanted pregnancy and infection

Certain methods of contraception are increasingly used for two separate reasons: to protect against unwanted pregnancy and to reduce the spread of Sexually Transmitted Infections (STIs), including HIV/AIDS, through the use of barrier methods.

Dual protection is needed if a woman and a man have sexual intercourse, do not want a pregnancy, and at least one of them has been at risk of acquiring HIV or another STI.

Excluding HIV infection and hepatitis B, there are approximately 350 million new cases of STIs worldwide per year. In order of frequency these are: trichomonas, chlamydia, gonococcal infections and syphilis. In addition, over six million new cases of HIV occur annually and this number is increasing rapidly.

This is the dilemma: ideally, methods used should protect against both unwanted pregnancy and infection. Only barrier methods protect against STIs, including HIV infection, but these methods are less effective than most other forms of contraception. In wealthier countries it is often possible to use two methods together, e.g.

Table 13.1   Family planning chart

Method	How	Advantages	Disadvantages	Who for?
Natural (rhythm)	No SI during the fertile days before and after ovulation. Calendar, (SDM)*, temperature and mucus methods help to try to detect those days	1. No supplies 2. No expense	1. High failure rate 2. Needs personal motivation 3. Difficult for those with irregular periods 4. Partner must be cooperative	1. Anyone well motivated 2. Useful for those unwilling to use other methods or with religious objections
Combined o/c pill (COC)	Take pill daily without missing	1. Very reliable if regular 2. SI at any time 3. Regular periods 4. Comparatively few side effects	1. Easy to forget 2. Reduces breast milk 3. Rare dangerous side effects – mainly in women who smoke or are very overweight	Any healthy women under 50 able to remember and not breastfeeding a baby 6 months old or less
Minipill (Progestogen only pill)	Take pill daily without missing	As with COC but periods may be very irregular	1. Easy to forget 2. Slightly less reliable than COC	Best used by women breastfeeding a child 6 months old or less, or above age 45 (otherwise effectiveness low; and bleeding problems)
Long-acting progestogen injectable contraceptive (Depo-Provera, DMPA)	Injection at least every 12 weeks	1. Simple and reliable 2. SI at any time	1. Periods may be irregular 2. May be delay to conceive after finishing	Any woman who prefers it especially if unreliable at remembering COC. Do not use within 6 weeks of child birth if breastfeeding, fine otherwise
Male condom	Rubber sheath placed on erect penis	1. SI at any time 2. Protection against HIV infection and STIs if used with care	1. Not very reliable 2. Some couples, especially men, dislike using them	Main use as barrier protection against HIV infection and other STIs. Pregnancy rate during typical use as sole method is 10–15%, so best used WITH another contraceptive in this Table

*SDM stands for Standard Days Method. Avoid SI on days 8 to 19 of standard cycle.

Table 13.1   Family planning chart (continued)

Method	How	Advantages	Disadvantages	Who for?
Female condom	Place within vagina before SI, with outer ring close against the vulva	1. SI at any time 2. Good protection against HIV and STIs if used with care 3. May be re-used after washing 4. It can increase sexual pleasure	1. Not fully reliable 2. Needs practice inserting	1. As under male condom 2. Women whose partners are unwilling to use male condom, or who want to control their own fertility
Vaginal foam (spermicide)	Foam placed in vagina, which kills sperm. Can be used with condoms	1. Few side effects 2. Easy to use 3. SI at any time	1. Not very effective if used on its own 2. The spermicide nonoxinol 9 should not be used where HIV is common	Any woman not willing or able to use other more reliable methods Any woman uncertain if she is pregnant
Copper-containing IUD	IUD inserted through vagina into uterus, left for 10 years (or, if fitted above age 40, till menopause)	1. SI at any time 2. New forms are as effective as sterilisation	1. Periods may be heavier and more painful 2. May cause anaemia 3. Less suitable for women who have not had children	Women with 1 to 4 children who want to delay having more. Avoid if high risk of pelvic infection or any tenderness, or if anaemic
Norplant subdermal implant or Jadelle (all contain levonorgestrel)	Inserted by trained professionals under the skin of upper inner arm	1. SI at any time 2. Very reliable 3. Can be left in place for 5 years	1. Has to be inserted and removed by health professional under sterile conditions 2 Removal can be difficult 3. Periods may become irregular	Especially useful for those not yet sure if they want sterilisation
Vasectomy	Cutting of male tubes (vas)	1. SI at any time 2. Effective, permanent	1. Occasional post-operative swelling/infection 2. Rarely, persisting scrotal pain	Stable couples with 3 or more children who don't want any more. Men with multiple partners should use barrier methods to prevent infection
Tubectomy or tubal ligation	Cutting of woman's tubes	1. SI at any time 2. Effective, permanent	1. As 1, under vasectomy 2. Significant failure rate	Any woman with 3 or more children definitely not wanting any more children

Table 13.1   Family planning chart (continued)

Method	How	Advantages	Disadvantages	Who for?
Lactational amenorrhoea	The period of low fertility in first 6 months after birth in mothers who exclusively breastfeed and have no bleeding at all	1. SI at any time 2. Quite effective for 6 months, less so from 6–12 months even if still no periods	After 6 months other forms of contraception needed	Those unwilling to use other methods or without access to them. Can be used with barrier method
Emergency contraception ('morning after' pill)	*Either* 2 COCs then 2 more after 12 hours, both doses within 72 hours, but can be up to 5 days of earliest SI, with less effectiveness *or* levonorgestrel 150 μcg all at once within 72 hours but as above can be up to 5 days of earliest SI (more expensive if the marketed product) *or* copper IUD insertion within 5 days – very much more effective, esp. beyond 72 hours and might then be continued as long-term method			

SI = sexual intercourse
A tip for bleeding problems with injections or implants: it may be helpful to try giving women 2 or 3 cycles of any available combined contraceptive pill as well, to give her 2–3 more regular bleeds. Then, when she stops the pill, she may find her bleeding pattern with the original method more acceptable.
STI = sexually transmitted infection (STD, VD)
Other forms of contraception are being used in some areas or being developed further. For example: monthly contraceptive injections, the progesterone vaginal ring, a T-shaped intrauterine system containing levonorgestrel (Mirena), and a monthly oral contraceptive pill widely used in China.

condoms for protection against HIV and the contraceptive pill to prevent unwanted pregnancies. For those in the poorest communities it may be difficult to use more than one method, but it is here that dual protection is most urgently needed.

In practice this means we need to:

- Remember the two possible reasons for using contraceptive methods.
- Think creatively about the best options for the people we advise, understanding the balance of their needs for preventing pregnancy and reducing infection.
- Provide choice wherever this is possible.
- Give skilled counselling to make sure the best options are explained for each couple so they can make an informed choice.

What we need to do

Decide whether to develop a programme

To help decide we must answer these questions:
1. **Is family planning a government policy?**
   Usually this is encouraged. Where it is not we should act cautiously. Where there is coercion we must act with justice.
2. **Is it a felt need in our target area?**
   Do the people actually want it? Have they asked us to provide supplies or arrange sterilisations? If not, we need to create awareness. Although most communities will have couples using some form of contraception, very few will be aware of the range available.

3. Can the programme be sustained?

Trained staff, reliable supplies, good planning, long-term commitment and effective community partnership are needed if the programme is to continue. So, too, is the finance to provide them, or better, a reliable locally available cheap supply.

> Family planning as part of reproductive health services is always a *real* need. In addition, the great majority of individuals and couples need to protect themselves against sexually transmitted infections.

Set aims and targets

These will vary and must be appropriate to the local area.

Here is one suggestion: an eventual aim if this fits in with the wishes of the community is to encourage a family norm of three children, spaced three or more years apart. This will take many years to achieve.

Specific targets for a community with low uptake might be:

1. **Years 0 to 3:**
   - To create awareness so that an increasing number of couples wish to use family planning services.
   - To provide family planning when requested.
   - To set up an effective mother and child programme that will help to stimulate demand.
2. **Year 3 onwards:**
   - To promote family planning more actively.
   - To set an actual target for the project area: *For example*: 30 per cent of eligible couples to have used a permanent method or be regularly using a temporary method after three years, 60 per cent after five years.

In nearly all areas of the world we need to maximise the use of condoms as dual protection both against unwanted pregnancy and to help prevent the spread of HIV/AIDS and other STIs.

A key target therefore will be to see annual increases in the use of condoms to promote safer sex.

These targets are usually incorporated in the logframe (see page 101).

Prepare the community

> An interest in family planning will usually develop when families know that children born to them are likely to survive. Family planning tends to grow naturally as primary health care begins to take effect.

But there will still usually be a need to create further awareness and above all to explain details of methods available.

Uptake and interest can be encouraged through:

- meeting objections through discussion, talking to parents in clinics, and so on;
- working through religious groups, priests or leaders;
- teaching through women's clubs, youth clubs, cooperatives and schools;
- training TBAs and CHWs to be FP motivators and suppliers;
- using national publicity campaigns, in particular radio broadcasts, details of which can be passed on to the community;
- including FP as a subject in literacy courses;
- HIV and STI awareness campaigns;
- the use of local HIV/AIDS support groups or home care teams.

Methods used for teaching must be appropriate for the culture, remove fears, answer questions and underline the many benefits in using FP.

> Benefits from family planning may include: more money, food and space for the family; no more worries about unwanted pregnancies; a better sex life; more peace and quiet at home; fewer dowries to pay.

Ensure supplies

It is better not to start a programme at all, than to start and run out of supplies. Community members must have confidence that repeat supplies are always available.

We should ensure, and if necessary advocate, for dependable supplies to be available locally at a reasonable price.

> Nothing destroys a promising FP programme so successfully as apologies from the health team that supplies have run out.

To ensure supplies:

- Identify two or more sources for each type needed.
- Obtain adequate initial stocks.
- Order well ahead.
- Protect supplies, especially condoms, pills and injections, from spoiling in storage.
- Set up a reliable system for moving supplies from central stores to clinics and other outlets.
- Encourage couples to use locally available good quality supplies often available through social marketing schemes, such as those set up by NGOs like Marie Stopes International.

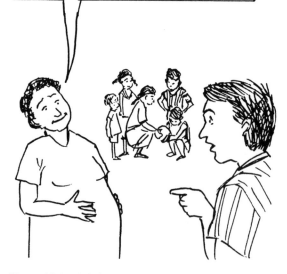

Figure 13.5 It is better not to start a programme at all than to start and run out of supplies.

Organise a family planning clinic

Although some activities, including distribution, take place in the community, the clinic usually remains the focal point of an FP programme.

Should the clinic be separate or combined?

Advantages of FP being part of a general clinic:

1. All health needs are met together, at the same time and the same place. This is especially convenient for patients travelling a long distance.
2. It reduces project time and resources if FP uptake is low.
3. It enables confidential advice to be given to women who may wish to keep their interest secret. (Generally couples, not individuals, should be counselled.)
4. When patients who may be eligible for FP come for other reasons, the need for FP can be raised with them, so increasing uptake.

Advantages of running separate FP clinics (which should always offer sexual health and STI services):

1. Staff can concentrate on family planning rather than trying to provide a range of MCH services as well.
2. Voluntary counselling and testing (VCT) can be offered and STIs can be diagnosed and treated. This can be done in a general or antenatal clinic, but is often best done in an FP context.
3. Equipment and supplies can be easily set up.
4. Family planning can be given the priority it needs. Without a separate clinic it can easily get squeezed out or forgotten because of more immediate needs.
5. Waiting time may be less.
6. Mutual support can be gained from fellow clients, so encouraging uptake.

   When a health centre first starts, a room can be set aside exclusively for family planning activities during an MCH or general clinic. As clinics develop and numbers increase, separate reproductive health, i.e. family planning plus STI clinics, can be considered.

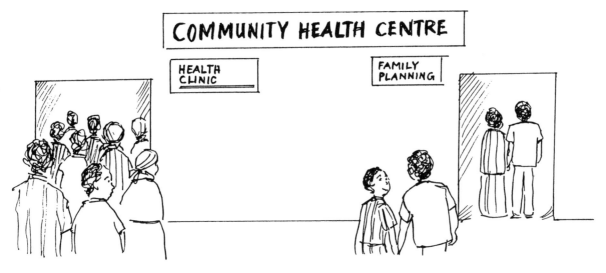

Figure 13.6   Family planning services must be convenient for clients.

WHO is involved in an FP clinic?

1. The Family Planning Provider (FPP), often a nurse who, except in large clinics, will also be in charge.
2. Assistants such as TBAs, CHWs, or responsible community members.
3. The visiting doctor.
   Jobs can include doing tubectomies and vasectomies on prearranged days, advising on difficult cases and giving training and supervision.

In one central African country, guidelines were drawn up about how a Family Planning Provider (FPP) should be selected, trained and used:

1. A member of the health team, usually a woman, is selected and sent for special training in FP.
2. The person chosen is acceptable to the community she will be serving, in terms of gender, age and personality.
3. The training takes place mainly within a well functioning family planning clinic, so that the trainee becomes familiar with all techniques used and advice given.
4. On her return, the FPP carries out family planning sessions at set times each week, during which she is not diverted into other primary health activities. Times of FP sessions are posted outside the clinic and made known to the community.

5. As soon as possible the FPP starts training another member of the health team both to share her work and to substitute when she is absent.
6. She avoids being rushed, trying to allow about ten minutes per patient.

> We must always remember how important it is for men to be involved in family planning, both at the family level and at the community (leadership) level. Our programmes must focus both on their needs and on their responsibilities.

What supplies and equipment are needed?

Supplies will depend on the types of family planning we will be offering (see Table 13.1). Plenty of reserve stocks will be needed in case of heavy demand, and careful storage to ensure supplies do not spoil.

Equipment will be similar to that listed for a community health clinic in Appendix B. If IUDs are used, additional instruments are needed including uterine sound, cervical tenaculum, sponge and artery forceps, curved, blunt and long-handled scissors. In the case of Norplant, doctors will need additional equipment for insertion and removal. Tubectomies and vasectomies will need correct equipment and very great care with hygiene and sterilisation of supplies.

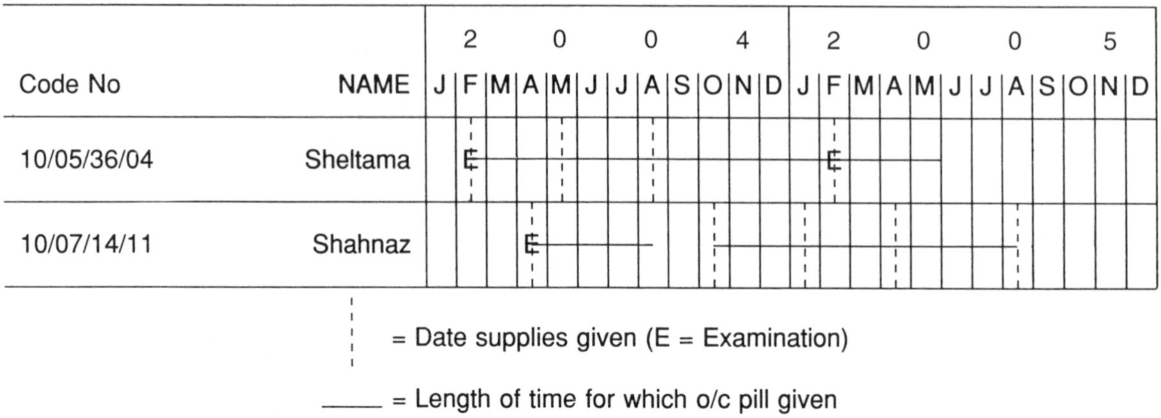

Code No	NAME	2	0	0	4									2	0	0	5								
		J	F	M	A	M	J	J	A	S	O	N	D	J	F	M	A	M	J	J	A	S	O	N	D
10/05/36/04	Sheltama	E												E											
10/07/14/11	Shahnaz			E																					

| = Date supplies given (E = Examination)

_____ = Length of time for which o/c pill given

Figure 13.7 Sample page from oral contraceptive pill section of FP register used in one project.

Instruction sheets for the *provider* on each FP method should be used.

Each sheet will include:

- indications for use;
- method of use;
- any absolute reasons they should not be used;
- any serious side effects;
- instructions to patient;
- type of examination needed if any;
- follow-up;
- treatment of any minor disease or infection discovered.

Instruction sheets for the guidance of the *client* will also be needed, in the local language and with clear illustrations.

We must make sure we do not put unnecessary medical barriers against the use of family planning methods because of rare dangers or side effects (see Further reading and resources below).

What records should be kept?

These could include:

1. Person's own self-retained card.
   Record the method (and number if OC pill used).
2. Family folder insert card.
   Record type, amount and date to be seen again.
3. Family planning register.
   For a sample page see Figure 13.7.

4. Some projects with a strong FP emphasis can give each client a special family planning record card.
5. The master register at project headquarters. Figures of FP coverage can be copied into the master register or project computer at regular intervals.

Arrange community-based distribution of supplies

Community-based distribution (CBD) refers to using ordinary members of the community as providers of family planning supplies. CBD is especially useful where contraceptive use is low, clinics are hard to reach (or intimidating) and where there are few qualified health workers.

Social marketing, though overlapping with CBD, has important differences. It refers to the commercial but subsidised sale of pills and injections with small profits made by a middle man. This means that users pay a small amount. Doctors may be involved in helping to set this up but should not usually be too much involved thereafter.

Keys to a successful programme

There are three factors necessary for any programme to be successful (see Table 13.2).

- **Support from three sources:** the organising health programme, the suppliers and the community.

Table 13.2   Factors affecting the success of CBD programmes

Support	Accessibility	Quality
Strong commitment of the sponsoring institution. Participation of members of the community. Adequate numbers of dedicated distributors. CBD is acceptable within legal, ethical and cultural norms. Financial and material support from the sponsoring institution, the community, and donor agencies. Plans in place to ensure the sustainability of the CBD programme.	Services offered at popular locations. Dependable supply of contraceptive methods. Travel time and cost required to reach service points kept to a minimum. Waiting time to receive services kept to a minimum. Services affordable to all potential users, including those on a low income. Services provided in culturally acceptable settings. Referrals offered for other family planning services.	Sponsoring institution adheres to standards and protocols for contraceptive distribution. Adequate training for personnel. Users receive all the necessary information to permit them to make informed choices. Contraceptives are medically approved, have not reached their expiry dates, and are locally known and trusted. Client-provider confidentiality is respected. A follow-up system exists to maintain contact with users.

Source: Community-based Distribution of Contraceptives: A guide for programme managers.
Geneva: WHO, 1995.

This will come about as we raise awareness, involve the community, respond to their suggestions and identify and train suppliers. Everything we help to bring about must be culturally and legally acceptable to the community, including influential religious leaders.

A large range of people can act as suppliers. Examples include shopkeepers, TBAs and traditional healers, VHC members, factory supervisors or workers, barbers and locally respected community members. There can be an overlap with those who act as DOTS supervisors in TB programmes and the use of ART in PLWHA as antiretrovirals become more widely used and available (see pages 281 and 299).

• **Setting up services and supplies that are accessible** (i.e. easy to make use of) and acceptable (i.e. do not cause offence).
Supplies appropriate for CBD include contraceptive pills, injections (by pharmacists or even storekeepers who have been adequately trained), condoms, spermicides, plus referrals

for IUDs or permanent FP methods to the nearest clinic or hospital.
It is obviously essential that any use of injectables has built-in safeguards against the use of unclean needles or unsterile practices, (see pages 196–8).

• **Quality of the services, including medical backup.**
We need to arrange well managed support to ensure quality, reliability of supplies and follow-up of users, also that all suppliers are trained and follow high ethical standards. Our CHP can provide checklists for new starters and protocols to guide suppliers about who needs medical backup or referral. We can also make sure that simple illustrated leaflets are available to explain choices to clients.

Family planning camps

In some countries special FP camps are organised by the government or by larger non-governmental organisations; vasectomies and tubectomies are carried out in the community, and supplies distributed.

This system can work well but may have dangers:

1. Patients may be coerced to have operations, especially if there are government targets to be met.
2. Standards of hygiene may be low, leading to postoperative infections. Inadequately sterilised instruments and needles may be used. This is especially dangerous when hepatitis B, C or HIV infection is common locally.

As long as government FP camps have high standards of hygiene and are popular with the local people, voluntary programmes can cooperate with them. They can help to motivate couples, they can assist during the camp and they can arrange follow-up afterwards. However, there is generally a move away from this approach in favour of more client-centred services, based on informed choice; also towards long-acting rather than permanent methods.

A summary of FP stages

FP provision includes these four stages:

1. **Motivation**
    - What is it?
      Helping the couple, or individual, to understand their need for FP so they actively request it.
    - Where does it happen?
      Anywhere (e.g. the community, clinic, advising over the family radio).
    - Who does it?
      Friends, other family members, CHWs, TBAs, trained attendants, other health workers, teachers, members of women's clubs, religious leaders, store-keepers, film stars.
2. **Counselling**
    - What is it?
      General explanation about different FP methods to help the couple or individual choose.
      Detailed explanation about the method chosen, including the way to use it, its

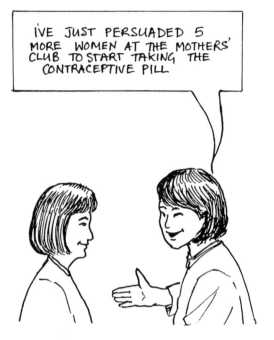

Figure 13.8 Satisfied customers make effective family planning promoters.

failure rate, side effects and follow-up. The counsellor must be ready to answer questions, and depending on the literacy of the client, should be able to supply good quality backup leaflets.
    - Where does it happen?
      The clinic, the hospital, the community.
    - Who does it?
      A health worker, nurse, trained attendant, TBA, FPP: the community distributor or sometimes store-keeper in the case of pills, injections, condoms and spermicides.
3. **Providing the service**
    - What is it?
      The initial FP service after counselling is completed, including giving the first supplies, injection or insertion.
    - Where does it happen?
      IUDs, injections, Norplant and sometimes the first pack of pills, usually in the clinic. Condoms and further pills in the community or clinic. Operations in the health centre or hospital.
    - Who does it?
      Doctors for operations. Family Planning Providers or nurses for IUDs, injections and

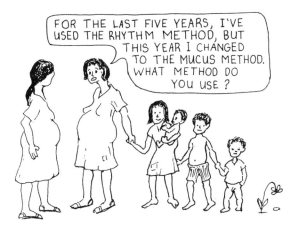

Figure 13.9

sometimes the first pack of pills; other health workers or community distributors for condoms and repeat supplies of pills.

4. Follow-up

* What is it?

    For operations: checking for wound infections or other side effects; answering questions.

    For IUDs: checking at least once after insertion and then with an 'open-house' policy but no set return dates until replacement needs considering every ten or more years.

    For injections: repeats at the prescribed intervals.

    For implants: no set follow-up necessary, but free to return especially for advice or help if there are bleeding problems.

    For pills: carrying out yearly checks.

    For all methods: an open-house policy so everyone knows they can always return with any problems or questions.

* Where does it happen?

    The clinic or community.

* Who does it?

    The least qualified health worker able to do it competently.

Include facilities for controlling sexually transmitted infections (STIs)

Before describing how we can do this for all sexually active men and women, we need to be aware of the overwhelming sexual health needs of young people in particular. Over one third of the world, i.e. about 2000 million people, are adolescents or children. They are, or soon will be, in the 'sexual marketplace'.

These young people arrive in huge numbers in the cities of the developing world only to find an almost complete absence of any sexual health services. If they need family planning advice they will probably be unable to find it. If they develop an STI they will not know where to find treatment. Many will have virtually no understanding of how to avoid or treat STIs, including HIV/AIDS. Even if they do have some knowledge, the situation in practice will often mean they fail to make use of the information they have. An increasing number, including older children, drift into commercial sex work because other employment is hard to find

The result of this migration to cities with no readily available services is fuelling an epidemic of sexually transmitted illness, backstreet abortions and increasing the spread of HIV/AIDS.

In addition, large numbers of babies with teenage mothers are born into urban situations with virtually no facilities or backup. (See Further reading and resources below, especially urban health and development.)

This is a situation where CBHPs need to think of effective ways of tackling this problem. In doing this we should make sure we work alongside any government-led services for adolescents that may have been drawn up but only rarely exist in practice.

To set up facilities for the control of STIs we need to consider first prevention, and second treatment.

1. Preventing sexually transmitted infection

In our programmes we should include the prevention of STIs as a normal part of our health teaching in home, community and clinic.

Because this is sometimes a very sensitive area, we should make sure that our approach is culturally sensitive and that the community knows that any personal counselling given will be completely confidential.

The prevention of STIs will tie in with many parts of our health programme and needs to be integrated with it. This will include:

- any HIV/AIDS programme we are involved with, including VCT;
- antenatal care;
- CHW training and the teaching by CHWs in the community;
- curative care in our clinics;
- part of our family planning programme.

We can use various approaches. Here are two important ones:

The ABC approach

A: abstaining from sex or delaying first sex for as long as possible

B: being faithful to one partner or minimising the number of sexual partners

C: Promoting male and, where appropriate, female condom usage.

The use of microbicides

These are substances that kill organisms which cause STIs. In the next few years they are likely to become an important part of our STI and HIV prevention programmes. They will be largely used in association with condoms, usually as intravaginal gels, or impregnated sponges. At the time of writing they are not widely available.

We need to make sure that, as soon as microbicides become available, affordable and acceptable we make full use of them in our programmes. See Further reading and resources below.

Microbicides must not be confused with spermicides such as nonoxynol-9, which kills sperm and therefore acts as a partial contraceptive but has no effect on disease-causing organisms. In fact, the use of this spermicide may actually increase the risk of passing on HIV.

2. Treating sexually transmitted infection

We will need to decide how much we are able to diagnose and treat STIs in our health clinic and how much we will refer these to other clinics.

In practice there are three reasons we should include this in our health programme.

The Five Cs of STI Control:

Compliance: ensure that patients complete their antibiotic course.

Confidentiality: ensure that staff understand the importance of confidentiality.

Contact tracking: gain patient's trust and understanding; be sensitive, but persistent in tracking down contacts.

Counselling: educate about sexual health and transmission of STIs

Condoms: educate about usage and provide easy access.

Source: Adapted from *Urban Health and Development*, Macmillan, TALC and Tearfund, 2001.

Figure 13.10   The 5 Cs of STI control.

1. STIs are common, dangerous and unless treated can have serious effects on past, present and future partners.
2. There will often be no practical alternative for our community members, especially in rural areas.
3. We can use what is known as the syndromic approach. This is a relatively easy way of treating symptoms or groups of symptoms with particular drugs, without needing to use a laboratory.
   Typical examples would be urethral discharge or genital ulcer. It works less well for vaginal discharge. WHO provides a series of charts that we can adapt and use in our clinics (see Further reading and resources below).

3. Evaluate the programme

At regular intervals we will need to evaluate the effectiveness of our FP programme. This will require baseline information before starting, which should include:

- **The Contraceptive Prevalence Rate (CPR).**
This is the percentage of eligible women, i.e. all women of reproductive age 15–49, who are using, or whose partner is using, a contraceptive method at a particular time:

$$\frac{\text{Number of women aged 15–49}}{\text{Total number of women aged 15–49}} \times 100$$
(or partners) using contraception

- **The Total Fertility Rate (TFR).**

This is the average total number of children to which women have given birth by the end of their reproductive period.

Both these figures can be calculated for communities from information on the family folder obtained at the time of the community survey. For information needed for the CPR viz use of contraceptives by the community, we might need to postpone asking questions until we had the full confidence of the people. One option would be to do a specific survey one year later or do a smaller sample survey.

We can monitor our programme yearly by checking the CPR according to the formula given earlier.

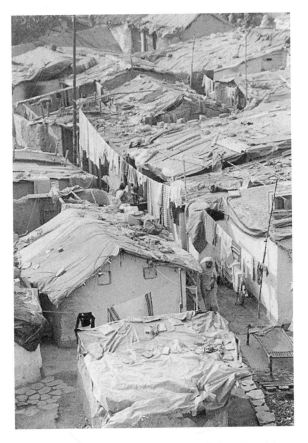

Figure 13.11 The price of failure: a drift to the cities and urban poverty.

Every three to five years we could resurvey the community and compare the new CPR to that at the start of the programme.

Every five to ten years we could in addition calculate the new TFR – the chief outcome indicator (see page 342), which takes longer to show any changes.

Summary

The world population is still increasing by a million every five days. Countries that have more people than their resources and services can provide for develop serious social problems. In conditions of poverty the children of larger families are at higher risk, especially when the space between children averages less than three years. In many countries mean birth rates are falling, largely because family planning services are more available but also sadly because of HIV/AIDS in communities that are seriously affected.

Each programme must decide how to develop FP in its partner communities, and which methods are most suitable. These will still include both permanent operations, but there should also be a variety of other long-acting reversible methods, which can increase child spacing and reduce family size. Family planning programmes need to bear in mind the dual protection many couples need – against unwanted pregnancy and against sexually transmitted infections, including HIV/AIDS.

Family planning is most successful when run as part of a primary health care programme because the guarantee of healthy children stimulates a wish to reduce family size.

A family planning clinic can act as the focal point of the programme and a health worker can be trained as a Family Planning Provider. Certain FP activities can also take place in the community, such as motivation, (especially through using the local radio for information) family planning camps, and the supply of pills and condoms. Such community-based distribution is becoming an increasingly key part of worldwide FP programmes, as are social marketing programmes of pills and injections.

Family planning is best seen as part of wider reproductive health services. An essential part of these is the prevention and treatment of sexually transmitted illness, including HIV/AIDS. We should try to integrate these services into our health programme.

FP programmes should be regularly evaluated in partnership with the community.

Further reading and resources

1. *Contraceptive Method Mix: Guidelines for Policy and Service Delivery*, PATH, 1992.
   A useful book including a detailed guide to different forms of contraception.
   Available from PATH. See Appendix E.
2. *Community-based Distribution of Contraceptives*, WHO, 1995.
   An extremely helpful practical manual giving detailed advice on how to set up commuity distribution.
   Available from: WHO. See Appendix E.
3. *Health Worker's Manual on Family Planning Options*, WHO, 2nd edn, 1998.
   An excellent field guide.
   Available from: WHO. See Appendix E.
4. *The Family Planning Clinic in Africa*, 3rd edn, R. and J. Brown, Macmillan, 1998.
   An extremely useful and practical manual relevant to all parts of the world.
   Available from: TALC. See Appendix E.
5. *Sexually transmitted infections*, A. Macmillan and C. Scott, Churchill Livingstone, 2000.
   An illustrated textbook.
6. *WHO Medical Eligibility Criteria*, 3rd edn, WHO, 2004, and
7. *WHO Selected Practice Recommendations*, 2nd edn, WHO, 2005.
   Both can be accessed via www.who.int/reproductive-health.
8. Website: www.unfpa.org.

Accessories

1. Flannelgraph on Family Planning STDs and AIDS.
   Available from: TALC. See Appendix E.

See Further references and guidelines, page 415.

14

Setting up a Community TB Programme

In this chapter we shall consider:
1. What we need to know
   - What is TB?
   - TB as a serious global disease
   - Methods being used to control TB

2. What we need to do
   - Decide whether to participate in a TB programme
   - Decide what type of TB programme to set up
   - Set aims and targets
   - Create awareness in the community
   - Identify TB cases (case finding)
   - Treat TB using DOTS programme (Directly Observed Treatment Short course)
   - Encourage adherence to treatment (case holding)
   - Understand some links between TB and HIV/AIDS
   - Control TB in the community
   - Evaluate the programme

What we need to know

What is TB?

Tuberculosis is a life-threatening disease that normally affects the lungs but can involve almost any part of the body.

The typical symptoms of TB are weight loss, chronic ill health and fever. Lung (pulmonary) TB also causes cough, often with sputum, sometimes with blood. Chest pain is commonly present. TB can mimic a wide variety of illnesses. Where AIDS is common the two diseases are often found together.

The cause of TB is a germ called *Mycobacterium tuberculosis* (also known as the acid-fast bacillus – AFB). Poverty, overcrowding, poor health and malnutrition make infection with the AFB more likely and more serious. So does HIV infection.

TB starts as germs enter the lungs, commonly in childhood, and multiply to form a patch with nearby swollen lymph nodes, together known as a primary complex. At this stage germs may enter the blood and spread to other organs. If the person is in weak health at the time of infection, the primary complex may enlarge at once to give active (primary) TB.

If the newly infected person is in good health, the disease may spread no further, but there is always the danger that later in life, especially during a time of stress, illness, poor diet or AIDS, the latent infection will become active and lead on to fully developed (post-primary) TB.

TB is spread from people with active lung TB when they cough, sneeze, talk or spit. The bacilli are then breathed in by others, who can become infected.

TB as a serious global disease

One third of the world's population is currently infected with the TB bacillus and 5–10 per cent of these become sick or infectious at some time during their life. Someone is newly infected with TB every second, and two million die from the disease each year. Left untreated, someone with infectious TB will infect between 10 and 15 people every year.

South Asia has the largest number of TB cases but Africa has the highest death rate. There are several reasons why TB has re-emerged as a major threat to world health:

- HIV/AIDS is the most important reason why TB is increasing.
- Travel spreads TB, especially through refugees, economic migrants and displaced people.

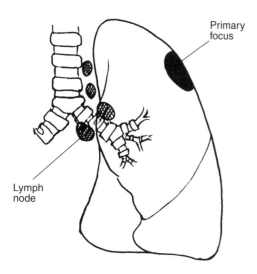

Figure 14.1   The primary complex (primary focus and lymph node).

- Resistance to commonly used drugs is increasing rapidly, especially in countries of the former Soviet Union and where HIV/AIDS is common. Poorly managed programmes and wrong treatment make the spread of resistance more likely.
- Poverty, both in developing countries and amongst any poor or marginalised group, is a major cause of TB.
  For example: A recent study from a poor urban area in Kampala, Uganda, showed that there were 9.2 new cases per 1000 population per year compared with an expected rate of 2 new cases per 1000. The finding that urban TB was over four times higher than expected suggests this is likely to be the case amongst urban poor in other countries, especially where HIV/AIDS is common. (WHO *Bulletin*, 2003, 81: 11.)
- Loss of health personnel is becoming a major problem especially where HIV/AIDS is common. WHO has warned that a TB workforce crisis is becoming a major problem in TB control.

To help combat TB and to coordinate treatment, WHO has set up the Stop TB partnership and is working with national governments to develop National Tuberculosis Programmes (NTPs). NTPs set up guidelines, plans and resources relevant to each country. Any TB programme we set up should liaise closely with the NTP and follow any guidelines they produce.

Methods being used to control TB

Millennium Development Goal number 6 aims to halve the prevalence and death rate of TB by the year 2015. This will be difficult to achieve, especially in areas with high resistance and where HIV/AIDS is common. Community based health approaches can make a big contribution in helping to achieve this MDG.

WHO and its partners through the Stop TB programme have set two key worldwide targets. The first is to detect 70 per cent of new infectious TB cases and the second is to achieve treatment success (this is treatment cure plus treatment completion) of 85 per cent. The second of these is the more important, but the first is the harder to achieve.

The most effective way of controlling TB is through using a DOTS programme. DOTS stands for directly observed treatment, short course.

At this stage it is helpful to be clear on our terminology. DOTS is the 'brand name' of the WHO recommended TB control strategy, which describes the five elements listed below. We can talk about DOTS programmes if they follow this standard.

DOT is just one of the five elements and refers to administering rifampicin-containing regimens under direct supervision and support (see point 1 below).

A DOTS programme consists of these five components:

1. **Direct observation of treatment (DOT)** is the key: trained observers ensure and observe that patients swallow their tablets for the full course of six to eight months, i.e. that patients take the correct drugs in the correct doses at the correct intervals.
2. **Microscopy services**: trained microscopists diagnose sputum-positive cases as near to the patient's home as possible.

3. **Drug supplies**: drugs must be high quality, accessible and always available, following national tuberculosis programme guidelines. Ideally some or all of these should be available as combined preparations, i.e. tablets containing more than one drug. This reduces the large number of tablets that have to be swallowed.

4. **Monitoring and recording**: this tracks the progress of each patient and therefore of the programme as a whole.

5. **Political will**: i.e. the commitment of the country and its national – and local – leadership to make this programme a priority and to give it public and financial backing.

Resistance to commonly used TB drugs, especially isoniazid and rifampicin is increasing worldwide. TB that is resistant to at least these two drugs is known as multi-drug resistant TB or MDR-TB. This is especially common in eastern Europe and central Asia.

Treatment regimes to treat MDR-TB are often known as DOTS plus. They include 2 or more drugs to which the particular strain of TB is sensitive. Total treatment lasts for 18 to 24 months and each dose taken must be observed. It is up to 100 times more expensive to treat MDR-TB with DOTS plus, than non-resistant TB with DOTS.

This underlines the huge importance of treating TB effectively so that MDR-TB does not develop. The key to this is to use a DOTS programme for all rifampicin-containing regimens.

Some programmes use a modified DOT approach that often depends on the 'self-supervision' of patients in taking their TB drugs, especially in the continuation phase of treatment (see below). Such programmes are not recommended by WHO, who consider self-supervision is never acceptable when rifampicin is being used. If we are involved in a programme that does not use a standard DOT strategy based on the observation of pills being swallowed, we must ensure that our programme is still achieving high treatment success rates. If it falls below 85 per cent in a pilot project we should switch to DOT or discontinue our programme. Experience shows, however, that it is difficult to change wrong practice once it has been introduced.

What we need to do

Decide whether to participate in a TB programme

TB, though usually a curable disease, is difficult to treat, requiring a great deal of time and commitment. It can be expensive unless there is reliable subsidy or free supplies. It is also complex to follow NTP guidelines, especially in areas where HIV/AIDS is common or there is a high proportion of MDR-TB. This means we should participate in a programme only after careful consideration. We must also remember that Stop TB is a worldwide initiative and that our responsibility is to work alongside any national programme and to follow its guidelines carefully.

However, there are still many areas without an effective TB programme and, if we wish to start in such an area, we must be sure to work in close association with the NTP.

Treating TB inadequately is worse than not treating it at all. A few patients may be cured but resistant germs will develop, making TB in the target area harder to cure in the future.

Before starting we will need to ask:

1. **Does the community wish to have a programme?**
   Will people work in partnership with us? Are they prepared to take on increasing responsibility for helping to manage the programme?

2. **Is TB common or important in our programme area?**
   We can usually discover this from national or official figures and annual rates of infection. If not, we could consider starting a programme if more than one per cent of people in our community survey were possible TB cases.

3. **Is TB already being adequately treated in the area?**
   Although the NTP may be functioning and private doctors treating many patients, effective programmes may not be present in the neediest areas, such as urban slums, or remote mountain or island communities.

As well as finding out what groups are involved in TB control, we will need to discover how much they are actually doing. Is there an effective and comprehensive programme that adequately includes the neediest members of the community?

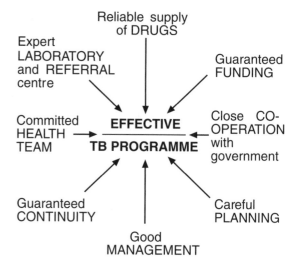

Figure 14.2   The essential ingredients in an effective TB programme.

Part of our assessment will be through meeting the District Medical Officer, or TB Officer, and directors of any other programmes involved in TB treatment in our project area. It is essential we work alongside and strengthen existing programmes rather than setting up alternatives. However, in areas with no effective treatment, we should be ready to set up DOT-based programmes following NTP guidelines and in agreement with local health authorities. We must have the resources to sustain our involvement.

4. **Have we the resources to set up a TB programme?**
   - A doctor to plan, advise, give clinical care and liaise with the NTP.
   - Health workers to identify cases, organise treatment and ensure follow-up.
   - Drugs, often difficult to obtain, whose supplies are reliable and subsidised.
   - Money, unless free supplies are available and guaranteed from the government or an aid programme for five to ten years.
   - A referral system for diagnosis and treatment, especially for complex cases, MDR-TB, or those with dual TB and HIV infection.
   - Effective management.

5. **Is our project likely to be long term or permanent?**
   Because it takes many years for a TB programme to be effective, we will need to make sure as far as possible that our programme will continue for a number of years.

Decide what type of TB programme to set up

There are two main choices:

A comprehensive TB programme

This is a programme where the project and community take full responsibility for case-finding, treatment and follow-up, in close association with, or as part of, the national TB programme.

If this is decided between project, community and NTP, we may wish to start TB control at the same time as setting up health centres. Alternatively, we can set up a general community health programme first, with health posts or mobile clinics, and a TB component later. Unless any members of our programme are very experienced, this is usually a better approach.

A selective TB programme

If a local programme already exists, we should work in cooperation with the agency running it, or take over responsibility for certain parts of the programme.

For example: The government (District Medical Officer) is usually responsible for the overall planning of programmes and the supply of drugs. However, at the community level, field work is often inadequate, giving voluntary programmes an opportunity to contribute. Specific tasks might include: case-finding, referral, providing and supervising treatment through a DOT approach, follow-up of defaulters, community education or BCG vaccination.

Set aims and targets

Our overall objectives in line with the NTP will be:

- To *detect* 70 per cent of existing cases of smear positive TB in our project area.
- To *treat* successfully 85 per cent of newly identified cases of smear positive TB.

An 85 per cent treatment success rate is the level at which TB usually starts to decline and less drug resistance develops.

From the start we should aim for an 85 per cent treatment success rate. However, achieving case detection rates is harder. Year on year, case detection rates should be improving.

The DMO or TB officer should help us in setting realistic targets and ways in which these can be monitored.

We will need to add targets to our logframe (see page 101). We must also remember that poorly managed programmes are likely to make the TB situation worse.

Create awareness in the community (see Chapter 3)

> Creating awareness is one of the key factors in eradicating TB. Once community members recognise their illness, believe it can be cured and ask for treatment, our programme is more likely to succeed.

We will need to understand local beliefs and customs, the difficulties faced by the poor both in getting diagnosed and in completing treatment. We also need to understand the role of private practitioners.

Local beliefs and customs

These vary from place to place but common fears include:

- TB can't be cured (this may well be true in their experience).
- Only the poor, low caste or those under a curse get TB.

- TB patients are unclean and should be distanced from their families or communities.
- A belief that TB is inherited (quite common in many African countries).
- If you have TB it means you also have AIDS (often true where HIV/AIDS is common).

In practice, patients may be excluded by their community, barred from marriage and face serious discrimination. This stigma may increase in areas where people assume that if you have TB you also have AIDS.

Difficulties faced by the poor

Imagine a poor villager or slum-dweller who starts to cough up blood. A frightening sequence of problems will have to be faced:

- 'Now I've caught the disease that has killed my close friends.'
- 'I don't have the energy to chase after a cure.'
- 'Can I trust the doctor or will I be cheated?'
- 'I've only enough money for four weeks of medicine: how can I afford six months?'
- 'I don't know who will take me to the clinic or pay for the journey.'
- 'I'm worried I will get AIDS if I have to have injections: perhaps I've caught it already.'
- 'If I can't go to work my family will starve and my children may die.'

In the case of a woman with TB, these problems are multiplied. Often her family may be unwilling or unable to spend money on her treatment. They may prevent her from attending doctors and hospitals when she should be busy at home, collecting firewood, or earning income.

Recent research from the Gambia has shown just how essential it is for health workers to understand the varied reasons why patients with TB do not seek treatment or discontinue treatment early. When we discover what the reasons are in our community, we can help people make plans to overcome these obstacles. (See page 415, ref. Harper.)

Private practitioners

Health workers often talk about health seeking behaviour. This refers to the action people take (or don't take) when they become ill.

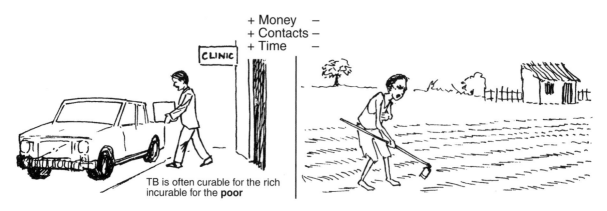

+ Money   −
+ Contacts −
+ Time   −

TB is often curable for the rich
incurable for the **poor**

Figure 14.3   TB in practice (1).

In practice, many people with symptoms of TB first seek out private practitioners. Usually the diagnosis and treatment they receive is inadequate and they may be charged high fees. Up to 50 per cent of TB patients in some Asian countries first see a private practitioner. Dangerous delays often occur before patients start taking appropriate NTP-based treatment.

One practical solution is to include and train private practitioners in any health programme with which we are involved. Some may be unwilling and many will need big shifts in their attitude. However, by including this huge group of 'unofficial' health workers we can help reduce delays to treatment and the use of wrong drugs. It may also help solve the shortage of trained health care workers in our programme area.

The use of public-private mix initiatives is another useful way forward and can evolve out of a defined cooperation with private health providers. Any initiative needs to standardise practice and report to the public TB control programme.

Identify TB cases (case finding)

Different forms of case finding

There are two main ways in which we discover which people have infectious TB. Passive case finding (or self-referral) refers to diagnosing patients who report symptoms – for example, to a heath centre, hospital, private practitioner, clinic or CHW. Active case finding refers to an active

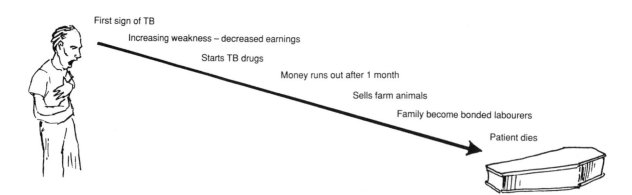

First sign of TB

Increasing weakness – decreased earnings

Starts TB drugs

Money runs out after 1 month

Sells farm animals

Family become bonded labourers

Patient dies

Figure 14.4   TB in practice (2): within one year this TB patient died and his family lost their farm, their money, their independence, their dignity and their future.

search for cases in the community – either those with symptoms who have not come forward or those who may be smear positive but do not have significant symptoms.

TB programmes should be based largely on passive case finding. Only when cure rates reach levels of at least 85 per cent should we actively be searching for new cases. *An exception to this is in people living with HIV/AIDS. As part of their treatment TB needs to be recognised and treated as soon as possible.*

There is a form of case finding midway between active and passive. We can call this opportunistic, though this is not currently part of WHO strategy nor a term that is officially used. It refers to discovering patients who come into contact with a clinic or health programme for reasons other than with symptoms suggestive of TB. *Here are two examples*: An elderly man who attends a clinic with severe toothache and is found on questioning to have a chronic cough: community members with possible TB being discovered in our community survey. In remote areas or amongst communities where TB patients are highly stigmatised, this can be a useful way of discovering additional patients through little extra cost.

Symptoms that suggest infectious TB

1. In adults and older children
- Cough and sputum for more than three weeks. Any people with these symptoms are considered 'TB suspects' or 'possible TB cases'. We will use the latter term, as the word 'suspect' is in danger of increasing stigma.
- Weight loss, fever, pain in the chest, or coughing up blood makes the diagnosis more likely. Often symptoms have a gradual onset. AIDS can accompany or mimic many of these symptoms.
- There are other forms of TB that affect different organs in the body. These patients should still be treated but usually, being non-infectious, are a low priority in terms of community control.

2. In younger children
TB can be very difficult to diagnose. The key is always to consider the diagnosis of TB in any child who is ill and does not get better.
Common symptoms include:

- Any of those found in adults, though children up to the age of 12 rarely cough up sputum (they tend to swallow it).
- Weight loss or failure to gain weight for four weeks or more with no obvious cause.
- Unexplained fever or night sweats with negative malaria smear or no response to malaria treatment.
- Large painless lymph nodes, most commonly in the neck, with or without discharge to the skin. (Other conditions can mimic this.)

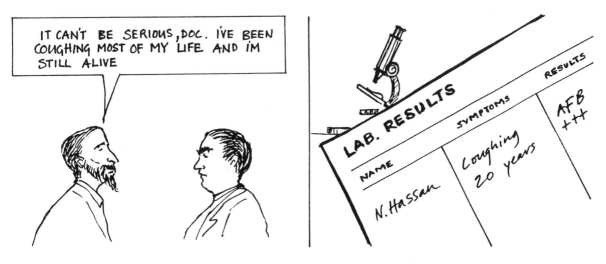

Figure 14.5   A dangerous source of TB germs: the elderly villager or slum dweller with a chronic cough.

How to make a diagnosis

1. **In adults and older children**
   - Carry out a sputum test by staining a slide and using a microscope. Wherever possible carry out three tests. If only one is positive, try to confirm with a further test. (See below and Figure 14.6.)
   - Only carry out an X-ray if three sputum tests are negative, TB is suspected because of the symptoms, and X-rays are easy to arrange and affordable. If the chest X-ray suggests TB and the patient is no better after a course of broad-spectrum antibiotics, TB is a likely diagnosis and we can start treatment.

   In areas where HIV/AIDS is common we must ensure people have access to voluntary counselling and testing services.

   There are many cases of chronic cough and usually only about 5–10 per cent of these will have positive sputum. We must take care not to overdiagnose TB, nor to treat patients for TB who have conditions with similar symptoms, such as 'smoker's cough' or chronic bronchitis.

   > Thousands of patients in poor communities have been made bankrupt by being incorrectly treated for TB when there is no evidence that they have it.

2. **In younger children**
   In developing countries children make up 15–20 per cent of all TB cases and many have dual infection with HIV. They are harder to diagnose than adults.

   We will normally have to treat according to a 'best guess' rather than through definite confirmation. If we suspect TB, the following will help guide us as to whether we should start TB treatment:
   - A chest X-ray, which may show typical changes.
   - A tuberculin test if available – a strongly positive test suggests TB.
   - Trials of two different antibiotics for one week each. Failure to respond makes TB more likely.

   We can follow the scoring systems or flow charts that should be available from the National TB Programme.

At the time of writing (2005), WHO had not fully agreed on an official community based algorithm for the management of TB in children.

Recording TB cases

In order to have consistent recording systems we should put any patient diagnosed with TB into one of the six categories used by NTPs:

- **New smear-positive TB case** = a patient who has never had treatment, or who has had anti-TB drugs for less than four weeks.
- **Relapse** = a patient who has been declared cured after one full course of treatment and has become smear positive again.
- **Treatment failure** = a patient who while on treatment remains, or becomes, smear positive again, after five months or more of treatment.
- **Treatment after interruption (TAI) or defaulter** = a patient who interrupts treatment for two months or more and returns with smear-positive sputum or strong evidence of active TB.
- **Transfer** = transfer in from another district or programme.
- **Chronic case** = a patient who remains or becomes smear positive again after completing a fully supervised retreatment course.

Although these categories may seem complex, it is important we follow them. They are based on a scientific system and give an accurate way of monitoring our programme

A note on sputum tests and laboratories

Sputum is most likely to give an accurate result if produced from a deep cough, preferably when first waking in the morning. It should be produced away from other people and placed in a clean, sealed, labelled container and taken or sent as soon as possible to the nearest laboratory able to carry out sputum tests.

Sputum testing through microscopes:

- **The first priority:** tests to be carried out by lab workers who have been adequately trained and carry out a sufficient number of tests for their skills to be maintained.

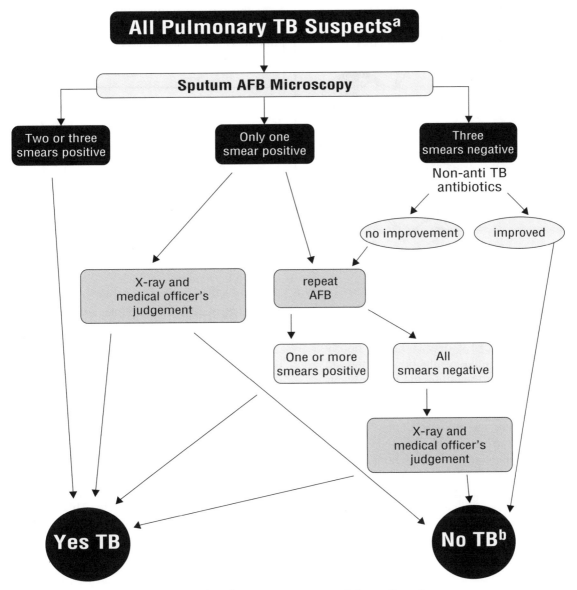

aScreening: cough >2–3 weeks. Diagnosis: clinical signs, symptoms, normal chest radiography.
bConsider other diagnoses.

Figure 14.6   Diagnostic procedure for suspected pulmonary TB. (WHO algorithm, see ref. 5 page 288)

- **The second priority:** to carry out the test in as convenient a location as possible for the patient, e.g. at the health post, clinic or primary health centre nearest to the patient's home. The further patients have to travel the less likely they will be diagnosed and treated. This means that the community based treatment of TB is an enormous advantage over many programmes based on distant health centres and hospitals.

- **A reasonable aim:** to incorporate sputum testing into the most peripheral health centre where standards can be guaranteed. In CBHC we should aim to include a well trained (and accredited) microscopist in our health team so that sputum cases can be examined quickly and conveniently (see page 153).

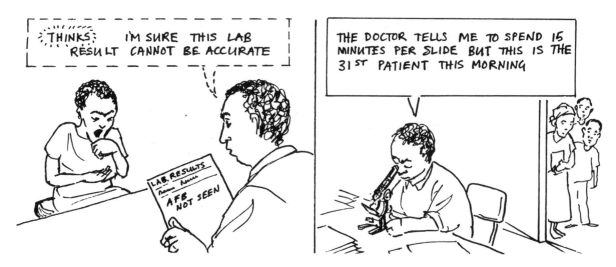

Figure 14.7 Results can be inaccurate if laboratory workers are overworked.

Lab workers need to be well trained, motivated and reliable. False negative results can occur when the microscopist is overworked or poorly motivated. False positive results occur when lab workers record what they think the doctor wants or expects.

Research workers are trying to make the diagnosis of TB quicker and more accurate. One way is to add sodium hypochlorite (NaOCl) to sputum, according to special instructions. Follow any guidelines from the NTP about this or other improved ways of examining sputums. Research is providing new possibilities for the future. *For example*: a blood test known as the Elispot is accurate but at the time of writing not generally possible at community level.

> No TB programme should be started unless reliable sputum testing is available: small TB programmes can be run effectively without X-rays.

Treat TB using DOTS (Directly Observed Treatment Short course)

As described earlier, we should aim to participate in a DOTS programme and make sure that each of the components will work in our community.

Some examples of programmes using DOT

1. In Bangladesh a programme set up by the NGO, BRAC, which uses community health volunteers, was shown to cost only half that of a government programme that was not community based. The BRAC programme for the same cost cured three patients for every two in the government system. CHWs in each village made the programme more convenient and in addition increased the number of women being cured of TB. This example shows that well managed community based programmes using CHWs are both cheaper and more convenient than government programmes that bypass this community involvement. (See page 415, ref. Islam.)

2. In many African countries treatment supporters or Community Volunteers (CVs), who are often neighbours or friends, are identified by the community after a new TB case has been diagnosed and referred back to the community. These volunteers provide DOT and effective support to patients often for no more than five minutes per day at no cost (because they live nearby and are usually known to the TB patient). Ideally, CVs and patients are regularly visited (e.g. every two weeks) by public health officers to monitor progress of treatment, and to supply new drugs, etc.

This approach works in areas where there are no CHWs but still depends on strong partnership with the community.

3. China originally covered a number of provinces in a programme supported by the World Bank with cure rates of 95 per cent (but case detection rates were much lower than the 70 per cent target): keys to success in cure rates included:
   - Free-of-charge diagnosis and treatment.
   - Financial incentives to village doctors.
   - Signing of contracts between village doctors and patients.
   - The use of blister packs for medicines.
   - Strong political will, management and reporting systems, which are relatively easy within the Chinese cultural and political system and which have enabled this programme to be replicated successfully in many provinces. (See page 415, ref. Chen.)

Successful DOTS programmes are far more difficult in countries where HIV/AIDS is common or in countries of the former Soviet Union where MDR-TB is widespread.

4. India has successfully expanded its DOTS programmes and there are several keys to success in areas where this has been achieved: reliable drug supplies, careful appraisal of communities before starting the programme, intensive monitoring and supervision, and expert advice and support, especially in the early phases of the project.

The message for us in CBHC is this: well managed programmes based on participation offer an excellent way of achieving high treatment success rates providing we work with the NTP and provide creative leadership. This is also the case if we are involved in scaling up existing programmes.

Who should supervise the treatment?

The observer or supervisor should be a responsible person, trusted by the patient and living nearby. Observers will need to be trained and helped to see the importance of what they are doing. Different programmes will use different observers. *Examples include*: responsible relatives and friends, teachers in the case of school children,

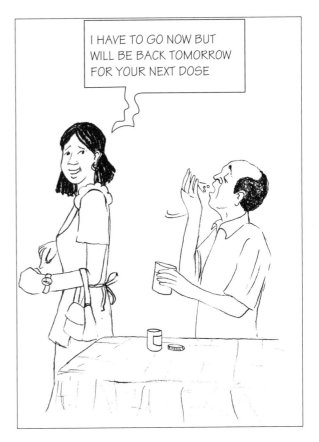

Figure 14.8

shop-keepers, CHWs, HIV/AIDS home care providers, priests, traditional health practitioners and health workers in a nearby health facility, providing they are not overworked or demotivated.

Observers will need to be answerable officially to the health programme, either NGO or government, and will need to keep confidentiality. In some cases they can be given some incentive or reward for the service provided, though many will do this out of goodwill.

The actual act of observation is not as important as the combination of trust and awareness that motivates the patient to visit the observer. WHO is encouraging the idea of patients' support rather than mere observation of treatment.

Direct observation of treatment is a cost-effective way of helping compliance. Nevertheless, we will still need a system for contacting defaulters who fail to attend their observer. This problem is less when the observer is a neighbour and there is good public health backup with regular visits.

What drug regimes should be used?

This will depend on the National Tuberculosis Programme, which will incorporate details of drug resistance, cost, availability of supplies and other factors. We should liaise with the District official responsible for TB, follow the NTP guidelines and work out a system of medicine supply and reporting that ties in with the NTP and works in practice for our programme.

> In practice, many programmes and private practitioners continue to use drugs that are not in line with national guidelines. This often contributes to the development of multi-drug resistant TB.

Most official regimes consist of two phases: an initial intensive phase using four drugs for two months followed by a continuation phase using two drugs for four or six months.

Two currently recommended WHO drug regimes for new cases are illustrated in Table 14.1.

Please note that these regimes are subject to change and there are variations between WHO recommendations and some other official sources. Follow your own NTP guidelines if in doubt.

There is an urgent need for new, effective and cheaper drugs.

Confirmation of treatment success

The key to this is repeat sputum tests:
- If possible two tests should be carried out. See Table 14.1 for when these should be done.

Table 14.1   Two currently recommended WHO drug regimes for new adult cases of TB

Medicine and dose (where possible as fixed dose combinations (FDCs)	Sputum test repeated at
1. *Common regime* Initial phase: duration two months: daily dosages of: Isoniazid 5 mg/kg Rifampicin 10 mg/kg Pyrazinamide 25 mg/kg Ethambutol 15 mg/kg	End of second month
Continuation phase: duration six months: daily dosages of: Isoniazid 5 mg/kg Ethambutol 15 mg/kg	End of fifth month In the eighth month
2. *Alternative regime* Initial phase: duration two months: dosages three times per week of Isoniazid 10 mg/kg Rifampicin 10 mg/kg Pyrazinamide 35 mg/kg Ethambutol 30 mg/kg	End of second month
Continuation phase: duration four months: dosages three times per week: Isoniazid 10 mg/kg Rifampicin 10 mg/kg	End of fourth month In the sixth month

Notes:
1. Twice-weekly dosages. These are not generally recommended because missing one dose can have serious consequences. A regime that depends on three dosages per week, especially in the initial phase, will need very strict Direct Observation.
2. For different categories, e.g. treatment failure, relapse, and special circumstances, e.g. pregnancy, different regimes are used: also for children's doses. See NTP guidelines.
3. People with AIDS and those HIV positive can use the standard regimes listed, but should not use any regime with thiacetazone, which some countries still include in treatment schedules.
4. WHO's DOTS–Plus strategy lists 2nd line drugs to treat MDR-TB (see ref. 5 page 228).

- Sputum tests are normally negative by the end of the second month. If they are not, the initial phase should be continued for a third month. If sputum tests are still positive at the end of the fifth month, this equals treatment failure.

Remember that treatment success means both achieving negative sputum tests and continuing treatment for the full duration.

Keeping records

For record keeping to be the same nationwide and globally we should record the outcome for each patient we start on treatment, under one of these six categories:

1. **Cure:** smear negative at completion of treatment and on one other occasion during treatment.
2. **Treatment completed:** patient has completed treatment without proof of cure.
3. **Treatment failure:** patient remains, or again becomes, smear positive at five months or later during treatment.
4. **Died:** patient dies for any reason during treatment.
5. **Treatment interrupted (default):** patient whose treatment is interrupted for two months or more.
6. **Transfer out:** patient transferred to another reporting unit and outcome not known.

The exact record forms we use in the project must tie in with the reporting systems needed by the NTP.

We should also record details of treatment on the patient-retained record card, and can also record data on family folder insert cards, or our own TB register. If the project is computerised, we can use Due Lists or computer-generated forms, for later data entry. However, we should keep records as simple as possible and avoid time-wasting duplication.

Encourage adherence to treatment (case holding)

There has been a shift in thinking, from trying to enforce adherence to treatment (also known as compliance) to working in partnership with patients (concordance). Treatment is supervised in a spirit of goodwill and cooperation, and in partnership with the patient.

In practice, however, we will still need a mixture of information, encouragement, incentive and discipline to encourage all patients to complete treatment, especially in areas where DOTS programmes are not used or cannot easily be started.

The CHW can be a very important person in this process, both as an observer in DOTS programmes, and in other supportive ways in programmes that depend on self-supervision. Here are some examples:

1. She should ensure medicine is being taken regularly.
   This is important throughout the course of treatment and absolutely essential in the initial phase.
   If patients are unreliable in taking medicines, the CHW can hand them out personally, daily in the first eight weeks, then three times weekly during the rest of the course. (See Table 14.1.)
2. She can collect supplies from the clinic either for all TB patients in the community or for those too ill to collect medicines themselves.
3. She can inform the senior health worker of any patients who are failing to take treatment.
4. She can encourage known possible cases to have sputum tests. She can accompany them to the clinic or even take a sputum specimen to the clinic for them.

In programmes using trained and motivated CHWs, it is their responsibility to make sure that every TB patient in the community who starts treatment takes medicine regularly until the course is complete.

From time to time a supervisor or MPW should visit TB patients in their homes along with the CHW.

Some ways of improving compliance are listed in the box.

Twelve practical suggestions to encourage compliance

1. Explain about TB carefully, and also give written instructions. Even if the patient is unable to read, a family member or friend probably can.
2. Understand local beliefs so that advice can be focused and appropriate.
3. If TB treatment is not reliably being supplied free, work out with patients how they will be able to pay for the whole course of treatment.
4. Consider asking patients for payment of a deposit at the start of treatment, returnable in full or in part on completion, and entitling them to medicines at overall reduced cost.
5. Explain about common side effects so patients will not be worried if they occur, for example, reddening of the urine with rifampicin.
6. Spend extra time with older sputum-positive men and women with chronic cough. They are often highly infectious, less willing to take treatment and need extra encouragement to comply.
7. Make sure members of the patient's family understand about treatment so they can support the advice given.
8. Set up a DOT supervision strategy that is acceptable and accessible for the TB patient, ideally home based.
9. Consider starting a TB support group – a regular meeting of those with TB who, helped by a facilitator, can encourage each other and share both concerns and practical solutions.
10. Learn to spot 'Hidden Defaulters'. These are those who claim to be regular but who forget or are untruthful about treatment.
11. Make sure health workers are both kind and firm.
12. Make sure supplies never run out. Have a standby supply of medicines in the community in case bad weather, floods or civil chaos prevent further supplies arriving.

Figure 14.9 TB advice sheet for patients, used in a Himalayan health project. Adapt this for the programme area and add appropriate illustrations. Information about DOT observers can be added.

A Message about Tuberculosis for TB Patients and their Families

The tests we have done have shown that you have TB. This is a very serious illness.

If you do not take medicine regularly, the TB may kill you. You will also spread it to others including children.

But you can be cured of TB if you take your medicine regularly for 6-8 months, according to what the doctor tells you. You must not miss even a single dose of medicines.

After you have been taking medicine for more than about one month you may start to feel much better and think that you are cured. You must still go on taking medicine for the full length of time. If you stop when you feel better then later the disease will come back much worse and it will be much harder to treat.

It is very important that you stop smoking and avoid too much alcohol. You should eat good nourishing food, including green vegetables, lentils, milk, eggs and meat if these are available. There are no foods that you should stop eating.

You should avoid getting too tired but you can continue to work unless you are advised not to.

When you cough put a hand or cloth over your mouth. This stops other people from catching your germs. Try not to spit in the house or when near other people. If you have to cough up sputum then put it into a cloth or small container and burn later, or bury it.

Also, if you are coughing a lot try to sleep separately from other members of your family – if possible in a different room until your cough has stopped. This will stop them from catching your germs, especially children.

Make sure that you bring any other people in your family or village who have a bad cough, to the clinic. We can check them to see if they have TB.

You can come back to the clinic or see the CHW any time you want, if you have anything you want to talk or ask about.

But remember, the most important thing is to be completely regular with your treatment, and never miss a dose. If you miss treatment or stop taking it, your TB will get worse. But if you are regular, your TB will get better and you will be cured.

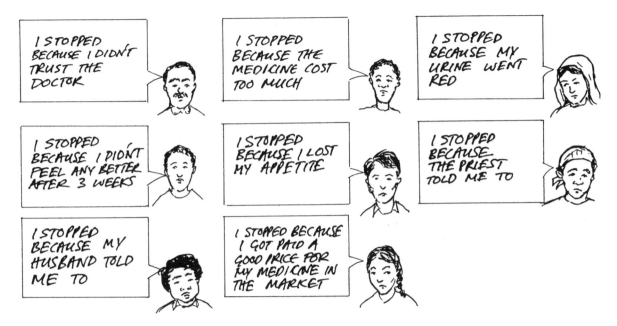

Figure 14.10   Reasons and excuses for poor compliance.

Understand some links between TB and HIV/AIDS

Here are some facts and guidelines if we are working in areas where HIV is common.

- **TB and HIV form a dangerous combination.**
  HIV is the main reason why TB has become more common in the past ten years.
  At the time of writing (2005) about one in three Africans who are infected with HIV also harbours the TB bacillus. Each year 5 to 10 per cent of these will develop active TB and up to half of them will do so at some point in their lives. Without TB treatment, HIV-infected people with TB usually die within months, though they usually respond just as well to TB treatment as those who are HIV negative.

  > We must therefore ensure that people living with HIV/AIDS have access to TB diagnosis and treatment, also that TB patients have access to voluntary HIV counselling and testing, and to antiretroviral therapy when indicated.

- **The use of a 'Double DOTS' strategy**
  With the use of antiretroviral therapy increasingly available for treating HIV/AIDS, a similar DOT approach as used in TB treatment can also be used for ART. This has been mainly pioneered in Haiti and Malawi and is likely to become a widespread approach.
  However, when patients are being treated for both TB and HIV, drug regimes are confusing, making careful supervision important. Drug interactions and side effects are common, making good medical management and clear guidelines essential.

- TB treatment regimes in PLWHA are generally similar in patients who are HIV positive and HIV negative. We should try to avoid using streptomycin because of the danger of spreading HIV further through unclean needles. The TB drug thiacetazone used in some continuation phase programmes can occasionally cause severe reactions.

- **Patterns of infection**
  In those infected with HIV, lung TB is still the most common form, though a higher number of infected cases are sputum negative, and TB in other parts of the body occurs more frequently. A classic presentation of TB is more common during early stages of HIV infection: atypical presentations are more common later when the patient's immune system has been seriously harmed by HIV.

- **Prevention of TB in those with HIV/AIDS**
  Isoniazid 300 mg daily should be given to PLWHA, providing active TB has been excluded. Evidence also suggests that children with HIV/AIDS, whether or not they have TB, should take the antibiotic co-trimoxazole, which increases survival rates. Adult HIV-infected TB patients should also take this drug.
- **Voluntary HIV counselling and testing (VCT)**
  VCT should be easily accessible and must be part of all TB control programmes except in areas where HIV is still rare. However, many people realise that, if diagnosed with TB, they may also be HIV positive and this can further increase the stigma of TB
- **In PLWHA we need to be strongly active** in TB case finding, through easily accessible TB testing and by raising awareness in the community.

Control TB in the community

The best method of reducing TB in a community is to cure infectious patients who have it.

TB will decline in a community if we succeed in two key objectives over a period of time:
- Treat smear-positive patients so that 85 per cent or more are successfully treated.
- Tackle the underlying causes of poverty.

In practice, most successful TB control programmes depend on the following:
1. Staff competence. Train programme staff in clinical, communication and management skills.
2. Management/planning. Excellent programme management is essential for long-term success.
3. Long-term commitment. Find ways in which the programme can be sustained and the cost of drugs be permanently affordable. This usually means accessing free supplies but advocacy and persistence are often needed for this to happen
4. Implementing a DOTS programme with its five programme components. If this is not possible, there are several options. These include admission during the intensive phase to a health facility or, usually easier, DOT

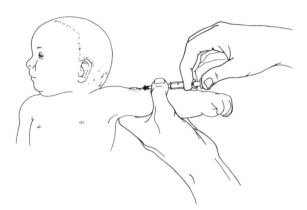

Figure 4.11   Giving BCG vaccine.

through a daily visit to the health centre. If the patient lives a long way from the centre, then simple community based DOT can be used as described earlier. If self-supervision is allowed, it is difficult to reverse later and usually brings less reliable results.
5. Giving BCG immunisation to all infants. This is best given at birth, or within a month, or within the first year (see page 195). BCG prevents TB meningitis but has only a small impact on reducing the number of TB cases.
6. Integrating the programme. Incorporate the TB programme into CBHC. Obtain expert advice and funding to back up the programme. Try to include (and train) private practitioners.
7. Following NTP guidelines. This includes treatment schedules, recommended practices reporting and ongoing liaison.
8. Continuity. If our programme fails or closes down we must ensure that we hand over all programme components for others to continue.
9. Using fixed-dose combinations of tablets (FDCs), which improve compliance.
10. Tackling underlying causes of poverty.
11. Integrating the diagnosis and treatment of TB and HIV/AIDS at programme level.
12. Prioritising nutrition. We should do everything possible to ensure reliable and adequate nutrition for the whole community, especially children and those known to have TB and/or HIV/AIDS.

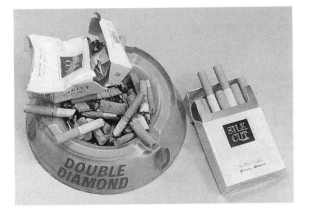

Figure 14.12   Part of TB control: reducing cigarette consumption.

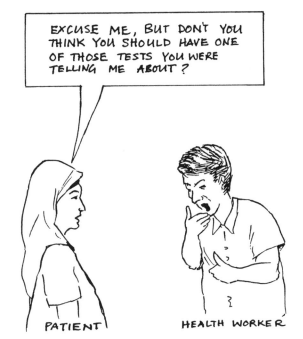

Figure 14.13   Health workers can get TB, too.

13. Reducing illiteracy and increasing the proportion of children and adolescents, in particular girls, who continue post-primary education.
14. Reducing air pollution from tobacco smoke and indoor cooking fires. This requires strong leadership, advocacy and persuasion to reduce the use of tobacco in all its forms.

Research has shown that smoking is associated with half the male tuberculosis deaths in India.

In practice, TB will only be eradicated from a community if over a prolonged period all sputum-positive cases are recognised and treated, and overall living conditions improve. In addition a high incidence of AIDS makes eradication impossible.

TB can however be controlled so that the prevalence of TB starts to decline.

As soon as all community members are sputum negative there will be no local source for infecting new contacts even though reactivated cases may continue to occur for many years. However, migration into the community or displacement of people can re-expose them to infection.

Evaluate the programme

As with any community health activity, we will need to evaluate our programme at regular intervals to see whether we are reaching the targets we set.

Each year we should record (as percentages):

1. **The numbers of new patients started on treatment.**
   We should use the categories defined on page 278, i.e. new smear-positive patients, relapse, treatment failure, defaulter, transfer in, chronic case.
2. **The outcome of patients on treatment.**
   We should use the categories defined on page 283, i.e. cure, treatment completed, treatment failure, death, default, transfer out.

From these figures we can monitor the success of the programme, in particular the number and percentage of newly diagnosed smear-positive patients in the community, and the percentage cure rate of patients started on treatment.

Other evaluations could include:

1. **BCG vaccination.**
   The proportion of children under one or under five who have a BCG scar.
2. **Community satisfaction with our service.**
   This might include comments on the side effects of drugs, ease of collecting medicines, whether drugs are affordable, health workers'

attitudes and convenience of DOTS strategies, especially Direct Observation.

85 per cent cure rate, at which point the incidence of TB declines in a community.

Summary

Tuberculosis kills more young people and adults than any other infectious disease, apart from AIDS; the poor are affected most, losing lives, health and livelihood because of the difficulties in obtaining treatment. HIV increases the incidence of TB.

TB can be cured; treatment is both expensive and long term. Dual infection with TB and HIV/AIDS makes diagnosis and treatment of TB and HIV/AIDS essential for long-term success, so these two infections always have to be considered together.

Before deciding whether to participate in a programme we must liaise with the District Medical Officer and enter into an informed partnership with the community. We must follow the National TB Programme (NTP) guidelines.

Sputum testing will be the main diagnostic method used before starting patients on treatment. Passive case-finding is usually the most cost-effective way of identifying patients but where HIV/AIDS is common we should follow a more active approach. Whenever possible, we should follow a DOTS strategy where each dose of medicine taken by the patient is observed, so as to ensure the best possible compliance.

Careful records need to be kept of categories of patients started on treatment and of treatment outcome. These statistics, which should be recorded according to national TB programme protocols, will form the basis of monitoring the success of the programme. We should aim for an

Further reading and resources

1. *Treatment of Tuberculosis: Guidelines for National Programmes*, WHO, 3rd edn, 2003.
    This is the key manual, which describes the correct ways of diagnosing, treating and recording TB. All programmes will need to have a copy of this book.
    Available from: WHO. See Appendix E.
2. *TB/HIV: a Clinical Manual*, A. D. Harries and D. Mahler, WHO, 2nd edn, 2004.
    A pocket-sized manual on how to treat patients with both TB and HIV.
    Available from: WHO. See Appendix E.
3. *Guidelines for the Management of Drug-Resistant Tuberculosis*, J. Crofton, P. Chaulet and D. Maher, WHO, 1997.
    With MDR becoming increasingly common, the details in this book will be needed by all projects.
    Available from: WHO. See Appendix E.
4. *Clinical Tuberculosis*, 2nd edn, J. Crofton, N. Horne and F. Miller, Macmillan, 1998.
    This practical and comprehensive book written by leading experts is especially designed for doctors, and any project involved in TB control should obtain a copy.
    Available from: TALC. See Appendix E.
5. Information from WHO on TB can be obtained from these websites: www.who.int/gtb and www.stoptb.org. Alternatively contact WHO at addresses in Appendix E.
6   *TB: A Global Emergency* is a picture card training pack available from TALC.

Slides

Natural History of Childhood TB TBNH (TALC)

See Further references and guidelines, pages 415–6.

15

A Community Development Approach to AIDS Care, Prevention and Control

Ian D. Campbell, International Health Programme Consultant
and Alison Rader Campbell, Community Development Consultant (HIV/AIDS and Health),
Salvation Army International Headquarters, London.

In this chapter we shall consider:

- Introduction – What is AIDS?
- A summary of our responses
- Carrying out a community appraisal
- What resources do we need?
- How is a response developed?
- What are the important principles for programme design?
- What are the entry points into the community?
- What are the elements of community counselling?
- The use of antiretroviral therapy (ART)
- How can we measure and monitor the effect of HIV/AIDS?

Introduction – What is AIDS?

AIDS stands for the Acquired Immune Deficiency Syndrome. This is a disease in which the body's immune system collapses, often leading to death within a few years. It is caused by the Human Immunodeficiency Virus (HIV).

Infection with HIV usually leads to AIDS. An individual becomes positive usually within three months of contact, but the time between seroconversion (i.e. becoming HIV positive) and the development of AIDS is variable, ranging from months to a number of years – for many about five to ten years. During this latent period the person infected with HIV is largely free of symptoms but is infectious to others.

AIDS is spread largely through sexual contact with an HIV-positive individual. In addition it can be passed on through blood transfusions, infected needles, breast milk and from mother to foetus before or during birth.

AIDS became generally known in the early 1980s, and since that time it has spread extremely rapidly, initially in sub-Saharan Africa and in the Asia-Pacific region. Some examples of countries with high or rapidly expanding rates within specific populations or parts of the country include Brazil, USA, Russia, the countries of Eastern Europe, India, China, Myanmar, Thailand, and Cambodia.

At the time of writing (March 2006) there are estimated to be 40.3 million people living with

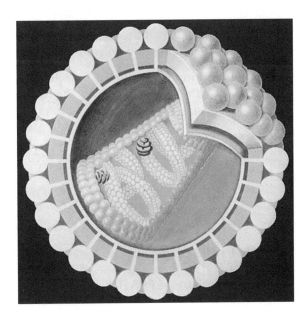

Figure 15.1 Structure of the human immunodeficiency virus (HIV).

HIV/AIDS worldwide. There were at least 3 million AIDS-related deaths in 2004, including half a million children. Sixty-four per cent of new infections occurred in Sub-Saharan Africa. Most people infected with HIV do not know they have the virus. Worldwide, the numbers increase each year (see Further reading and resources 16).

Although powerful drugs known as antiretrovirals can now prolong the life of many people infected with HIV, they are not yet generally available for community programmes in developing countries. Their cost is still high in many countries and side effects can be severe, meaning careful monitoring is needed. However, they hold enormous value in treating individuals and restoring hope to communities.

In many countries AIDS is becoming the number one health priority and there is a great and growing need for community based HIV/AIDS programmes to be established. These can be based in a variety of settings including hospitals and health centres, clubs and churches or in the homes of the community.

A summary of our responses

In HIV/AIDS community based programmes the four most important responses will be:

1. **Prevention through a variety of actions,** which will include the reduction of stigma.
   Experience in a community counselling approach shows that healthy choices regarding prevention can be made by the community and encouraged in the context of the community's long-term interests. They may choose these or other strategies. The key to success is that the community owns the decision and then long-term prevention is more likely to be sustained.
2. **Voluntary HIV counselling and testing** of individuals (VCT).
3. **Home-based care of PLWHA,** including their family members. Care is often carried out by relatives, friends and community members, usually as a team.

The ABC Approach to preventing the spread of HIV

A stands for **A**bstinence
B stands for **B**e faithful/reduce the number of partners
C stands for **C**ondom use: both male condoms, but increasingly female also.
We can add **D** for **D**iagnosis

The Lancet comments as follows:

All 3 elements are essential in reducing HIV incidence, though the emphasis placed on each varies according to the target population. Although programmes should include an appropriate mix of A B and C, each programme can promote the part(s) they feel most comfortable supporting.
Lancet, Vol. 364, Nov. 27, 2004, p. 1913

---

4. **Treatment with drugs** and in particular antiretroviral therapy (ART), sometimes known as Highly Active Antiretroviral Therapy (HAART), where available, affordable, and sustainable.

The ways in which we respond will vary greatly in different situations and will depend on the beliefs and cultures of both programme leaders and beneficiaries (community members). These activities are elements in a multidisciplinary strategy. Our overall aim is to encourage each of the above through a community based approach. This empowers people with information and confidence, so they can make informed choices and work together both to minimise suffering and to reduce levels of infection.

But before we make any response, we will first need to carry out an appraisal of HIV/AIDS within the community.

Carrying out a community appraisal

There are various ways of doing this, and some general methods are described in Chapter 5.

In the case of HIV/AIDS we can use a more specific approach.

We start by recognising that local communities can respond. Those of us based in hospitals, clinics or other organisations can and must learn

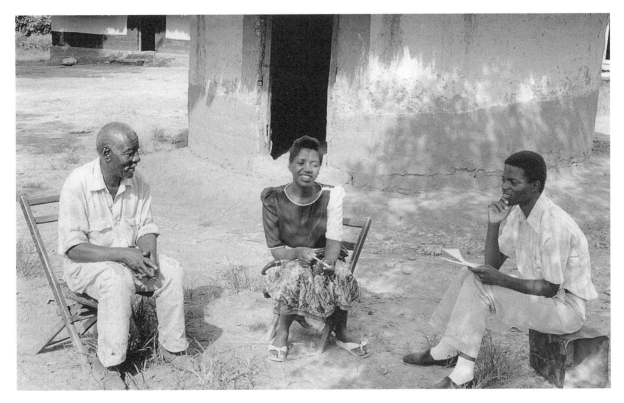

Figure 15.2   The headman of a village in Zambia works closely with community workers.

from local experience. We can help to bring about connections between all involved in prevention, care and treatment, so that understanding and vision spread more quickly. Policymakers need to be invited to learn from this local action and experience.

Whether a community based organisation, or a health programme team, our appraisal consists of two main areas: enquiring about concerns and understanding key local strengths.

Enquiring about concerns

Exploring deeply felt concerns is our first priority:

1. **Ask community members what they think** about the AIDS problem. Their answers usually include the way they feel as well as the way they think others feel. Here is an example of questions which can be asked:
   a) What do people know about HIV/AIDS?
      • How is HIV transmitted?
      • What do they think causes AIDS?
      • What are the symptoms and signs?
      • How does one talk to a person living with HIV/AIDS?
   b) What do people feel about AIDS?
      • Do they wish to avoid people living with HIV/AIDS, i.e. does their attitude *contribute* to stigma?
      • If community members are HIV positive or fear they might be, do they feel they must keep this quiet, for fear of what people will think, i.e. do they *experience* stigma?
   c) What do people believe about the behaviours that cause HIV/AIDS?
      • Can these behaviours be changed?
      • Do they have beliefs or opinions about whether abstinence, partner reduction or condoms might help to reduce spread?
      • Do they see how a safer future can be formed for their children and the next generation?

Collecting this information with community members will also help to build awareness that answers do exist. This in turn will help to build hope and stimulate action.

2. **Ask local health workers** – from hospitals, clinics or community based programmes – how they assess the problem. Those involved with Voluntary Counselling and Testing will often have a profound understanding of how the community perceives HIV/AIDS. The presence of VCT also helps to bring certainty and ideas of what actions are needed.

3. **Contact district and national health authorities** to seek information and guidance, and to explore partnership possibilities.

We need to respond not only to the present concerns and felt needs of the community but also to the needs recognised by health authorities, who can help to predict long-term trends and the solutions that are needed. But in turn we can help this process by giving the community a voice to the authorities. We can help people express their deep concerns, as many will feel too vulnerable to do this without our support.

Because the prevalence of the virus in the community is often not known, we need to realise that the existence of even one confirmed person with HIV usually means that many other community members will be HIV positive. Moreover, once the virus has entered a community the AIDS problem will grow. This means that it is usually only a matter of time before the community recognises the problem of HIV/AIDS and the need for an appropriate and robust response.

In these early stages we can build trust, which will become the foundation for an intentional HIV/AIDS programme in the future.

Understanding key local strengths

The way a community responds to HIV/AIDS can be thought of as four key concepts or strengths, which apply to all programmes. Just how they are expressed will be different for each project.

1. **Care.** This is best understood as 'being with' or 'standing alongside PLWHA' rather than just providing services. It includes sharing and support as well as encouraging prevention.

2. **Community.** This is best understood as 'belonging'. Home, neighbours and friends become the environment for care and risk reduction.

3. **Change.** Our task is to help community members make choices based on being well informed. This in turn helps to bring about behavioural change both in individuals and communities.

4. **Hope.** The experience of hope results in living fully and positively within family, community, culture and faith. Hope also helps to build confidence for the future and to sustain healthy changes in behaviour.

These four basic concepts are transferable. In other words they can apply in all cultures but we have to apply and develop them for our own situations. They need to be opened up and explored within specific settings. We can help people to do this by asking about their concerns and hopes. This includes understanding how communities respond when faced with difficult situations. Often we will find that local communities take charge of their situations, act for change, measure their progress (e.g. through mapping of risks, and community counselling) and then help other communities cope with the challenges brought about by HIV/AIDS. This shows that there is a great human capacity to respond to difficulty and to sustain hope. We can help and encourage communities in this situation but not impose our own understanding or interpretation.

For example:

At Kithituni, Kenya, a local church group was concerned about AIDS in the community. They developed action groups with women, youth, men and children. All met together every week. After a year, about ten other nearby communities had started to make responses. After two years at least 40 nearby communities were taking action. Linkage to local churches was developed and small amounts of government funding were raised to help communities network together and learn from each other's experiences. The Kithituni community is often visited by members of both government and NGOs. The impression is consistently one of astonishment that through 'coming together' such strength can emerge which leads on to such effective change.

What resources do we need?

- The most important resource for a successful programme will be a group of committed people who are concerned both for persons and for communities. Such a group can make decisions and gather ideas more effectively than persons working alone.
- In addition, we will need links to a referral hospital that does HIV testing, or can pass on samples to a testing centre, and which may also be a source for antiretroviral drugs. Local community members can be trained, supported and mentored by partner clinics or hospitals.
- As soon as HIV testing is known to take place, questions will arise within the community that will need to be answered, and counselling will become necessary. Indeed, HIV testing should always be accompanied by counselling, and this combined approach is usually known as Voluntary Counselling and Testing or VCT. In many parts of the world community volunteers are being selected and trained to carry this out, which if done sensitively can improve the community's response to the HIV epidemic. VCT needs to be combined with a follow-up plan that includes care, support and, increasingly, the option of using ART. In this situation, fear and stigma tend to lessen, more people come forward for testing and the whole response to HIV improves, often leading to lower infection rates.
- Suitable transport will be needed by HIV care workers, but many teams find that they can walk, use bicycles or motorbikes and, where convenient, public transport.

How is a response developed?

Many people who are concerned about AIDS will have neither formal health qualifications nor even any links with hospitals and clinics. This does not matter. The key stages in a response will include the following:

> An HIV/AIDS response can start with one motivated individual, whether based in a hospital, a clinic, a school, a village, or any other community structure.

Step 1: Form a team

This will comprise committed and caring people, drawn either from community members or health care staff.

A good starting point is to recruit people who are known to be doing well in their own jobs, but care needs to be taken not to detract from their existing tasks, and to make time for discussion and understanding with all involved.

Team members can work part-time provided their tasks are analysed, roles are defined, and the structure of the team is repeatedly examined.

For a hospital, it is relatively easy for a volunteer team to be formed, without hiring a single extra staff member. This can be an effective way of setting the programme in motion. Additional staffing, office facilities, funding and administrative details can all follow later on.

An important first step is to understand the way communities work together and solve problems.

> We may be tempted to impose our own solutions but it is better to discover the community's own beliefs and weigh up their own suggestions.

For example: 'SALT' visits can be arranged. This is a highly effective learning practice for health workers. A team learns by visiting a neighbourhood. This is done in a spirit of:

- **S**upport/stimulation
- **A**ppreciation
- **L**earning
- **T**ransfer of vision and action from one community to another

Any newly formed team should demonstrate from the beginning a willingness to visit local communities simply to learn, and appreciate, the situation, and understand the capacity of the local community to respond.

The SALT visit helps its members to realise that effective efforts do not depend on 'external' people.

Often, community members, because they are dependent on health services, believe they will not be able to manage at home. For this reason, reassurance about support needs to be given at an early stage. This is where home care can be helpful in building up strengths that have existed for a long time, and in promoting hope.

As early as 1987 an AIDS care unit was formed at Chikankata Hospital in the Southern Province of Zambia. This included a home care team. The decision to shift the emphasis from the hospital to the community was based on identifying community resources and listening to their requests. The community stated that:

- other health programmes should continue.
- the family is the greatest long-term strength.
- people prefer to die at home.
- people learn best by talking together.
- changes in behaviour are best achieved through activating traditional leadership and helping the community to take responsibility for care and prevention.

Step 2: Identify specific risk situations

It is not always obvious that the family and neighbourhood are the primary environment of risk in most countries. Specific risk situations may also include boarding-school children, youth culture, and the behaviour of those known to have AIDS or to be HIV positive.

For example: truck drivers are a potential high risk group and frequently a means of introducing HIV into previously unaffected communities. Each truck driver will have a friend, wife or partner somewhere else, and most commercial sex workers also have some form of family life. The challenge for the team is to discover an entry point, ideally by invitation into these less visible family relationships.

Step 3: Help communities learn together

Community-to-community visits can be arranged by health-care staff who will themselves learn in the process and speed up the useful learning that emerges. Communities can help set the pace in the expansion of home care, ways of preventing HIV/AIDS from spreading and reducing stigma by increasing openness. The health programme can give the support that helps the community to build confidence.

Step 4: Develop community care and counselling

The objectives will include:
- Drawing on information from our Community Appraisal mentioned above and also from any information gathering as described in Chapter 3.
- Caring for patients at home and helping local people to do the same.
- Supporting families, through family counselling and home visits.
- Promoting discussion within the wider community. This is best done through a facilitative approach that helps people to reflect and consult, then to clarify and apply their response.
- Helping to prevent the spread of HIV through:
  - Community discussion, which in turn leads to community action, one simple example from Uganda being the change in opening times for bars.
  - Community counselling, which stimulates people to change their behaviours, one important example from countries in southern Africa leading to discouraging the belief that HIV can be prevented by ritual cleansing, e.g. by sleeping with a virgin.

Step 5: Link the community's response to HIV/AIDS with general processes of treatment and management within the hospital or health centre

This will include:
1. Acceptance of a multidisciplinary approach. The HIV/AIDS hospital or clinic programme will involve medical, nursing, laboratory, education, counselling, administration and pastoral care staff. Part of a community led response will be making a link to a hospital or clinic. Now that antiretroviral therapy is becoming more widely available, these links are becoming essential. Close cooperation between the community based organisation, e.g. church, the clinic and the community itself will be key to the reliable use of ART (see Further reading and resources 7).

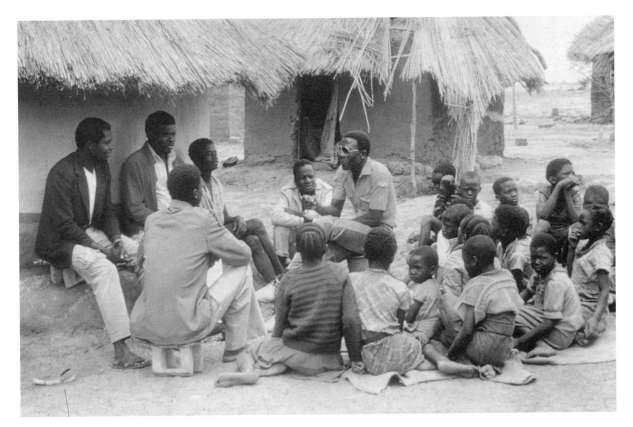

Figure 15.3   Community counselling helps people to take responsibility for changing their behavioural patterns.

2. Setting up a hospital management plan, which in turn should include:
   - A diagnosis/counselling/treatment regime (see guidelines on antiretoviral treatment – Further reading and resources 7).
   - Planned discharge, with family involvement.
   - Liaison with the community and home care team.
   - Access to hospital care when required.

Step 6: Obtaining additional funds

This is deliberately placed as the last in the steps because many of the earlier activities so far mentioned can be done on relatively small budgets. However, as the programme develops, expenses can rise dramatically. We should by this stage be working alongside or participating in any national HIV/AIDS programme and funds and resources may be available from them.

But extra funding will usually become necessary in addition. Chapter 4, pages 61–5 describes in more detail how we can obtain funding for CBHC programmes.

In the case of funding for HIV/AIDS programmes, the project proposal does not need to be a complicated document. Help can usually be found from donor agencies, national AIDS organisations or from within other departments of the institution or organisation.

When writing a project proposal for an HIV/AIDS programme, certain aspects need to be mentioned and highlighted, as described below.

Writing an HIV project proposal

A summary statement at the beginning of the project is useful, outlining the main concept. The vision should emphasise an expanded community response to HIV/AIDS. This then justifies activities proposed such as visits by health teams to communities, skills training and learning between communities. This is best followed by an outline of the project background, giving a picture of HIV/AIDS in the district and its possible impact on other areas of development. Then should follow a statement of concerns, goals and objectives. The donor needs to know about activities, and a schedule for implementation. There needs to be a budget (separating capital and recurrent expenditure). The proposal needs to comment on ways in which the community is involved, and the strategy of linking home care to prevention in a participatory and relational way. This enables ART to be used more effectively for more people, with access to drugs, monitoring of side effects and compliance being given top priority.

Ensure the proposal shows how the health organisation will network with district, provincial and national levels and other providers.

What are the important principles for programme design?

The steps outlined above will tend to follow in order, though some will be running together and the order may sometimes need to be changed. But underlying all programme stages are the following principles, which are necessary for successful outcomes.

Human resource development

Good programmes will depend on well trained individuals and on teams that function effectively.

Communities and health staff need to strengthen skills, activities and systems. The human capacity to care is central but workload and timetables need to ensure that people are not overloaded, leading to discouragement, burn-out and feeling overwhelmed. There need to be steps in place where people can share problems and griefs, and gain strength from each other or from specially trained counsellors or mentors.

Integration

An approach is needed that combines home care, community development, VCT, the use of ART and hospital support. This is the basis for the integrated management of HIV/AIDS.

Such an approach produces a framework for care in which genuine interest will result in action, and hope stimulates plans for prevention by communities. Care is one vital entry point.

This principle of integration is expressed in many ways. *For example*: within the institution it means a coordinated approach amongst the following disciplines:

- Clinical/nursing/laboratory;
- Education;
- Pastoral care;
- VCT;
- Reliable access to drugs;
- Monitoring side effects of treatment.

Outside the institution it means a community-driven partnership, supported by government and non-governmental organisations, religious groups, field workers and policy makers.

The heart of integrated management is the link between two processes: caring for people and change of attitudes and behaviours in the wider circles of people connected to those receiving care. It requires health staff to integrate themselves into local realities by visiting and understanding homes and neighbourhoods and being willing to learn from them as in the SALT method mentioned above (see Further reading and resources 15).

Partnership between community and government

To be successful, AIDS responses need to be decentralised and grounded with the community, but we will still need to follow national policy, allow our programmes to be supported and to make use of supplies, including ART, that may be available. Indeed, we may need to advocate for more involvement of government support and supplies for our programme, while at the same time guarding our particular approach. When the voices of people suffering from HIV/AIDS are effectively heard, policy can change.

Organising and mainstreaming

We need excellent systems and high quality management in order for the huge workload of HIV programmes to be as effective as possible. The actual structures can be part of existing primary health care departments, or can co-exist with them. Whatever the arrangement, an HIV/AIDS response will eventually need a specific allocation of people, skills and resources, for prevention, care, treatment and monitoring.

However, every department in a hospital, clinic or health programme needs to engage with HIV/AIDS – this is often known as mainstreaming. Health staff and community workers should be encouraged to share in different activities, learn leadership skills and remain multipurpose within the response. SALT visits as described above can help to keep all team members in touch with realities in the community, so increasing both their understanding and their compassionate response.

Training and expansion

Continuing training of all staff members is important both to encourage the team and to make sure it is well informed about the issues involved in HIV care and control. The use of ART is complex and all team members will need to know the basic principles and be able to answer questions from community members.

As experience grows, other groups needing help may visit the health facility, project or community based organisation. Later, more formal learning programmes can be set up if the numbers of interested visitors grow. These will need to cover home care, community counselling, networking, monitoring, hospital linkages, team building and the use of ART.

What are the entry points into the community?

Because HIV/AIDS is usually surrounded by ignorance and fear, especially when it first appears, communities will often be protective or suspicious of those wishing to enter this 'new world'. This means we need to find entry points into the community in a sensitive way.

Communities are made up of relationships. It is these relationships that will bear the strains caused by HIV/AIDS. When HIV is known to be present in a community, changes begin to take place immediately. This works through a ripple effect from the person who is infected out to his/her closest relatives and friends, then almost invisibly to the surrounding community.

Communities become aware of something happening. There is uneasiness. Curiosity masks anxiety. Information becomes a source of fear and speculation, as other ideas become attached to the 'facts'. There is a shared secrecy, which produces stigma. Yet often many people in the same neighbourhood, family or group share and learn together because it is known that AIDS is everybody's problem. This is part of what is known as shared confidentiality: when the community knows what is going on inside it, without saying it aloud in so many words.

It is with communities involved in this process that we need to gain entry points. These must be based on trust, which means first establishing a caring relationship. This can be done in various ways. *For example*: There may be existing programmes in the community, e.g. for health, teaching, or worship. There may be institutions that have links with the community. The time will come when a household will welcome a home visit, which is usually best carried out by a team of two or three people.

Home visits may start as an expression of care for members of the community. They soon help to normalise the situation and act as a means of encouraging others to share their concerns for other community members.

Soon will come an entry point for community counselling (see the next section). The use of both these forms of care (home visits and community counselling) has a greater impact than either alone, provided each is carried out with sensitivity, in the same geographic area.

Confidentiality is of great importance. Within the home it is about individuals and their HIV status. It is therefore person centred. Within the context of community counselling, confidentiality is more about issues raised and felt, and the community's response to them. This is known as issue-centred confidentiality. Both forms of

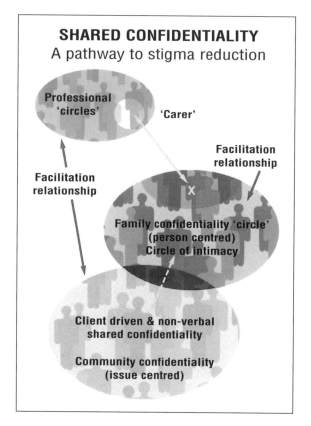

SHARED CONFIDENTIALITY
A pathway to stigma reduction

Professional 'circles'

'Carer'

Facilitation relationship

Facilitation relationship

Family confidentiality 'circle'
(person centred)
Circle of intimacy

Client driven & non-verbal
shared confidentiality

Community confidentiality
(issue centred)

Figure 15.4   How shared confidentiality works.

confidentiality must be maintained and respected outside their particular circles.

What are the elements of community counselling?

Community counselling is a conversation-based activity that focuses on groups and communities. It enables the whole community to take responsibility for care and change. Community counselling includes the following:

- Building relationships, especially between the counselling team and the community.
- Community identification of problems and exploring solutions.
- Decision-making by the community, including the planning of strategies.
- Implementing any actions decided upon.
- Evaluating the response together, and exploring any additional problems.

Chapter 2 has more details about similar approaches used in other aspects of CBHC.

These elements are explored within a timescale with which the community must feel comfortable. This may be faster or, more commonly, slower than we expect. Our aim as health workers is to facilitate and not to press for quick solutions or to impose our views.

> Once sufficient trust has been established so that discussion about HIV and related issues can take place, the community must set the pace.

However, the facilitators still need to help move the group towards making decisions and planning strategies. Sometimes this will mean narrowing down from a range of options that the community needed to explore first.

If the facilitator is too anxious to reach a conclusion, some deeper issues may not be faced. So, although each meeting should conclude with the question 'What next?', the answer at times may simply be to meet again.

This whole process, though not very costly financially, does take a great deal of energy, time and teamwork. It can and must involve a wide range of people who are not health staff. It is a key to sustained and expanded care and prevention.

The volunteer community counsellor

The role of the community counsellor can include the following:
1. Opening up concerns in the context of the community's own responsibility, strength and capacity to respond.
2. Linking the community and the health services.
3. Helping to implement community-specific strategies.
4. Referring patients to hospital when necessary (and working as a treatment supporter for those who are receiving ART).
5. Counselling in bereavement and other stress times in the community.

Community name..   Date...

Issues/concerns discussed	Strategies discussed	Decisions made	Action taken	Results	How do they know? (Indicators)
Youth and sexual activity; they seem unaware of risk Men travel for work Lack of local employment	We need to teach our young: • Grandmothers should resume their traditional role in this • Teachers could organise • Talk to youth for their point of view More employment by way of income generating projects	Talk to the youth: one community counsellor and a group of grand-mothers will gather the youth for a discussion	Discussion with youth was held on (*put in date*)	The youth are very interested (*see reports of youth discussion on date*)	They want to meet with this group to discuss further They are also forming their own strategies and want to keep meeting themselves

NOTES ON TONE OF MEETING: Several people *(put in their names)* were trying to shift the discussion to the topic of economic development, saying that nothing could be done without jobs and money. Others in the group, especially *(put in their names)* strongly challenged this view. After three hours, agreement was reached on the specific action to be taken.

Figure 15.5   An example of 'Summary Documentation' (see page 302).

As community counsellors carry out these functions they will try to:
• Involve every member of the discussion group.
• Reflect the discussion back to the group by summarising at regular intervals what has been discussed or agreed upon.
• Keep the discussion on the agreed subject.
• Encourage positive relationships between group members.
• Take care to be seen as a facilitator rather than the person in control.
   See also pages 22–6.

Widespread HIV/AIDS control will only happen if care and counselling teams in one community are prepared to share their skills with other communities.

It is exciting to see that effective steps in dealing with any aspect of the HIV/AIDS challenge can begin with any community member. But a realistic strategy for an HIV/AIDS response also needs to contain strong community and political leadership from the 'top'. This is an area where programmes and community members can help to advocate for change and effective support from both politicians and government health departments.

In summary, we must remember that helping a community to change its behaviour is very different from trying to control behaviour. This 'facilitation of behaviour change' is the most effective AIDS control measure.

The use of antiretroviral therapy (ART)

Antiretroviral drugs are now becoming available more widely and at more affordable prices. These drugs slow down the development of AIDS by acting against the virus. The use of antiretrovirals is becoming an increasingly important part of AIDS treatment and control. But they need to be used in the context of well managed programmes, where HIV testing is available and 'DOT' style supervision of treatment is possible (see pages 272–3, 280–1). In such situations, they can prolong life, reduce suffering from secondary infections, and minimise mother-to-child transmission.

A number of approaches are being used by different governments and NGOs. For those involved in HIV programmes, it is important to keep up to date with the latest information from sources listed below.

Programmes that are successfully managed with high rates of compliance can prolong life and help to reduce the levels of HIV in a community, if used as part of an integrated approach. However, poorly managed programmes where people start and stop treatment without adequate support and monitoring are likely to cause increasing drug resistance, which will make HIV/AIDS even harder to bring under control.

The Salvation Army (see Further reading below) has summarised the key roles of each person involved in the use of ART. These are listed in the box below:

Role of the person living with HIV/AIDS
- Adherence and self-care.
- Note side effects.
- Live responsibly.
- Stimulate response in others.
- Have a secure place to store drugs – e.g. a cupboard with a lock.
- Have a means of accurate timing to take drugs – sunrise and sunset if this is regular, a watch, clock or radio.
- Have 'treatment supporter' – friend or relative – who will monitor drug adherence.

Role of family
- Primary care and support.
- ART's safe keeping and storage.
- Administration of ART.
- Encourage adherence.
- Observe side effects.
- Documentation.
- Family members trained in monitoring and administration of ART (Treatment Supporter (TS)).
- Family member able to collect ART if patient cannot collect them.
- Support/supervision of drug taking and monitoring adherence to treatment schedule.

Role of church/community organisation
- Secondary care and support.
- Church/community organisation facilitation team to stimulate response in partnership with Community Care and Prevention Teams (CCPT).

- Stock and distribute and monitor ART where the clinic is too far away.
- Accompany people with HIV in maintaining treatment and prevention through home based care.
- Participate in community conversation and transfer.
- Can be a place for storing ART for stable PLWHA already receiving ART when the clinic or hospital is too far away, or too expensive to reach regularly.
- Provide a trained person with responsibility for distribution and storage of drugs.
- Monitor adherence through a pill count system, and follow up when the person on treatment does not collect drugs, or cannot adhere to the treatment schedule.

Role of neighbourhood
- Secondary care and support.
- Care and Prevention Teams (CCPTs), home-based care support for adherence and prevention.
- Supporting and advocating for community based voluntary counselling and testing (VCT).
- Support documentation.
- Ongoing community conversation for dealing with issues arising, and updating information about ART.
- Transfer of concepts and action to other issues and communities.
- Know where to obtain ART.
- Ensure there is a 'treatment supporter' to offer support and encouragement to the person on ART.
- Ensure that there are community members trained and motivated to link between the clinic and treatment support (a Community Helper for ART (CHART)).
- Encourage adherence, especially when the person on treatment gets physically well and returns to normal activities.

How can we measure and monitor the impact of AIDS?

Collecting information about the activities we carry out can be relatively easy, and is valuable provided it is systematic.

At district hospital level, the information that can be easily collected is listed as it applies to

Experience from the field

'When I found out that I was HIV positive, I encouraged the rest of my family to go for VCT.' *Man living with HIV, Chikambola September 2004*

'Since I started ART, I feel a lot better and I have encouraged 17 people in the last three weeks to go for VCT.' *Man on ART from Chikambola, September 2004*

'In this community we care for our sick and look for transport. We want the medicines at our clinic here so that people can easily access them.' *Village Headman, Zambia, 2004*

'In our work in the village, some villagers have been taking the ARTs for a few months. We found they were very confused with the use, effects and complications of it.'

'We found one woman [who] shared that she had had a strong reaction, but she persisted for three months and gained full strength. We asked her to share more of her experience, and she continues to do this in the village.'

'Why do we have to get drugs from the hospital? It is a long distance; we can get them from the clinic, here'. *Chikambola, Zambia*

Impact on the hospital

If we work in a hospital or health centre, the impact of AIDS on the institution needs to be observed. An example can be the number of people found to be HIV positive (tested because they have symptoms) listed year by year, for all patients, and for specific groups (such as antenatal patients).

Financial impact

The financial impact on hospitals and clinics can be followed to some extent by calculating costs for the following:

- Safety precautions (gloves, needles, plastic bags, etc.);
- Inpatient care days;
- Drugs;
- Test kits;
- Administrative charges.

Home care as it affects health programmes will cost money, mainly for transport, extra training for team members and community care teams, and essential handouts to the seriously impoverished.

Community impact

This is most easily measured by ongoing operational research in homes and neighbourhoods. Some of the figures in Table 15.1 can be discovered in this way. Responses are gathered according to expressions of care, behaviour change, income generation, transfer of vision and responses from one community to another. For examples of protocols, see Further reading and resources 14 and 15.

A way of documenting team activity

Home care and community counselling are effective settings for measuring both motivation and behavioural change in the community.

The community may find it helpful to allow documentation to be done by the team itself, or it may suggest a community member should be

some programmes in Africa and Asia. However, it is even more useful if we find ways to measure and learn from the patterns of response of local communities and of organisations. The Human Capacity Development core indicators are one way of doing this (see Further reading and resources 12). A useful tool for tracking progress as teams is the self-assessment tool for AIDS competence (see Further reading and resources 13).

Table 15.1 outlines field and hospital data that can be collected by simply counting the numbers of people participating in various situations.

In local communities, mapping by community members is a reliable way of self-measurement (often one part of participatory appraisal, see Chapter 5). The self-assessment tool for AIDS competence (see Further reading and resources 13) is a tool for communities and health teams to assess and share progress.

Table 15.1   Types of data that can be collected easily

Administration	• total persons seen • new persons seen • total families seen • new families seen • patients preferring home care to periodic checks at hospital
Clinical care	• number with pre-AIDS • number with AIDS • number asymptomatic • number persons or families/friends with nursing care felt needs
Laboratory	• total contacts tested • number contacts HIV+ • results from all sources (inpatients, outpatients, etc.)
Mortality	• total persons known to have died • number died at home • number died in hospital/readmission

Education	• number of persons (friends, families) applying what they know in
	    – action for prevention (self reported)
	    – involvement in home care
	    – helping others to know what to do for care and prevention

Pastoral care	• number funerals attended • number times pastoral care required in the form of prayer, scripture, counsel
Counselling	• number children of HIV+ persons • number families with HIV+ primary breadwinner • number families headed by HIV+ single mother • number families with abnormal atmosphere due to disease • number persons, family members, friends, communities acknowledging lifestyle changes in social activity, family life, sexual behaviour
Transfer	• members of PLWHA who motivate others to respond • how many others respond (as a result of the influence of a PLWHA) • how many families transfer response to other families • how many families are responding as a result of the action of PLWHA • how many communities transfer • how many communities are responding as a result of transfer from a community by PLWHA

responsible or take part. The counselling team can be both observer and participant.

Documenting team activities is important for accountability and should be seen as an open commitment with the community. Records should be kept and be available to any community member who wishes to see them.

Figure 15.5 is an actual example of what is known as 'Summary Community Counselling Documentation'. This particular one summarises a community counselling session (see Further reading and resources 2).

For programmes that reach a sufficient size we should consider using some of the specific indicators for monitoring programmes that have been set up by WHO/UNAIDS. These are listed in a box on page 345 of Chapter 18 on Monitoring and Evaluation.

Health programmes need to measure and monitor the human impact of AIDS so that strategies can be remodelled to meet ever-changing and growing needs. Information for this can be gathered from health institutions and from the community.

Unless we express care for people living with HIV and AIDS, we will have little chance of preventing transmission of the virus. Care creates hope and, as the communities with which we work sense this, they will be motivated to work towards preventing the spread of HIV infection.

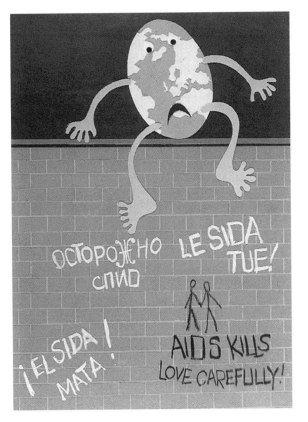

Figure 15.6   A fragile world teeters on the brink of a 'great fall'. Only a worldwide effort will stop it.

Summary

The key to a successful HIV/AIDS response is the participation of the community in a response to HIV/AIDS. Home care and community counselling are two essential components. They are best implemented by teams. Together they encourage the community to reflect and respond in positive ways. The concept of 'facilitating behavioural change' emerges as one key method of reducing the spread of infection. Volunteer community counsellors can play a leading role. The use of antiretroviral therapy has opened up great opportunities for treatment but also causes big challenges, including reliable access to drugs, monitoring of side effects and helping PLHWA to continue treatment long term.

Further reading and resources

1. *Strategies for Hope* series, Action Aid/AMREF/ World in Need, 1990–2005.
   These excellent and practical booklets grew out of field experience in Africa. The most recent are still available and are published in English and French. Videos and films are also available. New titles are added regularly.
   See the Strategies for Hope Foundation, www. stratshope.org, from which these and other community HIV/AIDS resources are available.
2. *Community Counselling: A Handbook for Facilitating Care and Change*, The Salvation Army, 1998.
   This is part of an integrated response to HIV by the Salvation Army.
   Available from: The Salvation Army International Headquarters (Health Services), 101 Queen Victoria Street, London EC4P 4EP, UK. Fax: +44 (0)207 489 1410.
3. *The AIDS Handbook*, 3rd edn, J. Hubley, Macmillan, 2003.
   This excellent book is written for those involved in AIDS education and community work.
   Available from: TALC. See Appendix E.
4. 'HIV Counselling in Developing Countries: the link from individual to community counselling for support and change', I. Campbell and A. Rader, *British Journal of Guidance and Counselling*, 23, 1, 1995.
5. WHO publishes a number of titles on AIDS. It is also a partner in the Joint United Nations Programme on AIDS, UNAIDS, which produces useful resources.
   See www.who.int/topics/hiv_infections/en and www.unaids.org.
6. *Primary HIV/AIDS Care*, C. Evian, Macmillan, 2005.
   This is a highly recommended practical manual for the primary health care level.
   Available from: TALC. See Appendix E.
7. 'The Salvation Army Guidelines for community-led ART through a Human Capacity development Approach', far-reaching guidelines for establishing

community-led antiretroviral therapy – a key area of need in HIV/AIDS programmes. The Salvation Army International Headquarters, April 2005: email: IHQ-IntHealth@salvationarmy.org. Website: www1. salvationarmy.org/health.

8. *Zambia National Facilitation Team – A case study of a human capacity development initiative*, A. R. Campbell, S. Mphuka, S. Lucas and I. Campbell, The Salvation Army, London, 2002. Email and website as for No. 7.

9. *Human capacity development: learning from local action and experience*, S. Lucas, A. R. Campbell, U. Duongsaa, S. Mphuka and I. Campbell, The Salvation Army, London, 2002.
Email and website as for No. 7.

10. *A short note on AIDS competence*, Ian Campbell. Notes on HIV/AIDS competence prepared November 2001. The Salvation Army International Headquarters, London.
Email and website as for No. 7.

11. *Expanding Community Action on HIV/AIDS: NGO/CBO Strategies for Scaling Up*, International HIV/AIDS Alliance, 2001.
Extremely useful principles and case histories on scaling up community health programmes.
Available from: International HIV/AIDS Alliance, Queensberry House, 104–106 Queens Road, Brighton, BN1 3XF, UK. Email: mail@aidsalliance.org. Website: www.aidsalliance.org.

12. 'Measuring Human Capacity Development for an Expanded Response', I. D. Campbell, A. R. Campbell and S. Lucas. Poster presented at the XVth International Conference on AIDS, Bangkok, 11–16 July 2004.

13. Self-assessment tool. Website: www.unitar.org.

14. 'Participatory action research on community response to HIV/AIDS', Claire Campbell, Susan Lucas, 2004. The Salvation Army International Headquarters, London: April 2005:
Email and website as for No. 7.

15. 'Palliative and home care in relation to HIV/AIDS – perspectives on going to scale through nurturing community determined shared confidentiality', I. D. Campbell and A. R. Campbell, The Salvation Army International Headquarters, London, October 2002.
Email and website as for No. 7. Subsequently published in the *Compendium on Palliative Care Toronto – palliative care proceedings*.

16. UNAIDS statistics. Website: www.unaids.org.

17. ARV Treatment Fact sheets written in the clearest way possible are available from the Interrnational HIV/AIDS Alliance or can be downloaded from www.aidsalliance.org.

18. *Responding more effectively to HIV and AIDS: A Pillars Guide*, A. Carter, Tearfund, 2004. An effective way of helping uninformed communities understand and respond to HIV/AIDS. Available from Tearfund. See Appendix E.

19. *HIV, Health and Your Community*, R. Granich, J. Mermin, Hesperian Foundation, 2006.
Another excellent publication from the Hesperian. See Appendix E.

Other resources

A number of slides, CD ROMS, Videos/DVDs and accessories are available from TALC. See Appendix E.

See Further references and guidelines, page 416.

16
Setting up Environmental Health Improvements

In this chapter we shall consider:
1. What we need to know:
   - Why environmental health improvements are important
   - Water supply and water sources
   - Methods of waste disposal
2. What we need to do:
   - Help the community to recognise its needs
   - Understand the culture and beliefs of the people
   - Assess what resources are available
   - Choose what improvements to make
   - Work through a community action group
   - Help the community take action on other environmental hazards
   - Evaluate the programme

What we need to know

Why environmental health improvements are important

WHO estimates that four people out of ten do not have access to basic sanitation (that is 2.6 billion people of whom 1.5 billion live in China and India). Two people out of ten do not have access to clean water.

The 7th Millennium Development Goal is to ensure environmental sustainability, and targets include halving the proportion of people living without clean drinking water and the proportion of people without sanitation by 2015 (see pages 12–13). These priorities have put water and sanitation (WATSAN) high on the global agenda.

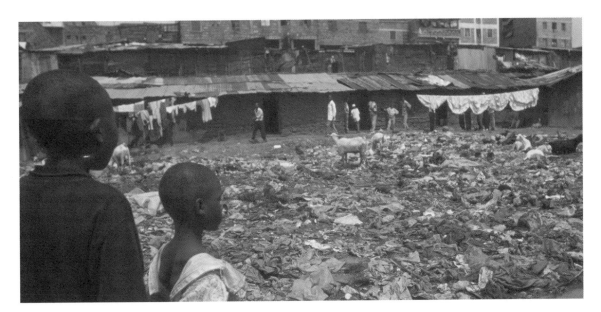

Figure 16.1 Fifty per cent of the population of developing countries lives in urban areas, many in unimproved slums.

Many diseases are caused by water that has been contaminated by human faeces. Environmental health measures are directed towards keeping human and animal waste separated from water used for drinking and washing.

Every day, 3900 children die as a direct result of unsafe water or absence of basic sanitation. Countless more suffer from diseases that are directly linked.

Diseases associated with poor WATSAN include diarrhoea, dysentery, typhoid, cholera, hepatitis, intestinal worms, trachoma and bilharzia. Quite apart from those who die, many million, especially children, are weakened by repeated infections.

Success in reaching this MDG target would enable people to lead healthier and more productive lives and would improve the economies of all the poorest nations. To reduce these diseases of poverty, three actions are essential:

- Improving the quality and availability of water.
- Disposing of human waste, especially faeces.
- Improving hygiene – at personal, household, school and community levels

These three components have been described as the legs of a three-legged stool. Unless all legs are present, the stool falls over.

This chapter concentrates on water supplies and waste disposal. See pages 217–8 for the essential third part of the three-legged stool, i.e. how to improve the hygiene of individuals and communities.

Recent research has shown just how vital this is: regular hand-washing with soap can reduce diarrhoea by almost half. (See page 416, ref. Curtis.)

In Community Based Health Care (CBHC) we can empower community members to make significant improvements at household level and to make more widespread improvements through advocating or working with government departments.

It is worth emphasising that any technology that is not affordable by the community will not be sustainable.

Nearly all government funded or subsidised investments in capital works fail in any handover. There are rarely sufficient government funds – or political will – for proper maintenance.

This means that, for any government linked programme to be successful, there must be full community involvement from the start in deciding what improvements should be made, in management, in maintenance and in community financing. The community must have ownership of changes and improvements from the very beginning.

Ways in which this can occur in both water and sanitation projects are described more fully in *Urban Health and Development*, see Further reading.

Water supply and water sources

Why clean water is needed

Water is needed for two main reasons: to drink and to wash. Many diseases, such as diarrhoea and cholera, are caused through drinking unclean water or eating food contaminated by dirty water; others such as scabies and trachoma are caused by having insufficient water for washing clothes, bodies and faces.

This means that each community will need a small supply of very clean water for drinking and a much larger supply of adequately clean water for washing.

Some health experts believe that the number of water points per 1000 population is a better guide to the level of health care than the number of hospital beds.

As an approximate guide, communities should aim to have available 20–30 litres per person per day within half a kilometre of the home or settlement.

Surface water (rivers, lakes, ponds, etc.) is often highly contaminated both with germs and from pesticides and fertilisers. Groundwater, (stored in permeable rocks more than 100 metres underground), is usually of higher quality and safe to drink unless poisoned by minerals such as arsenic or fluoride.

Before looking at any structural improvements we can make at community level, it is important to realise that simple improvements at household level can make a huge difference.

Studies have shown that improving a water supply can reduce diarrhoeal disease by up to 21 per cent. Regular handwashing with soap and water can reduce such disease by 35 per cent; handwashing plus point-of-use disinfection of water plus safe storage can reduce diarrhoeal episodes by 45 per cent. (See www.rehydrate.org/facts.)

We should therefore concentrate on simple community based measures, including behavioural change, and only spend our time and energy on improving water supplies (or constructing latrines) when we have consistently improved community behaviours and introduced simple household improvements.

Water sources – improving those that already exist

> Improving a water source is often within reach of a community health programme. However, it involves much more than the building and engineering, which can become part of a community project. As well as health behaviours needing to change, the community needs to learn how to use and maintain the improved system. Unless we work with the community to ensure this happens, the whole project is likely to fail.

Springs

Spring water is usually clean when it emerges from the ground but may quickly become contaminated. It can be made safer in the following ways:

1. By erecting a fence with a gate around the spring area to keep out animals.
2. By building a ditch to allow water to drain away.
3. By building a stone wall or 'box' around the spring itself, through which a pipe is led.

Wells and boreholes

Wells come in a variety of forms, including step wells, open wells from which water is collected by rope and bucket, and tubewells from which water is raised by a hand pump. Open wells may be covered and fitted with hand or mechanical pumps.

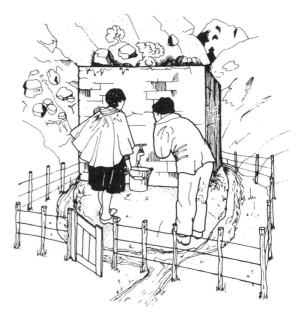

Figure 16.2   A properly protected spring.

Well water can be made safer by:

1. Fixing a removable cover.
2. Building an outward-sloping apron wall around the well, 0.5–1 m high. The wall prevents dirty water from running into the well and acts as a shelf where waterpots can be

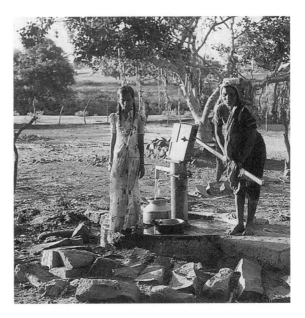

Figure 16.3   A tube well with hand pump, sunk in the low caste area of a village in western India.

placed. The slope helps water to drain and discourages people from standing on it.
3. Building a concrete drainage channel around the outside of the wall.
4. Providing one container to draw water.
This container with its fixed rope is allowed to rest only on the apron wall, never on the ground. Those using the container clean their hands before use and touch only the outside of the container and handle, never the inside.
5. Ensuring that no one uses the well for washing.
6. Encouraging the community to set up its own system for keeping the surrounds clean, repairing the well each year, keeping the hand pump in good repair, and chlorinating the well at regular intervals.

An important example: reducing the dangers of arsenic

In several countries of the world, arsenic contaminates well water. This is worst in Bangladesh, where about half the population is affected.

Arsenic poisoning leads to skin pigmentation, bronchitis, high blood pressure, liver problems and cancer, but these effects take up to ten years to appear. Recent research shows that arsenic has doubled the risk of death from liver, lung and bladder cancers in Bangladesh.

If we know or suspect this is happening in our area, we must get experts to carry out measurements. We then need to find other sources, such as treated surface water or rainwater, well-switching to less contaminated sources, and rainwater harvesting. Other techniques are being developed such as using packets of chemicals, in particular iron sulphate and calcium hypochlorite, added to sand, to act as a filter.

Women traditionally do most of the fetching and carrying of water. The further away the water source, the greater the time and energy spent in carrying. This in turn means less time is available for looking after children, caring for the home and fields, and earning money. A reliable water source near the home therefore has both health and economic benefits for the family.

Ponds and watering holes

Although widely used, water from these sources is dangerous and can spread a variety of diseases, including bilharzia (especially in Africa).

Pond water should not be used for drinking unless there is no other supply available. If there is no alternative, it should be boiled or sterilised before drinking. Any pond used as a water supply or for washing should not also be used for washing or watering animals.

Small ponds can be protected by a surrounding fence.

Rivers and streams

Water from most rivers is contaminated. If river water has to be used, we should ensure that:

1. Water is collected from the river above the village, preferably through a sand filter, infiltration gallery or, in the case of hill communities, a gravity flow system.
2. Bathing, washing and the watering of animals take place only below the village.

Water from standpipes or other piped systems

Water from a tap is not always clean. It may come from a dirty source or become contaminated in the pipes.

Tap water can be made safer by:

1. Checking the source is not dirty or contaminated.
2. Checking the pipes to make sure there are no leaks or joins where germs can enter.
3. Keeping the surrounds of a standpipe (standpost) clean and well drained.
4. Building a concrete or wooden platform on which to rest buckets.
5. Constructing a fence to keep away animals.
6. Encouraging the community to set up a system for checking source, pipes, tap and surrounds and keeping them clean and in good repair (see pages 317–20 'Setting up a Community Action Group').

Rainwater tanks

Water, though clean at first, may quickly become dirty on storage. It can be made safer by:

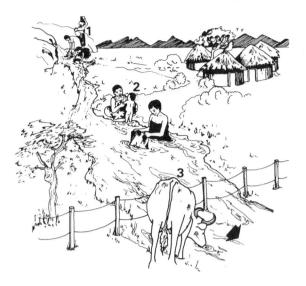

Figure 16.4   River water: 1. Draw water from above the village. 2. Bathe and wash downriver from the village. 3. Exclude animals where possible.

1. Cleaning the tank and entrance pipe before the rainy season.
2. Placing a filter or screen where the water enters the tank to keep out insects, leaves and other dirt.
3. Placing a sealed cover over the tank to keep the water clean and to prevent mosquitoes from breeding.
4. Ensuring that taps alone are used for withdrawing water.
5. Allowing the first heavy rainfall of the season to run through without being used.
6. Chlorination.

Water sources – developing new ones

Larger projects or those working in areas where improved water is a strongly felt need can help their communities develop new sources or make major improvements in storage or transport. Outside experts or resources will usually be needed to give guidance in this.

Examples might include:

1. Installing pipes from water sources to suitable sites in the community or into each house.
2. Drilling tube wells or building new 'open' wells. If arsenic is thought to be present in ground water, call in experts to test levels.

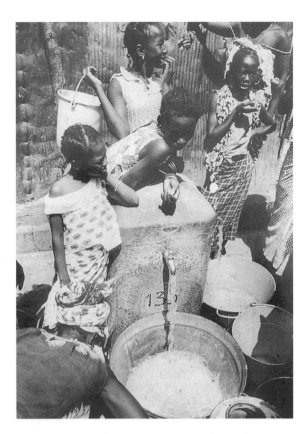

Figure 16.5   A clean water source in Senegal.

3. Installing hand pumps to existing wells.
4. Building community water tanks, such as those made of ferrocement. These are also suitable for individual houses or groups of houses to collect rainwater from roofs.

For example: One poor sheep-rearing village in southern Asia with a single spring at an inconvenient site below the village, decided to construct a large storage tank with multiple taps within the village itself.

Capital costs were obtained from the health project to buy a diesel pump and piping for lifting water from the source into the water tank. The community built the tank and was taught how to maintain it. All members now have easy access to clean water throughout the day.

Projects on this scale need careful planning and coordination between community, project director, government departments and donor agencies.

Water storage

Water may be dirty when collected, or become contaminated in transit or storage, especially in hot climates, crowded conditions or from distant sources.

Containers can be made of almost any suitable material. Earthenware or clay pots are suitable but should not be placed on dirty surfaces where germs can 'leach in'. No storage container should be used that has ever contained pesticides or dangerous chemicals.

Storage can be improved if containers are kept off the floor and away from animals and children, covered, and cleaned regularly, e.g. with bleaching powder. They should have narrow openings.

Water sterilisation

There are various ways of reducing the number of germs in water. They include the following:

1. The three pot method (see Figure 16.6).
2. Filtration – there are various methods such as that shown in Figure 16.7.
3. Disinfection with chlorine or bleach is highly effective. Although the best place for this to be done is at community level, for example in the

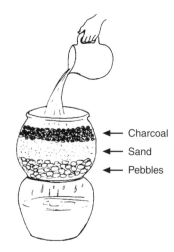

Figure 16.7   Charcoal filter: 1. With a sharp instrument, punch holes in the bottom of the container. 2. Place pebbles, sand and charcoal in the container to make a filter. Set this on top of the receptacle. 3. Pour water into the top filter and collect drinking water from the bottom filter. (PATH adaptation from *Peace Corps Times*.)

storage tank or well, it can also be done in each household. One cup (about 250 ml) of household or laundry bleach is mixed with three cups of water to make one litre. Three drops of this solution are then added to one litre of water and allowed to stand. If the water is badly contaminated, six drops can be used.
4. Boiling. Boiling for one minute will kill most germs. Boiling is the most effective way of killing germs but is costly on fuel and human energy.
5. Exposure to sun – the 'SODIS' method. Place water in transparent containers in the sun. Plastic bottles that contained soft drinks or bottled water are ideal. Leave them in full sun, e.g. on the roof of the house, for at least five hours. Their lower half can be painted black or they can be placed on black-painted corrugated iron or plastic sheets to aid heat absorption (see www.sodis.ch).
6. New technologies are regularly being tried out and developed.
For example: The treatment system, Pur Water Purifier, involves mixing a sachet into a container of dirty water to separate the contaminants from the water, which is then filtered through a cloth. This reduces the number of

This simple system will provide cleaner water. It will not provide pure water but will reduce the risk of infection.
Day 1: Collect 1 pot of water and leave it to settle for 1 day.
Day 2: Pour off the clear top water into a clean pot and use this for drinking water. Use the remainder for washing. Collect another pot and leave it to settle for 1 day.

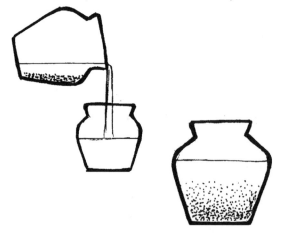

Figure 16.6   The three pot system.

germs in water, including viruses, and cholera, to almost undetectable levels.

Boiling drinking water is not usually a practical option and should only be done if this is suggested or fully agreed by the community. Boiling is only appropriate if there is an adequate supply of fuel nearby, a water source that is highly contaminated, and time and energy available for fuel collection.

Water usage

Even if water is clean at the time of storage it can become contaminated at the actual point of use, usually by dirty hands or implements being put into the container.

Water usage can be made safer if we can teach the community to:

1. Cover the container.
2. Use a container with a tap or spigot.
3. Tip water into a cup or glass or
4. Dip with a long-handled dipper that is touched only above the level of the container. This should be used for pouring, not for drinking from direct.

We need to make sure that improvements at the point of use tie in with what the community is familiar with or what works easily in their situation

For example: An improved container used in a refugee camp in Malawi has proved popular and has reduced diarrhoea by one third in children under five. It can hold 20 litres, has a lid with a hole just large enough to fill from a hand pump; also a handle and spout to aid pouring. For more information on environmental health in emergency situations see Further reading below.

Methods of waste disposal

It is helpful to think of waste under four headings: liquid waste, solid household waste, human waste and household smoke. We will look at different ways of disposing of each.

Liquid waste disposal

Liquid waste includes all household waste water, including that used for washing clothes and utensils.

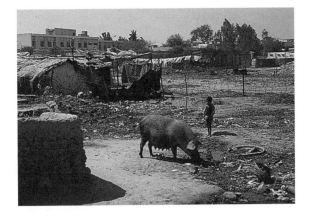

Figure 16.8   Sanitation: an urban health priority.

Where washing takes place outside, run-off is usually less of a problem. Where washing takes place inside with use of an exit pipe, pools of stagnant water quickly develop by the house or in the street.

Community hygiene can be greatly improved when stagnant waste water is removed. Diarrhoeal diseases, malaria and dengue fever become less common.

Waste water can be disposed of in various ways:

1. Through a kitchen garden where it can be used to water vegetables (see pages 188–9).
2. In a soakage pit. This can be constructed below ground outside each house, by making a cubic hole with sides 1.5 m, lined with brick or stone.
3. A biogas (gobargas) plant.
   Waste water can be piped into this or taken by bucket. In practice, biogas works effectively in very few areas.
4. A simple communal drainage system of covered drains (or pipes). This is effective if well constructed and regularly cleaned. It is the method of choice in poor urban areas.

Household solid waste disposal

This can be disposed of all together in a household or community tip, or in cities by putting pressure on the civic authorities to arrange refuse removal. In rural areas, waste can be separated:

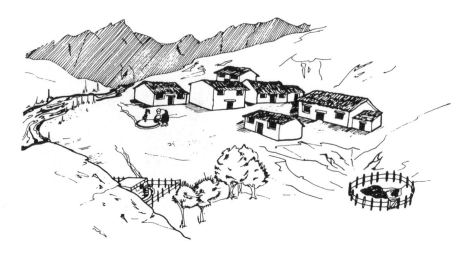

Figure 16.9   A well-placed community pit, at least 20 metres from the nearest house, 100 metres from the river, well or spring.

1. **Material suitable for burning**, such as paper, which can be incinerated well away from homes at appropriate times.
2. **Solid matter for burying**, which can be done by each household digging its own hole at least one metre deep, or by the community making a communal rubbish dump. This must be at least 20 metres from the nearest house and 100 metres from any river or water source. Any rubbish tip should be covered with several inches of earth to reduce flies, and protected by a fence or enclosure to keep out animals. Needles, syringes and other waste from health centres must not be disposed of in this way. It is the health programme's responsibility to make sure it is incinerated.
3. **Organic (vegetable matter) for composting**, which, along with animal dung, can be rotted down and used as fertiliser after four to six months. A shallow pit is dug and kept covered by a few inches of soil. Wooden posts can be inserted as 'chimneys' to help take air into the pile, which speeds up the decay.

Human waste disposal

Faeces, in particular those of children, are highly infectious and can remain so for some time. In urban areas or wherever there is overcrowding, virtually everyone, especially playing children, will become contaminated by the faeces of other people. This effect is multiplied when open spaces are used for defecation, children's play, agriculture and communal gatherings.

> Studies have shown that safe disposal of children's faeces can reduce diarrhoeal disease by up to 40 per cent.

Understanding all this helps us to see why it is so essential to dispose of faeces so that others are not infected. In addition, this reduces the chance of flies having access to faeces, which in turn helps to reduce the incidence of diarrhoea and other infections also.

For example: Trachoma, a severe infectious eye disease affecting many millions of the poorest communities, is spread by a fly called *Musca sorbens*. This fly seeks out human eyes but breeds in human faeces. Building latrines that are regularly used has been shown, on its own, to reduce the frequency of trachoma, but regular hand- and face-washing reduces this still further. (See page 416, ref. Emerson.)

WHO and other international agencies have set up a web-based information service called Sanitation Connection (see Further reading and resources).

Methods of human waste disposal

1. **The traditional open field system.**
   This system can be improved if the community is not ready to build latrines.

- The site should be appropriate. It should be a safe distance from any house, at least 10 metres from any water supply, and away from any paths.

  For example: in many parts of the world, but especially in south Asia, paths are used as the public toilet. This is an effective way of spreading germs throughout the community. The health team, supported by the CHW and health committee, can raise community awareness and help to set up alternative sites.

- Shoes should be worn. This reduces the risk of hookworm and other infections.

- A small hole should be dug with a stick or simple digging implement and the faeces placed inside and covered with earth. This will help to keep off flies and animals. Sunny areas should be used rather than shady ones, which helps to reduce germs.

- Young children should not normally go alone.

- The open field system is only appropriate in rural areas with relatively low populations.

2. **The simple pit latrine** (also known as the sealed-lid latrine, Figure 16.10).

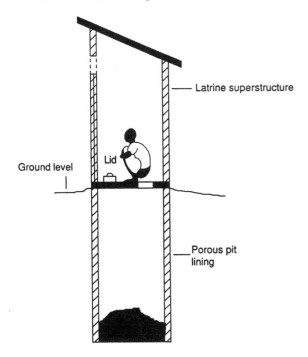

Figure 16.10   Simple pit latrine with sealed lid and single pit.

This is most suitable where bulk materials such as paper, stones or corncobs, rather than water, are used for anal cleansing, as in much of Africa.

The most basic type of latrine consists of a pit in the ground 2–3 metres deep, lined by bricks, blocks, concrete rings or by making use of an old oil drum.

If the soil is hard and firm throughout the year, only the top 0.5 to 1 metre needs to be lined. In all cases the lower part of the lining should have small holes so liquid can seep out. The pit is covered by a slab, ideally made of concrete at least 80 mm thick with 6 mm iron bars every 150 mm in both directions to prevent it from collapsing. The size of the slab should extend right up to the lined side of the pit, or beyond it if an oil drum is used. The squat hole should be shaped like a key-hole, 400 mm long, 100 mm wide at the narrow end, 200 mm wide at the larger end. This size and design is safe for all but the smallest children. The hole is fitted with a tight-fitting cover with a handle. A wall can be built for privacy, using wattle, grass, mud or brick.

The twin problems of flies and smells are reduced by ensuring the cover is always replaced and by scrubbing the slab regularly with soap and water. However, these problems are more effectively solved by using VIP or water-seal latrines.

Children are often frightened to use latrines. Adults can accompany them for reassurance to start with, and can help clear up faeces. Also we must make sure that, when children defecate into a container in the home, the parents empty this into the latrine, not outside the home.

Remember that the faeces of young children are often more infectious than those of adults. Make sure either that children are happy to use the adult latrine, or construct smaller, child-friendly versions where they feel safe.

---

3. **The VIP latrine (Ventilated, Improved Pit)** (Figure 16.11).

   This is basically the same design as the simple pit latrine, but contains a ventilating pipe with screened exit to reduce smells, flies and mos-

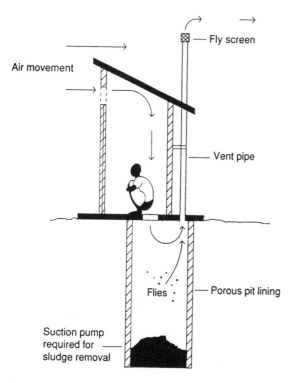

Figure 16.11   VIP latrine with single pit.

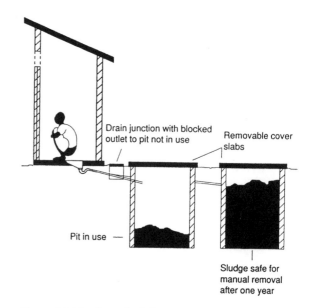

Figure 16.12   Pour-flush latrine with twin pit.

quito breeding. The pipe must be high enough above the roof to ensure good air flow and be at least 150 mm in diameter. The screen should be made of fibreglass or stainless steel to prevent corrosion. The squat hole should not be covered. The shelter should keep the latrine fairly dark and, ideally, the door should face the direction from which the wind normally blows. These measures help to kill flies (which are drawn up the vent pipe), and to improve ventilation.

The shelter should have no holes in the door or walls, otherwise young women in particular may not have the confidence to use it.

4. **The pour-flush latrine** (Figure 16.12).
Pour-flush latrines are more expensive but also more hygienic. They are appropriate only in communities where water is used for anal cleansing, as in much of Asia, or in other areas where there is a demand for them. There must also be a regular source of sufficient water.
Any latrine used can have either a single pit, or double pit, as shown in Figure 16.12. All latrines must also be used and sited correctly.

Consider also whether a simple low-cost improvement, the Sanplat (see below and Further reading 5) is worth using.

The correct use of latrines

Although we should encourage the building of latrines, they are of no value unless they are well used, well maintained and well cleaned, and unless the population, including children, has been carefully taught how to use them.

Soap and water must be kept near the latrine for handwashing, and leaves, paper or water kept in the latrine for anal cleansing according to custom.

An effective way of spreading diarrhoeal diseases is to build public latrines, give no health teaching, forget the soap and arrange no maintenance. Such buildings quickly become the most serious health risk in the entire community.

The correct position of latrines

Latrines should be near the home, but on ground lower than any nearby water source or river and at least 15 metres away from them.

The use of the Sanplat

This is a specially designed concrete platform that can be installed in existing latrines and supported by a floor of logs and clay. It uses much less concrete than the standard slab, meaning more people can afford it (see Further reading 5).

What we need to do

As we look at practical ways forward, we must remember that the most effective programmes combine three components: increasing access to clean water, providing basic sanitation and encouraging personal hygiene, all of which we need to integrate into our action plan.

It is also worth quoting a UN official definition of basic sanitation because hidden amongst its words (in bold) are principles and objectives that should be central to our programme.

> Basic sanitation is the **lowest-cost option** for securing **sustainable access** to safe hygienic and convenient facilities and services, for excreta and sullage disposal that **provide privacy and dignity** while ensuring a **clean and healthful living environment** both at home and in the neighbourhood of users. (See www.populationenvironmentresearch. org.)

Help the community to recognise its needs

Water supplies

The community may identify problems such as:
1. Supplies are too distant: in some communities women and children may spend up to 2–3 hours per day in collecting water.
2. Supplies are intermittent: water sources may dry up completely at certain times of year meaning more distant sources have to be used. In the case of piped supplies, water may only flow once or twice per day (or per week).
3. Supplies are contaminated: the community may not always understand the need for clean water or may feel their existing supplies are sufficiently clean.
4. Supplies are only available for the rich, the high caste or the dominant tribal group. The poor may have to use a more distant or more contaminated source.

The community, especially women, will already be aware of any need to improve water supplies, in particular the time taken for collection. It will often be a strongly expressed need in our first meetings with the community.

Sanitation

In contrast to water supplies, the community may see no need at all to change existing patterns of waste disposal. Often practices will be strongly tied in with traditions, and there will need to be a convincing reason for people to want any changes. Creating awareness is therefore an important part of any sanitation programme.

Where community members want their own latrine, this is usually for one of two reasons: either they hope to improve the health of their family or more commonly they expect a latrine will give them extra status in the community, or especially in urban areas increase the value of their property. In fact, a social marketing approach for the use of latrines is often the most effective. We can promote them as a sign of being modern, trendy and educated, as a home improvement rather than for reasons of health. This will work especially well when we target younger members of the community.

> Whatever the motivation, it is generally better to wait until a family is ready to build its own latrine and pay for all or a large part of it themselves, rather than providing the latrine and its construction free of charge.

Revolving loan funds may help to make this possible.

Understand the culture and beliefs of the people

> In both water and sanitation projects we need to help the people identify their own needs and suggest their own solutions.

Most communities have strong beliefs about waste disposal and traditional rights over use of water. The knowledge, attitude and practice of the community must be understood before any plans are drawn up.

For example (1): In many parts of the world, especially the Middle East, northern Africa and central Asia, there is a severe lack of water. This means that any increase in water use by one family or community may mean less for another. Local and regional conflicts can develop as a result of this.

For example (2): In parts of Latin America it is sometimes believed that women who use the same latrines as men may become pregnant.

For example (3): In parts of east Africa, daughters are forbidden to use the same latrine as their fathers. In Madagascar some communities believe that squatting over a pit can cause a miscarriage or that angry visitors will place bad medicine in a pit to bewitch a family. In one such community latrines became popular once the Tangalamenas (traditional leaders) tried them in their own yards with good results (no bad luck, fewer flies and less smell).

More commonly, social embarrassment, especially amongst young women, is the major community concern.

Assess what resources are available

We will need to ask the community the following questions, while being aware of what support there might be from the government or a voluntary WATSAN agency.

- What is the level of interest?
- How much time will be available to make changes and at what time of year?
- What skills are present, including both technical and managerial skills?
- What materials are available?
- What sources of funds are available?
- What degree of cooperation is possible between the different groups who will need to work together?
- How will the community be motivated about using the new facility?

We should encourage the community itself to contribute as many of its own resources as possible. See the logframe on pages 103–5 as an example of planning a programme.

Choose what improvements to make

This should be done by the community with guidance from the health team. Any improvements chosen should be culturally acceptable, and be affordable for most of the people.

In choosing what improvements to make, the following have to be 'matched up':

1. The priority needs of the people.
2. Resources available.

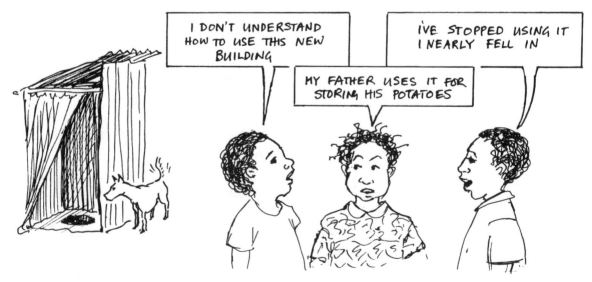

Figure 16.13   Awareness raising, joint planning and ownership are the keys to successful sanitation.

3. Ability of the community to manage the project and ensure upkeep afterwards.
4. Methods used successfully in nearby areas, either by government or other voluntary agencies.
5. Government or national guidelines. These should be followed where they exist. Funding may be available if they are.
6. In the case of sanitation – the type of system that ties in with the culture of the people.
7. In the case of water supplies – a method that does not interfere with traditional water rights or cause anger in a neighbouring community.

In practice it is wise to start with small, simple schemes such as improving existing systems.

For example (1): In the case of latrines. The International Committee of the Red Cross carried out a latrine improvement scheme in Kabul, Afghanistan. This included either constructing a new latrine or renovating an existing one to ensure the following: adequate faecal storage (2.1 cubic metres), an underground soakage pit for urine, venting with a nylon mesh and using a removable door to make faecal evacuation easier.

These improvements led to a reduction in the deaths of children under 11 years of age and was found to be equally, or more, cost effective as other programmes targeting children's health with which it was compared. (See page 416, ref. Meddings.)

For example (2): in the case of water: Demonstrations should first be given on ways to improve water storage, simple systems of composting or, as appropriate, a more hygienic use of the open system for defecation.

Later, larger-scale improvements could be carried out such as the protection of an existing water source, e.g. a spring or a well, or the building of a latrine in the local primary school with teaching on how to use it.

Later still, a new water source could be developed or a community latrine building programme be set up.

By progressing from smaller projects to larger ones several advantages occur:

1. Success is more likely. Without this the community will quickly lose its confidence and trust.
2. Experience is gained – both by the health team and by the community.

3. The community learns how to manage at levels within its ability.

Any large-scale improvements should be piloted first.

Work through a Community Action Group

The Community Action Group (CAG) is in effect a committee but is more likely to get things done if given a dynamic name. This is what we can help to facilitate:

1. **Setting up the CAG.**
   We can use an existing health committee provided its members have proved themselves effective in getting things done. We should also aim to include at least one CHW, one or two older school children and a representative of any coordinating agency. Above all, women must be strongly represented.

Eleven guidelines for planning an improved sanitation programme*
1. Aim for a sustainable programme which makes long-term improvements. This will not happen quickly – it may take many years to be achieved.
2. Find an appropriate latrine design for the area. It should be technically able to provide adequate sanitation, affordable for most people and culturally and socially acceptable.
3. Discuss all you are doing and planning with the future users of the sanitation – especially the women and community representatives or leaders. Work with people. Don't aim to do the work for them.
4. Don't offer to give people latrines or to subsidise them. The desire to achieve rapid results often leads to serious problems. A credit scheme, or revolving loan fund, may help many people build a latrine while leaving them fully responsible.
5. Promote latrines so that people desire to have one – don't threaten people that they 'must get a latrine or else…'.
6. Use any means possible to promote improved sanitation. Convince community leaders, local officials, teachers, primary and village health workers and encourage them to assist in the promotion work.

7. Either encourage people to build the latrines themselves or privatise the construction of latrines, by training local builders.
8. Make sure all latrine construction is backed up with full health and hygiene education and help on how to use and clean the latrine properly.
9. Coordinate the work with those aiming to improve the water supplies or other forms of sanitation.
10. Keep the programme costs as low as possible and keep staff numbers low. This will help the programme keep running for a longer period.
11. Encourage and help schools, churches, clinics and other institutions to improve their sanitation. This has a good demonstration effect on everyone seeing them.

*Reproduced, with permission, from an article by Isobel Blackett in *Footsteps*, December 1991, published by Tearfund.

It has often been shown that water and sanitation programmes work best when women are involved in planning them and carrying them out.

The reason for this is quite obvious: water projects bring greatest benefit to women, who now spend much less time in fetching water than before. Also women usually take greater interest and responsibility than men in matters of family hygiene.

2. **Ensuring that the CAG is informed, motivated and trained.**
We will need to train the group:

- To understand why changes are being made.
- To realise the felt benefits it will bring in terms of convenience, time and money saved.
- How to act as motivators and agents of change.
- How to set up and organise the programme.

In training the CAG, we can use interactive teaching, visits to other programmes, and discussion with community members to generate ideas. Elders, opinion formers, teachers, religious leaders, traditional healers, and children should all be included.

For example: One successful programme in Bangladesh has used children as the main agent of change. Local school children were carefully taught by the committee about the value of latrines. Children in the school which encouraged the most families to install latrines won a prize. Children also helped other family members to see the benefits the latrines would bring. They then set an example by using them after they had been installed.

In all projects, teaching on water and sanitation needs to be given to school children, and school latrines need to be built. The community can help advocate for the government to carry this out but will need to be involved in its management and maintenance.

3. **Enabling the CAG to manage the programme.** This will involve careful forward planning, communicating about all programme stages with the population being served, involving members of outside agencies, and coordinating the process through an action plan.
A simple, unaltered task analysis sheet from Marakissa in the Gambia in Figure 16.14 shows a method used in a small successful latrine-building programme.

4. **Empowering the CAG to maintain any new community facility.** This is a key and permanent function of the CAG.

It has been estimated that in many poorer communities between 35 and 50 per cent of water and sanitation systems break down and become useless after five years. Many communities are littered with the wreckage of disused water tanks, broken pumps and abandoned equipment, which now lie unrepaired and unusable while community members return to their traditional practices.

Sometimes this is because the community never wanted a new system in the first place. Often too it is because no one has been given either the training or responsibility for keeping equipment in working order. A new combined approach known as PHAST (Participatory Hygiene and Sanitation Transformation) is proving successful in both rural and urban communities. See Further reading for more details.

Marakissa Latrine Plan

Things to be done	When	By whom
– Meet with village leader re Community Health Nurse working in village.	August	M.P.
– Meet with village leader re CHN to do survey of every compound. – Training for CHN to do survey work – population breakdown, latrines, health education (worm flip chart).	Sept	M.P. & F.C. M.P. & F.C.
– Survey of village.	Sept/Oct	CHN
– Meet village leader and heads of compounds re incentives for latrines & de-worming all compounds with latrines. – Analyse results of survey – how many interested in having new latrines?	Nov	F.C.
– Arrange for Health Dept. to make cement slabs for latrines. Give nos.	Dec	M.P.
– Organise transport of slabs from Banjul to Marakissa.	End Jan	M.P.
– Arrange for Mr Jobe, Health Inspector, to visit Marakissa. – Meet heads of compounds again to discuss details. – Mr Jobe to inspect siting of latrines with reference to well sites. – Arrange for Govt. Info. Office to show film 'How to Dig your Latrine' at the village Independence Celebrations. – Flip chart worm/latrine talk – Primary School, classes 4, 5 & 6. – Showing of film.	Early Feb Early Feb Mid Feb	M.P. M.P. Mr Jobe M.P. Fatou Film unit
– Latrine construction – holes to be checked before slabs issued. – Issuing of slabs.	Feb–May	I.S. & clinic compound man
– Deadline to finish.	May	
– All compounds to be visited. – Inform Mr Jobe of total no. new latrines.	June	F.C. M.P. I.S. Fatou
– Contact Mr Fal (Health Dept.) re no. of slabs still required after rice harvest for others wanting new latrines. – Photograph new latrines with owners. – De-worm compounds with new latrines.	July June–Aug	M.P. M.P. F.C. & Fatou
M.P. = Marilyn Pidcock; F.C. = Fansainey Colley, I.S. = Ibrinia Sabally		

Figure 16.14 Marakissa latrine plan.

> The upkeep of equipment should be the sole responsibility of the community. The key to this is a sense of ownership; we all know in experience that most people will only take care of things that belong to them.

In order to bring this about we should:
1. Ensure responsibility for upkeep is in the hands of the community from the very beginning. The CAG takes charge and in turn can select, arrange training for, supervise and pay an individual to carry out regular maintenance and cleaning.
2. Identify suppliers of spare parts and other materials needed for upkeep.
3. Ensure that training is given by outside experts in how equipment can be maintained. This should be during an active project phase

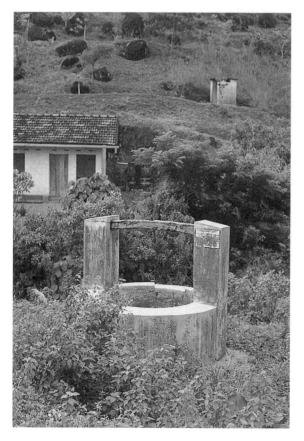

Figure 16.15 $600 of unused well.

when interest is high. The CAG should coordinate this.

Help the community take action on other environmental hazards

There are many other hazards that can affect the health and well-being of a community.

An important one is household smoke, which arises mainly through tobacco smoking, and through cooking inside without an adequate chimney or ventilation. Wood, dung, coal or cropwaste are especially harmful, and are used by over three quarters of the population in most African and Asian countries. Charcoal is less polluting, but should not be obtained by cutting down or raiding indigenous forests. Sources of irritating smoke make lung, heart and eye diseases worse. Indoor air pollution seriously increases the dangers of TB.

We can discuss with the community the building of smokeless hearths, see pages 355–6, and ways in which cigarette smoking can be reduced.

Figure16.16 gives various ideas on how we can tackle dangers and nuisances in an urban environment.

Evaluate the programme

The simplest way to evaluate any improvements is to discover if:

1. The system is still functioning after a given length of time.
2. The quality of life has improved, e.g. percentage of families with clean water source 15 minutes' walk or less from the house has increased.
3. The community is still actually using the system, e.g. percentage of families regularly using latrines.
4. The community prefers the new system to the old.
5. There are measurable improvements in health, especially reduction in the frequency of diarrhoeal episodes amongst children and/or improvements in the average weight of under-five children.

Evaluations can be carried out by the community, through inspection, questions and surveys. Often the answers will be obvious and visible.

Summary

Many serious diseases are spread through water that has been contaminated by human or animal waste. Many other conditions become worse through lack of water for adequate washing. Improvements in both water supply and waste disposal, if carried out successfully, can greatly improve community and individual health. We should make sure we first concentrate on behavioural change and improvements at household level before starting more major projects. Unless the whole community alters its hygiene practices, such as regular handwashing, no programme will have much effect.

Water supplies can be made safer both at source, during transit, in storage and at the time

Ways of minimising risks from environmental hazards	
Solid waste	• Educate community on ways to dispose of household waste and show them what should not be done • Organise a campaign to increase proper disposal of household waste • Install garbage bins that prevent entry by animals • Learn rights and laws about municipal cleaners, garbage bins, and garbage collection vehicles • Press municipality to collect garbage regularly from community collection sites • Hire and supervise street cleaners, ideally from the community, to keep streets and footpaths clean • Consider organising the collection of solid waste into three types: items for recycling, waste that generates fertiliser (composting), and unusable waste • Organise a campaign to remove mosquito-breeding sites in the community • Investigate possibility of whether there is chemical pollution from near-by industries
Flooding hazards	• Ensure that authorities inform slum when upriver dams are released • Weigh advantages and disadvantages of relocation
Electrical hazards	• Press for legal electrical connections for community households • Monitor existing wiring
Fire hazards	• Press for legal hook-ups to natural gas lines for the community • Check illegal hook-ups to gas line for leaks • Monitor homes for flammable chemicals
Vehicular accidents	• Avoid unnecessary risks when travelling on roads • Avoid travel during rush hour • Avoid begging/selling at traffic lights • Travel on less busy streets (unless a security risk)
Workplace hazards	• Avoid drinking alcohol before operating machinery or travelling • Obey safety rules when operating dangerous machinery • Advocate for safe working conditions in factories
Air pollution	• If possible, cook with clean fuel (natural gas or electricity) • If not possible, install smokeless cooking stove/chimney or cook outdoors • If not possible, provide ventilation if cooking indoors • Stop smoking tobacco inside the house and preferably stop completely • Avoid travel during rush hour • Take less travelled streets
Noise pollution	• Encourage setting radios, tape players at low volume • Advocate for ear protectors when working with loud equipment

Figure 16.16   Source: Urban Health and Development, Table 17.4, p. 324, (see Further reading and resources).

of use. Health programmes can help to improve existing systems, and as needs dictate and resources allow, help communities to develop new ones.

Similarly, help can be given to improve sanitation. This will cover all forms of household waste, and most important of all the effective disposal of human faeces through the building of latrines.

To ensure success, communities themselves must identify their needs and suggest solutions. These need to be in line with cultural patterns, matched with resources available and guided by national health plans.

Health projects can act as facilitators in this process by creating awareness, coordinating personnel, and teaching management skills. All these activities should be coordinated through a community action group. Small-scale improvements can be made first, and as experience and confidence grow, the scale of programmes can be increased.

From the very beginning communities should take full responsibility for maintaining equipment and carrying out necessary repairs. Programmes initiated and carried out by governments and larger NGOs, which are then handed over to the people, nearly always fail. Community involvement must be present from the beginning and be central in all programme stages.

Evaluation is necessary at regular intervals, especially as large sums of money can be wasted on programmes that bring little benefit.

Further reading and resources

1. *Urban Health And Development: A Practical Manual For Use In Developing Countries*, B. Booth, K. Martin and T. Lankester, Macmillan, 2001.
   This has a large section on environmental improvements from an urban point of view.
   Available from: TALC. See Appendix E.
2. *Healthy Villages: A Guide for Communities and Community Health*, Howard et al., WHO, 2002.
   The book to buy if working in rural areas.
3. *A Guide to the Development of On-site Sanitation*, R. Franceys, J. Pickford and R. Reed, WHO, 1992.
   A book providing detailed, practical advice on all aspects of sanitation, including how to build different types of latrine.
   Available from: WHO. See Appendix E.
4. *Developing and Managing Community Water Supplies*, J. Davis, G. Garvey and M. Wood, Oxfam, 1993.
   Available from: IT Publications and Oxfam. See Appendix E.
5. *Latrine Building: A Handbook for Implementing the Sanplat System*, B. Brandberg, IT Publications, 1997.
   Details on how to carry out this effective, low-cost method.
   Available from: IT Publications. See Appendix E.
6. *Low-cost Urban Sanitation*, D. Mara, Wiley, 1996.
   Available from IT Publications. See Appendix E.
7. *Reaching the Unreached: Challenges for the Twenty-first Century*, ed. J. Pickford, IT Publications, 1997.
   A selection of papers on all aspects of water and sanitation.
   Available from: IT Publications. See Appendix E.
8. *PHAST Step-by-Step Guide: A participatory approach for the control of diarrhoeal diseases*, S. Wood, R. Sawyer and M. Simpson-Herbert, WHO, 1998.
   All projects involved in water/sanitation should obtain this.
   Available from: WHO. See Appendix E.
9. The journal *Waterlines* is published four times per year and is devoted to low-cost water and sanitation improvements. This is recommended for all projects planning to get involved in public health improvements.
   Available from: IT Publications. See Appendix E. Can also be read online.
10. *Tobacco: A Global Threat*, J. Crofton, Macmillan, 2001.
    The dangers of tobacco and how to take action.
    Available from: Macmillan. See Appendix E.
11. Sanitation Connection. Website: www.sanicon.net or details from WHO. See Appendix E.
12. *Environmental Health in Emergencies and Disasters: A practical guide*, B. Wisner and J. Adams, WHO, 2002.
    This book and all others on water and sanitation from WHO can be downloaded free from www.who.int/water_sanitation_health/hygiene/emergencies.
13. Solar Disinfection of Water: see www.sodis.ch.
14. Handwashing: see www.globalhandwashing.org.
15. UN Millennium Project Task Force on Water and Sanitation Final Report, abridged version, United Nations, New York, 2005 also available from www.unmillenniumproject.org/reports/tf_water-sanitation.htm.
16. *Encouraging Good Hygiene and Sanitation*, I. Carter, a Pillars Guide, Tearfund, 2005.
    Valuable information for individuals and groups at community level.
17. GWSI – Global Water and Sanitation Initiative; www.ifre.org/what/health/water.
18. Institute of Water and Environment; www.silsoe.cranfield.ac.uk/iwe.

See Further References and Guidelines, page 416.

PART IV
Appropriate Management

17

Using Medicines Correctly

In this chapter we shall consider:
1. What we need to know
   - The dangers of misusing medicines
   - The idea of a rational drugs policy
   - Poor access to life-saving medicines
   - The difference between medical care and health care
   - How medicines are wrongly prescribed
   - Know about expiry dates
2. What we need to do
   - Make an Essential Drugs List
   - Train the health team
   - Create community awareness
   - Use the correct medicines in the correct way

What we need to know

The increasing number of effective medicines is one of the most significant events in the past 50 years. It means that most infectious diseases can be cured and many non-communicable diseases can be controlled. This makes it all the more important that we help communities gain access to essential supplies, that we learn to use medicines in the most effective ways and that good practice becomes embedded in our health teams and in our communities.

The dangers of misusing medicines

The dangers of using too many injections and too much medicine are becoming a very serious problem in all countries.

Too many injections

Each year more than 16 billion injections are given worldwide. In some countries more than 10 injections per person per year are being used. One project in south India calculated that on average 150–200 injections were given each morning by a single nurse in each of the primary health centres studied. Figures from Ghana have shown that 17 prescriptions out of 20 include an injection.

Unsafe injections

Of these 16 billion injections, about 95 per cent are used for curative care, many by traditional healers or private practioners. Immunisations account for only 3 per cent. Many of these injections are entirely unnecessary and many are carried out in an unsafe manner. WHO estimates that unsafe injections cause 1.3 million early deaths each year, many of these from hepatitis B, C and AIDS. (See page 416, ref. WHO injection safety.)

Wastage and dependence

The price of treating these illnesses, along with the cost of inappropriate injections and staff time, is wasting huge sums of money each year. In addition, injections cause dependence.

> Patients come to believe the dangerous myth that only an injection or an intravenous drip has any effect.

Almost as serious as the overuse of injections is the use of far too many medicines that are wrongly prescribed, ineffective or dangerous

Most patients are prescribed (on average) three medicines per prescription, up to five per patient in some countries. About half of all prescriptions contain one or more antibiotics.

For example (1): It is estimated that 60 per cent of antibiotics in Nigeria are prescribed unnecessarily.

324

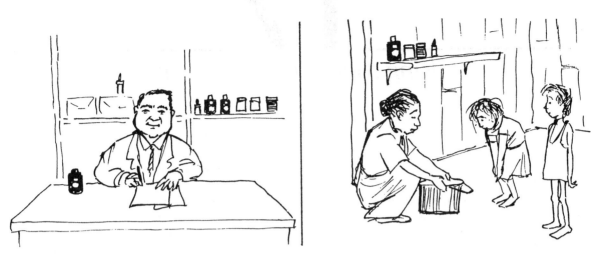

Figure 17.1   PPNN: a Pill for every Problem, a Needle for every Need.
An effective way of robbing the poor to pay the rich.

For example (2): One project in Garwhal, north India, showed that 77 per cent of all patients presenting to the government hospital outpatients received an antibiotic and 90 per cent an anti-inflammatory drug (NSAID).

For example (3): The author once witnessed a patient collecting 21 separate medicines and injections from an urban pharmacy. They had been prescribed by a local doctor, and included three different antibiotics. They were all for the use of the one patient, who was sufficiently strong to load these into a large carton and carry them out of the door.

Substandard and counterfeit medicines

A growing and deadly problem is the use of substandard and counterfeit medicines. Substandard medicines are of such poor quality that they may be ineffective or dangerous. Counterfeit medicines are fraudulently manufactured and labelled, but do not contain the active ingredient they claim to possess. It is estimated that 25 per cent of medicines used in poor countries are counterfeit or substandard. This is another reason for limiting the medicines we use to those that are really essential.

Self-medication

It is also reckoned that, in many poorer countries, patients buy or obtain half of all medicines without seeing a health worker. This is known as self-medication.

Side effects and drug resistance

This misuse of medicines causes not only dependency, but also serious or fatal side effects. When antibiotics are misused there is an even greater danger – drug resistance. This resistance of antibiotics to increasing numbers of dangerous germs is developing rapidly. Some diseases are becoming very difficult and expensive to cure. Multi-resistant TB is just one example (see page 273). Another is the development of Methicillin Resistant Staphylococcus Aureus (MRSA), a dangerous infection spread mainly in hospitals with poor hygiene control.

Wastage leads to poverty

The combined effect of all these bad practices also leads to enormous wastage. Drugs absorb up to 40 per cent of national health budgets. At the grass-roots level, overprescribing increases poverty. Those who are poor and uneducated are charged for injections and medicines they often don't need at all. Manufacturers and suppliers of these medicines often make profits at their expense. The poorest may have no money left when they really need essential drugs.

The idea of a rational drugs policy

These multiple effects from wrong prescribing have led experts to develop the idea of a rational drugs policy, in part driven by WHO estimations that almost half of all medicines used globally are used irrationally. Guidelines are laid down for appropriate treatment, manufacture and quality control. The use of ineffective and dangerous drugs is actively discouraged.

WHO drew up the first Model List of Essential Drugs in 1977, and this is now regularly updated, and comprises a formulary giving details on each drug listed. Different countries use this list to draw up their own national drugs policies and essential drugs lists. One government that has been successful in doing this, thanks to strong medical leadership, is Bangladesh. However, the pressures against developing these policies and carrying them out are extremely strong.

Each year drug manufacturers, especially multi-national corporations, are developing new and more effective ways of persuading ordinary people that a whole range of medicines and injections is necessary. With more countries opening up to the free market and having weaker central controls, the situation becomes more and more unsatisfactory. Although many medicines are of good quality, an increasing number, especially those made locally without careful checks, can be poor quality, altogether fake, or dangerous and contaminated. Beware of products that lack clear information or are poorly packaged.

Two examples illustrate the pressures against rational drug use. *Example (1)*: recently one drug company offered Peruvian pharmacists a bottle of wine if they ordered three boxes of its cough and cold remedy. *Example (2)*: another company told doctors to suspect *Giardia* or amoeba in all cases of diarrhoea and treat it immediately with metronidazole. In fact, this drug is only needed in a very small proportion of diarrhoeal cases.

For us in Community Based Health Care (CBHC) these trends have two main implications. First, we ourselves must follow rational drug policies and use only drugs on an essential drugs list. Second, we must help members of our community to be 'immunised' against the promotional efforts of any unethical drug companies.

One important footnote: although some pharmaceutical companies are guilty of unethical advertising, most are not. We should try to build contacts with drug manufacturers and suppliers as this can reduce our costs and make it easier to maintain regular supplies of essential medicines.

Poor access to life-saving medicines

The UN Millennium project estimates that approximately 1.7 billion people have no access or inadequate access to life-saving drugs. That is nearly one person in three. There are many reasons for this, which include insufficient drugs being manufactured, high price, trade tariffs, corruption, the collapse of health systems and no local access because of distant or understaffed health centres.

The 6th Millenium Development Goal aims to halt and reverse the spread of HIV/AIDS, TB and malaria by 2015 (see pages 12 and 13). The 8th Goal also relates to rational drug use.

> In our health programmes we must ensure that all community members have access to life-saving drugs and that we tackle any causes that prevent this from happening.

The most important life-saving drugs for most areas of the world include antibiotics, first-line treatment for tuberculosis, artemesinin combined therapy (ACT) to cure malaria, and antiretroviral therapy (ART) to treat HIV/AIDS.

One of our roles in CBHC is to make sure these drugs are available and this may involve us in advocacy at local, district or even national level. Often the most effective way for us to get involved is to join and add weight to existing campaigns that aim to ensure these drugs are both available and affordable at local level.

The difference between medical care and health care

Most health workers enjoy using medicines and many will expect to relieve symptoms and cure diseases simply through prescribing medicines and giving injections. This is medical care as opposed to health care. It is summed up in the slogan: PPNN: a Pill for every Problem, a Needle for every Need.

CBHC follows a different model. It aims to promote good health and to prevent ill health mainly through raising awareness in the community. Medicines are still used but only when necessary. This is health care as opposed to medical care.

Those who are more interested in profit will wish to continue a medical model of care. In CBHC we will be actively opposing this.

> One of our main tasks as community health workers is to educate the people about the correct and incorrect use of medicine. If we succeed, communities will become healthy and self-reliant. If we fail, communities will become poorer, more exploited and more dependent.

How medicines are wrongly prescribed

There are two main faults in prescribing:
1. Using too much of what is not needed – overprescribing.
2. Using too little of what is most needed – underprescribing.

Using too much of what is not needed

Here are some common *reasons* for overprescribing:
1. Health workers have been wrongly trained: they have learnt a medical model, not a health model. This is later reinforced by drug company representatives who encourage high prescribing.
2. They get a feeling of satisfaction from prescribing, or a free handout from the drug company, the more they prescribe.
3. It is easier to prescribe for each symptom than to discover and treat the illness and its cause.
4. Those lacking in knowledge or confidence will use several medicines in the hope that at least one will work.
5. Many CHWs and some village doctors, for example in China, often receive payment

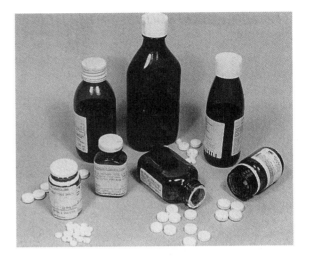

Figure 17.2   Avoid overprescribing.

according to medicine prescribed: the more they prescribe the more they earn. We need to find a different way of reimbursing CHWs.

> However, the commonest reason why doctors overprescribe is this: Patients expect many medicines and an injection. If they don't receive them they seek out another doctor willing to provide them.

If patients fail to receive the medicine they want or expect, they will often try to obtain it from another source.

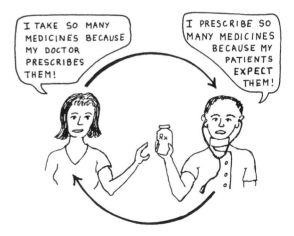

Figure 17.3   The vicious circle that leads to the overuse of medicine.

Here are some common *results* of over-prescribing:

1. Patients become dependent on medicines and doctors. This in turn means:
   - They spend more and more money on medicines.
   - They don't know what to do if no medicine is available.
   - They develop a demanding attitude.

   For example: One project decided not to pay money to its CHWs but instead to provide free medicines both for the CHWs and their families. The heads of these families soon came to realise they could obtain a profit by reselling such medicines. Encouraged by their families, the CHWs demanded ever-increasing amounts, refusing to cooperate when medicines were refused. The project was forced to close down.
2. Patients fall into debt to pay for medicines.
3. People take no interest in disease prevention.
4. Patients pass on consumerist thinking to their children.
5. When essential medicines are really needed, supplies have run out.

Using too little of what is really needed

Here are some common *reasons* for underprescribing:

1. Medicines are not available.
   They may be hard to obtain, be delayed in transit, or not ordered in advance. Stocks may have been used up because of overprescribing when supplies last arrived. There may be a severe lack of supplies at country and international level for a variety of reasons.
2. Patients may not be able to afford the full course of the medicine nor understand why they need to complete it.
3. Health workers may not follow the correct treatment schedules.

Here are some common *results* of underprescribing:

1. People die from curable diseases such as malaria, pneumonia and TB.
2. People lose faith in the hospital, health centre or programme when they fail to get better.

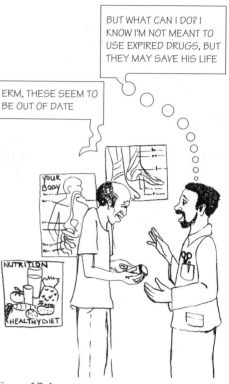

Figure 17.4

3. People waste money and endanger their health by buying useless substitutes.

Know about expiry dates

Medicines can only be kept a certain length of time before spoiling. This is known as the shelf life. Usually a printed expiry date shows when the shelf life has been reached.

What happens to a medicine after the expiry date?

1. It may become less effective: the case with many antibiotics.
2. It may become more toxic: sometimes the case with tetracyclines.
3. It may become more likely to cause an allergy: sometimes the case with penicillin.
4. It will often continue for a time to be both safe and effective. Drug companies may record early expiry dates to protect themselves from legal action if adverse effects occur.

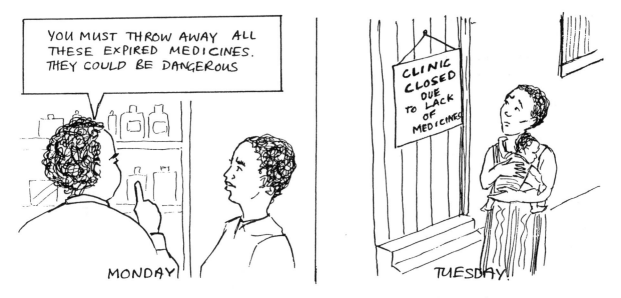

Figure 17.5   A common dilemma where medicines and good management are in short supply.

How can we know if a medicine may be spoilt?

The normal way is to see if the expiry date is passed. However, some medicines, under bad storage conditions, may spoil before their expiry date.

Check all medicines to make sure they are not:

- damp or sticky;
- discoloured;
- broken.

In addition, check certain drugs and supplies for specific problems, for example:

- tetracycline, which turns brown when ineffective;
- aspirin, which may smell unpleasant;
- condoms, which may dry out;
- vaccines, which must be kept cold (see pages 198–9);
- ergometrine, which needs to be kept in the fridge and protected from light;
- epinephrine (adrenaline), which has a very short shelf life.

How can medicine be prevented from spoiling?

We can help medicines last longer by:

1. Keeping them in a dry place at even temperature out of direct sunlight. These means that any store room will need to be shielded from direct sunlight and have adequate ventilation.
2. Making sure containers are airtight and lids are firmly closed.
3. Using sugar-coated or foil-wrapped tablets where cost allows.
4. Packing medicine carefully to reduce breakages in transit.
5. Storing supplies in peripheral health centres for as short a time as possible.
6. Maintaining the 'cold chain' for all vaccines.
7. Buying only high quality medicines, which helps to preserve their active life.

Should expired medicine still be used?

Reasons against using expired medicines:
1. Supplies may be less effective or unsafe.
2. If discovered, it may anger the local people; we may be accused of dumping on the local community unwanted or expired foreign medicine that no one else is prepared to use.

Reasons in favour of using expired medicines:
1. There may be no other supplies available.
2. It may mean throwing away supplies that are desperately needed. Large sums of money may be wasted if supplies are discarded.

3. Many expired medicines still work and are still safe.

Some suggested guidelines:
- Only use medicines past their expiry dates when absolutely essential, i.e. when no alternatives are available.
- Never use medicines that show signs of having spoilt.
- Order the right amounts of medicines in plenty of time so as to have sufficient in-date supplies.
- Check expiry dates on arrival, first using any with an early date.
- Use a storage system in both stores and clinic to guarantee that old supplies are used up first (see Chapter 8, page 157).
- Be sensitive to the community's beliefs about expired drugs. Some will be greatly concerned, others will not mind at all.

What we need to do

Make an Essential Drugs List (EDL)

What is an EDL?

An EDL is a list of important drugs needed for the cure of serious diseases and the relief of major symptoms.

CHWs may need approximately 12 essential drugs (see Chapter 7, page 125). Clinics and hospitals will need more.

The EDL will be different for each country, each region and each project. For this reason each programme should draw up its own Essential Drugs List, Standing Orders, Protocols or Treatment Schedules that incorporate these. When involved in national programmes such as Stop TB, Roll Back Malaria or the Integrated Management of Childhood Illness we should always use the nationally recommended essential drugs.

What are the ideal features of an 'Essential Drug'?

The drug in Figure 17.6, clearly labelled with its generic name, strength, and expiry date, in locally used language or script.

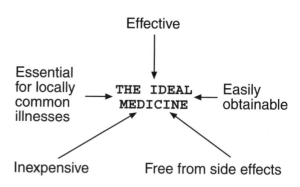

Figure 17.6   The ideal medicine.

Whom should we consult?

1. The project doctor or medical advisor.
   Their suggestions, though valuable, may include more drugs than are actually needed.
2. Other projects working in the area.
3. The District Medical Officer, who may have a national EDL or a list recommended for primary health centres.
4. The latest WHO Model List of Essential Drugs, from which all our drugs should be selected.

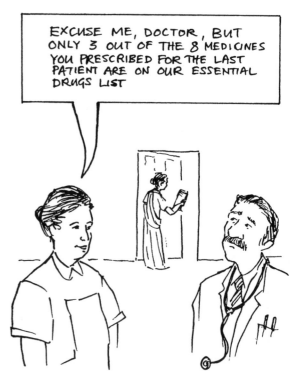

Figure 17.7   Doctors must be accountable.

We will need only a small proportion of these at community and health centre level.

5. The health official responsible for any national programme mentioned above, who will both guide us in what medicines to use and help us to obtain supplies.

> The final EDL should be worked out between the director of the project (who will know how much drugs cost) and the medical officer (who will know which drugs are necessary).

A suggested list is given in Appendix C.

Train the health team

All those who will be prescribing need careful instructions on the following subjects:

1. **The dangers of overprescribing.**

    We will need to correct any wrong knowledge, attitude or practice in the health workers and point out the extent and the dangers of overprescribing that are probably already taking place.

    For example: To show the extent of overprescribing we can arrange a simple survey. Sample homes are visited to find out what medicines have recently been used and where they have been obtained. Alternatively, patients who come to the clinic are asked which medicines they have been prescribed in the last few months from other practitioners. Often wads of old prescriptions or bills will be produced.

> Unless the whole health team understands and practises the appropriate use of medicines at all times, community members will never be taught how to change their expectations.

2. **The methods of correct prescribing.**
    These include:

- Understanding and using the project EDL.
- Knowing the correct amount of the correct medicine for each condition.
- Writing the prescription correctly.
- Being aware of possible side effects.
- Knowing the approximate cost of each drug.

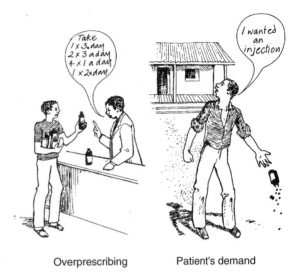

Overprescribing   Patient's demand

Figure 17.8   Spend time in correcting expectations.

- Giving the right advice with each drug.
- Using prescribing aids such as the EDL, Standing Orders, Protocols or Treatment Schedules.

Those learning to use drugs need careful supervision until they do it correctly. Although classroom and book teaching are important, the most valuable way of learning is on the job. At the beginning, the trainer sees the patients while the trainee watches how the diagnosis is made and medicines are used. As soon as possible, the trainee sees the patients under the trainer's guidance.

In some countries it is illegal for anyone other than accredited pharmacists and doctors to prescribe.

One effective way to help rational prescribing in children is to use the protocols set up by the Integrated Management of Childhood Illness (IMCI). One study from Nigeria has shown that treatment costs are five times higher using traditional ways of prescribing compared to guidelines laid down by IMCI. (See page 416, ref. Wammanda.)

> No health worker should prescribe without supervision until he/she has been tested and shown to be accurate.

Create community awareness

The correct use of drugs is one of the most important subjects for the community to understand. Among health workers and practitioners there will often be a hidden struggle between followers of the medical model – those who want to prescribe as many medicines as they wish – and followers of the health model – those who want to prescribe medicines only when they are essential. Both sides will be trying to win the hearts of the community.

> It must be our aim to create awareness in the people so successfully that, when tempted by glossy advertisements or TV commercials promoting the latest health tonic, they refuse to buy it.

In creating awareness we can use a variety of methods as listed in Chapter 3. Drama is one of the most effective.

For example: we can help our health workers or community members to write a play that contrasts two mothers: the wise mother who develops a healthier and wealthier family by following good health practices and using a few essential medicines; the foolish mother who sees many doctors, takes many medicines, falls into debt and whose children remain sick.

Use the correct medicines in the correct way

Here are some Dos and some Do nots.

> **Some Dos:**
> 1. **Do** use as few medicines as possible.
>   Fight the belief that, if one pill is good, more must be better. Some patients will need no medicine at all; few will need more than two or three varieties.
> 2. **Do** spend time explaining rather than prescribing.
>   Explain why medicines are not always necessary. Simple advice may not only cure the problem but prevent it from recurring.
>   *For example*: A doctor working in North Africa, frustrated by the large number of patients demanding medicines for minor problems, decided that instead of prescribing

for every symptom he would spend time giving advice instead.
>   The new method seemed to work well until a tribal chief appeared with headache. When refused tablets, he angrily left the clinic, warning all the waiting patients that the doctor was useless.
>   A few days later the chief reappeared, smiling. He explained how the headache had gone when he followed the doctor's simple advice. He would now encourage other patients to do what the doctor suggested.
> 3. **Do** treat causes rather than symptoms.
>   If the illness is cured, the symptoms will soon improve. If symptoms alone are treated, the disease may continue as before.
> 4. **Do** usually use single generic preparations and not combinations of drugs.
>   There are a few important exceptions to this, e.g. iron and folic acid in pregnancy and fixed dose combinations in TB, antiretrovirals to control HIV/AIDS, and artemesinin combined therapy (ACT) in malaria.
> 5. **Do** buy good quality drugs at the cheapest possible prices.
>   *First choice*: reliable, quality-tested local manufacturer. *Second choice*: multinational company making good quality, inexpensive drugs in-country or in-region. *Third choice*: obtain from outside, e.g. from NGO low-cost good quality supplier.
> 6. **Do** try to obtain drugs from government sources for any national programme in which the project is involved, e.g. Stop TB. These will usually be quality assured.
> 7. **Do** make sure that all project members and doctors use the project's Essential Drugs List.
> 8. **Do** avoid wastage: through assessing supplies needed, bulk buying, checking supplies on arrival for breakage and discoloration, using older stock first, and ensuring safe storage and transport. Set up good management systems (see pages 67–9 and 155–7).
> 9. Do discourage self-prescribing.

> **Some Do nots:**
> 1. **Do not** give injections when medicines by mouth will work as well.
>   Each time we decline to use an injection we will need to explain gently why a medicine by mouth is more appropriate.

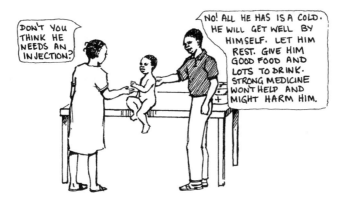

Figure 17.9   When medicines are not needed, take time to explain why.

2. **Do not** give drugs or injections for common colds. They don't help and they can be dangerous.
3. **Do not** give antibiotics unless they are really needed, such as when a child has pneumonia (see pages 221–2).
4. **Do not** give intravenous glucose for dehydration unless the person is unable to drink.
5. **Do not** use tonics or enzyme mixtures. Only use vitamins if the patient is dangerously ill or malnourished. Give nutrition education instead.
6. **Do not** give medicines just because the people want them, expect them or say they will go somewhere else if we don't provide them.
7. **Do not** be discouraged if this advice seems hard to follow: health workers throughout the world are all facing similar problems.

Each time we refuse to prescribe an unnecessary medicine it is another small victory for the people's health and a defeat for the forces of greed and profit.

spend money they cannot afford. We must oppose the misuse of drugs by supporting the practice of a rational drug policy and the use of an Essential Drugs List.

CBHC should aim to use a health model rather than a medical model. In promoting good health and preventing illness health workers should prescribe only medicines that are really essential.

Two mistakes are commonly made in prescribing – using too much non-essential medicine and using too little essential medicine. Health workers need to be taught correct prescribing and communities shown that good health comes from a healthy lifestyle, not a dependence on pills and injections.

Each programme needs to draw up its own Essential Drugs List, which all those prescribing should follow. When we are involved in national programmes such as Stop TB, Roll Back Malaria or IMCI, we should use only the medicines recommended in our national programme. When a community understands the correct use of drugs, initial objections give way to improvements in health and widespread satisfaction.

Summary

Far too many injections and medicines are being used worldwide. Unclean needles from unneeded injections spread hepatitis B, C and HIV infection. Increasing numbers of medicines are substandard or counterfeit. Excessive use of medicines wastes money and leads to serious side effects. Unnecessary injections and medicines cause resistance to antibiotics and force the poor to

Further reading and resources

1. *WHO Model Formulary 2005*, based on the 14th Model List of Essential Medicines, 2005 WHO.
All projects will need the latest Model List, which is regularly updated. WHO is also publishing a series of model prescribing-information manuals on a range of different illnesses, e.g. parasitic diseases, STIs and HIV, skin diseases. They publish the *Essential Drugs Monitor*. See www.who.int/medicines/publications/essentialmedicines.

All these are also available from: WHO. See Appendix E.

2. *Medical Supplies and Equipment for Primary Health Care*, M. Kaur and S. Hall, ECHO International Health Services Ltd, 2001.
   Essential for all health programmes.
   Available from TALC. See Appendix E.

3. *Essential Drugs Practical Guidelines*, J. Maritoux and J. Pinel, 2nd edition, Médecins sans Frontières, 2002.
   Available from TALC.

4. *Where There is no Doctor*, D. Werner, Macmillan, 2003.
   A variety of editions and languages is available from TALC and Macmillan. See Appendix E.

5. *Medicinal Plants in China*, WHO, 1989.
   Lists and describes Chinese herbal remedies.
   Available from: WHO. See Appendix E.

6. *The British National Formulary (BNF)*, BMA and RPS, 2005 and updated annually.
   Clear and precise details of which medicines to use for which conditions. Also useful for doctors involved in hospital medicine.
   Available from: TALC. See Appendix E.

7. *Drug doses*, F. Shann, 12th edn, 2003.
   Doses of every drug commonly prescribed for adults and children.
   Available from TALC.

8. *Primary Diagnosis and Treatment: a manual for clinical and health centre staff in developing countries*, 2nd edn, D. Fountain, Macmillan, 2006.
   A valuable book.
   Available from: Macmillan and TALC, see Appendix E.

Slides

The following teaching slides are available from TALC. See Appendix E.

Cold Chain   CoV
Essential Drugs   DAP

CD ROMS and websites

WHO Medicines Bookshelf CD-ROM. Available free of charge from EDM Documentation Centre, WHO, see address in Appendix E or email: edmdoc centre@who.int.

WHO Essential Medicines Library: mednet3.who.int/eml. (Restricted access.)

MSF Access to Essential Medicines Campaign: www.accessmed-msf.org/index.asp; www.who.int/medicines.

The Safe Injection Global Network (SIGN): www.injectionsafety.org.

See Further references and guidelines, pages 416–7.

18

Monitoring and Evaluating the Health Programme

In this chapter we shall consider:

1. What we need to know
   - The meaning of monitoring and evaluation
   - Who benefits from monitoring and evaluation?
   - Who should carry it out?
   - Some pitfalls to avoid
2. What we need to do
   - Choose what to monitor or evaluate
   - Select the best indicator
   - A sample monitoring and evaluation chart (Table 18.1)
   - Act on the result

What we need to know

The meaning of monitoring and evaluation

Monitoring and evaluation (M and E) are the techniques we use to find out how well our health project is achieving what it set out to do.

Our programme will have set original objectives (i.e. the results we will want to achieve) for the various programme activities we wanted to cover. We will probably have recorded these on the Logical Framework (logframe) (pages 103–6). M and E enables us to see how effectively we have reached those objectives: it is one measure of our success.

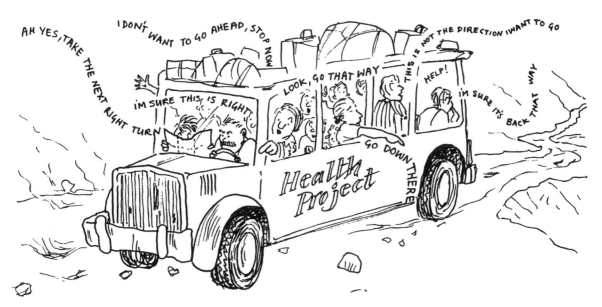

Figure 18.1 Evaluation helps everyone to see what they are doing and where they are going.

Although these terms are often used together and sometimes cause confusion, each has a specific meaning. *Monitoring* refers to the regular, e.g. yearly, assessment of our progress. It should be part of the normal programme management we originally set up. It is usually done by project members and uses the basic record systems we have built into the project.

Evaluation refers to a more systematic review of the project, or certain features of it, after a period of time, e.g. three or five years. It often involves outsiders and usually uses other methods of assessing progress in addition to the information from our normal recording systems.

> If regular monitoring is well carried out, evaluation can be less frequent and will be easier to do.

Our project development follows the pattern outlined in Figure 18.2.

Who benefits from monitoring and evaluation?

The programme itself

We will often start with good ideas and ambitious objectives. As time goes on these often become lost or buried in day-to-day activities or problems.

M and E helps the project to know whether it is still on the right road, how far it has travelled and how far it still has to go.

> Regular monitoring will help us to identify problems early so they can be corrected, and to suggest improvements so they can be incorporated.

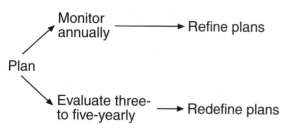

Figure 18.2   Monitoring and evaluating the health plan.

The planning cycle

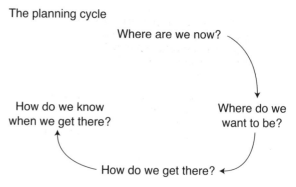

Figure 18.3   The planning cycle.

The main purpose of monitoring is for the benefit of the programme itself – both health team and community.

The community

M and E will help the community to see how the programme is working, and help to explain the benefits it is bringing. Community members will be involved with us as participants in this process. We will also feed back information to them at the end as beneficiaries. Findings and results will need to be presented in such a way that, first, the community sees the benefits (and problems) and, second, is motivated to work with us to bring about improvements.

Donors and sponsors

In practice, evaluations are often carried out because donors want confirmation that their money is being well spent. But all stakeholders – programme, community, donors and government – should benefit from evaluation if it is well planned and sensitively carried out.

Government

Governments will want to know what results the programme is achieving and especially if it is reaching national and district targets. If we are involved in specific programmes such as Stop TB, Making Pregnancy Safer or Roll Back Malaria, their coordinators will need our results.

NGOs involved in Community Based Health Care (CBHC) are often able to achieve more

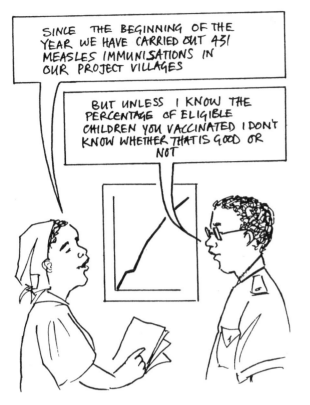

Figure 18.4   Know the percentages.

effective results at community level than government workers. Evaluation (and the return of key annual figures through our regular monitoring) will help us to demonstrate this and to increase our credibility. This in turn will enable CBHC as part of civil society to be entrusted with an increasing number of health tasks in national health programmes. This will be to everyone's benefit.

Some useful definitions of words used in monitoring and evaluation
The following definitions each have an example from a well building programme:

Activities What is actually done
• Building of wells
• Hygiene education

Evaluation An assessment, at a specific time, of the effects of a programme
• Assessing whether water use in the village has changed and whether the wells have influenced household hygiene and sanitation

---

Monitoring Continuous process of observation to record, reflect and use information regarding progress
• Use of resources, progress of activities, changes towards meeting programme objectives

Indicators Evidence or signs that change has taken place
Quantitative indicators are those which can be measured or counted
• Number of people collecting water from the wells
Qualitative indicators are those gained by observation and perception
• Local people's views about the changes caused by the wells

Goals Long-term aims for impact
• To improve health in target population

Objectives Results and outcomes the programme is expected to achieve
• To increase the amount of clean water used in village households

Outputs What is produced as a result of completed activities
• Completed wells producing clean water

Inputs Physical and human resources used within the programme
• Tools, bricks, labour …

Impact Long-term and sustainable change resulting from an activity
• Long-term effects on the health of local people, social relationships in the village and the position of women

Outcomes The effect on the original situation due to the programme
• Increased use of clean water in households

Adapted from CSSDD Project Yangon, Myanmar

Who should carry it out?

Monitoring is usually done by the health team, working closely with the community, as already described.

Evaluations can be done by project and community members alone. To be effective these 'insider evaluations' need to be relatively small scale and analyse a limited number of project activities. The team would need to possess the necessary skills, and good monitoring systems would need to be in place.

In practice, evaluations usually involve the use of outside experts who come to work alongside the health team and community.

The success of using outsiders depends on several conditions:

- **The evaluation must be planned in advance.** It may last one or two weeks, and will need to be done at a time of year when neither the health team nor community is overworked, nor the weather too extreme. Essential project activities should continue, not least because evaluators will want to observe the programme at work.
- **The evaluators must have clear terms of reference**, i.e. know exactly what they are meant to be doing, and also what they are not meant to be looking into. They should be sensitive to the local culture, and have an affirming attitude to the health team and community. Terms of reference should be agreed between evaluator, project and any donor agency who is involved. Evaluators should be carefully briefed both by donor and project before starting to work.

The advantages of using outsiders include:
- **Expert advice:** those with special skills will be able to design effective methods, and give advice on how to carry out the evaluation.
- **Lack of bias:** results may be more accurate as outsiders will not have such a strong personal interest in the achievements of the programme.
- **More accurate feedback from the community**, whose members may be more ready to share with outsiders the way they really feel than with health team workers with whom they are working each day.

The disadvantages of using outsiders include:
- **Cost in terms of time and money**, though a donor agency often funds the evaluation.
- **Visiting experts may not know the local customs**, language or situation. It is therefore helpful if evaluators are familiar with the country, region and type of project.

If the evaluation includes any research that may be written up, this must be clearly discussed beforehand. Material from evaluations or visits is sometimes published in a way that is politically insensitive or unhelpful to the community.

Some pitfalls to avoid
Programmes monitor too little

Many projects go from year to year without proper monitoring or evaluation. Annual reports are still written, and numbers listed of patients seen, immunisations given or procedures carried out. Such figures may accurately record the amount of work being carried out, but have little to say about the impact the project is having on the community.

In practice it is quite easy for a project to get 'out of control'. We get overwhelmed by challenges in the field, overcome by needs and our record systems and reports turn into a nightmare. Obviously this is a serious condition and we need to take action, including being open with any agency that is helping to fund the project.

The list of questions in Figure 18.5 was specifically designed by one funding agency to help programmes who were in this situation to focus on some key issues on which to report and to guide their forward planning.

This is not a permanent substitute for the systems described later under 'What we need to do'.

Programmes monitor too much

Some programmes go to the opposite extreme especially if very bureaucratic, or run by managers with a special interest in statistics or a love of computers!

In these situations collecting figures and producing good 'results' can become more important than working in partnership with the community for long-term improvements.

Sometimes projects have to provide huge numbers of records and reports. This happens particularly if they are involved in several separate programmes such as EPI (childhood immunisation), Stop TB, or Roll Back Malaria. We must therefore help donors to request only information they really need, and only agree to evaluations that are genuinely useful for the project. We need to prevent programmes from becoming driven by the donors, also from spending too much time

Informal Evaluation Questions

Project impact on local community

What effect does the presence of the project have on the local community? (If the project did not exist, what would happen?) A story may help to show the project impact.

Disease prevalence and project impact

What do project staff consider the three most common diseases in the project area? What effect has the project had on the prevalence of these diseases during the last three years? (Is there any statistical evidence?)

Community involvement in project

Is the local community involved in this project? If yes, how is their involvement facilitated e.g. through village health committee, community volunteers, etc. How often do project staff meet with community members? If there is no community involvement, why? Are there any plans to increase this? If not, why?

Community volunteers

Do volunteers from the community work in the project e.g. as voluntary health workers (VHWs) or HIV/AIDS home-based care workers (HBCWs)? Approximately what number are there currently active and newly trained in the last year?

Current project problems and challenges

What are the three most serious problems which have a negative effect on the running of the project? How have these problems been addressed? How successful have these efforts been? What do project staff consider would be needed to solve them?

Do you expect any future changes in project area?

e.g. economic or political changes, climatic changes, staff 'brain drain' e.g. to rich countries, or changes in disease prevalence e.g. HIV/AIDS, etc.

Future plans and priority objectives for the next year

What are project staff's 3 priority objectives for the project? What may stop them implementing these objectives? How do they plan to overcome these problems?

Thank you for completing this form.

Figure 18.5   Informal evaluation questions for struggling projects.

recovering from the last evaluation and preparing for the next.

The real needs and opinions of the poor are ignored

Especially when gathering 'soft' information, the articulate and well-off usually do most of the talking, while the poor have little chance to express their opinions or describe their needs. Sometimes the overall health of a community may improve but the health of the most vulnerable may stay the same or even decline.

Differences in health improvements between the rich and the poor can be highlighted by keeping separate figures for the better-off majority (e.g. the high caste or members of the dominant tribal group), and for the worse-off minority (e.g. the low-caste or landless). Similarly, we can keep separate figures for men and women, or for different language or ethnic groups.

> We must ensure that any evaluation clearly shows the impact of the programme on the poorest subgroups.

Results of the evaluation are not used at all or are wrongly used

If an evaluation shows up negative findings, these should be shared openly and honestly with the team. Only then can everyone face up to the issues raised and make improvements. At the same time, blame, criticism and discouragement must be avoided. Any positive features should be shared with all, especially with those who are mainly responsible.

In some circumstances it is prudent for the project leaders to shoulder any blame, and for the community, government or political leadership to receive any praise.

What we need to do

Choose what to monitor or evaluate

There is a very large list of programme activities we could monitor or evaluate. Usually, however, we will want to look at a few key activities of our programme.

Most chapters in this book set out aims and targets for various project activities and give ideas of what to evaluate. Table 18.1 includes many of these and lists some more.

If our programme is larger and well established we will need to be aware of the indicators used for the Millennium Development Goals that are related to health. And if we are involved in any national programmes such as Stop TB, we will need to follow the indicators set up by these programmes. Some of these indicators are included in Table 18.1.

Whatever the size or scale of our programme, at the start, we must be careful to set up simple but accurate recording systems for the topics we wish to measure. In turn these systems will lay the foundation for a more comprehensive evaluation in the future.

We will probably have constructed a logframe, (see pages 103–6) and this can be used as a guide or template to help monitor progress towards the objectives we set. We can then make adaptations to the logframe based on the results of our monitoring. The logframe will need to be carefully revised after more formal evaluations.

> In M and E we need to select a few key targets that are important to monitor, easy to record and helpful for planning and management.

Select the best indicator

Having chosen which programme activities should be evaluated, we must now decide on the most appropriate measurement tool. This is known as an indicator. An indicator is best defined as a measure or evidence of progress towards an agreed target.

It is helpful at this stage to distinguish between two different types of evidence. The first is *quantitative, numerical or 'hard'* evidence and the second is *qualitative, descriptive or 'soft'* evidence. For the first we will need indicators that measure numbers, rates and percentages. For the second we will need descriptive indicators to help provide evidence on knowledge, attitudes and practice. Both types are important in CBHC.

Five finger planning method

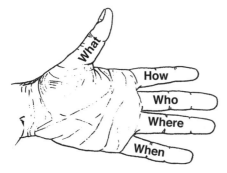

What is the purpose of the evaluation and who is asking for it?

How will information be gathered?

Who will be involved and what resources will they need?

Where will the work be done?

When will it take place?

Figure 18.6   The five finger method for planning evaluation.

An example of indicators measuring hard information:

We want to evaluate our DPT immunisation programme over the past year as in Table 18.1. (See also the example of measles immunisation as written on the sample logframe on page 106.) The indicator chosen must give the most accurate measurement of what we really want to know.

Here are some possible indicators we could use:

a) The total number of DPT injections given during the past year.

b) The total number of children under five who received DPT injections during the past year.

c) The total number of children under five who completed courses of DPT during the past year.

d) The percentage of children under five who completed courses of DPT during the past year.

We can see how moving from a) to d) the indicator is becoming increasingly useful.

The indicator commonly used in annual reports is a) but has only limited value. What we really want to know is how completely we have immunised our target population, the figure given by the lower indicator d). This is therefore the most appropriate, even if it takes a little longer to calculate.

These four (**a** to **d**) are all examples of *input indicators* – in other words, they measure the amount of work we have actually put in.

But we could use a very different indicator. We could measure: number **e)** or percentage **f)** of children who suffered from the diseases diphtheria, pertussis and tetanus during the past year.

These are examples of *output* or *impact indicators* and measure the effectiveness or impact of the immunisation programme. Because our ultimate aim is to eradicate these three diseases from the target population, f) is therefore the best indicator of all.

Indicators are more useful still if we use them for comparisons.

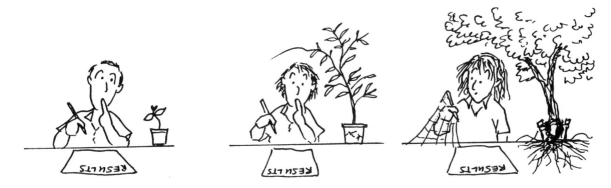

Figure 18.7   Write up the results of monitoring and evaluation before they are out of date.

Table 18.1   A sample monitoring and evaluation chart

Subject	Examples of indicators	Possible sources of information
Child nutrition (Chapter 9)	Percentage of under-5s who are underweight	Child's growth card
	Percentage of children between 1 and 5 with MUAC under 13.5 cm	CHW notebook MUAC Charts Family folder insert card IMCI returns
Immunisations (Chapter 10)	For each immunisation, especially measles, percentage of children under 5 who have completed course (in past 1, 3 or 5 years)	Immunisation register Family folder and insert card
	For BCG, percentage of under-5s with BCG scars	Special survey
	For tetanus toxoid, percentage of women at delivery who have had 2 or more injections	Mother's Home-Based Record Card Immunisation register CHW/TBA records Returns from Making Pregnancy Safer Initiative
	Incidence rates of some immunisable diseases	Disease Register Clinic and CHW records Special survey
Control of malaria (Chapter 11)	Percentage of children 5 or under sleeping under bed-nets	Sample survey or Roll Back Malaria records
	Percentage of patients seen with positive malaria slide	Clinic records
Maternal heath (Chapter 12)	Percentage of mothers attending for 4 or more antenatal checks in clinic or with TBA	Mother's Home-based Record Card TBA/CHW records
	Percentage of newborns weighing 2500 g or above or with MUAC of 8.7 cm or above	CHW/TBA records Mother's Home-based Record Card
	Percentage of babies delivered by midwife or trained TBA or Trained Attendant, using sterile delivery pack	CHW/TBA records Mother's Home-based Record Card Returns from Making Pregnancy Safer Initiative
Family planning (Chapter 13)	The Contraceptive Prevalence Rate	FP Register Family folder and insert cards
	Average space between children	Family folder
Control of TB (Chapter 14)	Follow the National TB Programme Aims and Targets (page 275), Recording TB cases (page 278) and Recording outcomes (page 283)	

Table 18.1   A sample monitoring and evaluation chart (continued)

Subject	Examples of indicators	Possible sources of information
Curative care (Chapter 7)	Percentage of all patient attendances seen by CHW	CHW records Clinic attendance register
	For diarrhoea, percentage of families using ORS as first line treatment	Special survey
Use of essential drugs (Chapter 17)	Percentage of CHWs or health centres with regular supply of essential drugs, e.g. antibiotics and antimalarials	Inventories Spot surveys CHW and clinic records
	Percentage of population with reliable access to affordable essential drugs	Special surveys
Abuse of tobacco, alcohol, drugs	Percentage of population aged 10 and over who admit to use*	Family folder
Use of clean water (Chapter 16)	Percentage of families using clean water source within 15 minutes' walk from house	Family folder
Waste disposal (Chapter 16)	Percentage of families with all family members using latrine*	Family folder

Note: the section following is more complex and many of these topics will only be possible to carry out in larger projects with good outside support and technical help.

Infant Mortality Rate	This is: $$\frac{\text{Number of deaths under 12 months}}{\text{Number of live births}} \quad \frac{\text{per year}}{\times 1000}$$	Vital events register Family folder CHW records
Under-5 Mortality Rate	This is: $$\frac{\text{Number of deaths of children under 5}}{\substack{\text{Total number of under 5 children} \\ \text{at mid-year}}} \quad \frac{\text{per year}}{\times 1000}$$	Vital events register Family folder CHW records
Maternal Mortality Rate	This is: $$\frac{\substack{\text{Number of maternal deaths with} \\ \text{pregnancy-related cause (during} \\ \text{pregnancy, delivery and up to} \\ \text{42 days after delivery)}}}{\text{Number of live births}} \quad \frac{\text{per year}}{\times 1000}$$	Vital events register Duplicate mother's home-based record Family folder and insert cards Clinic and hospital records
Adult or Female Literacy Rate	This is: $$\frac{\substack{\text{Number of adults (or women) aged} \\ \text{15 or over who can read and write}}}{\substack{\text{Total number of adults (or women)} \\ \text{aged 15 or over}}} \quad \times 100$$	Family folder Special survey

Table 18.1   A sample monitoring and evaluation chart (continued)

Subject	Examples of indicators	Possible sources of information
Work of the CHWs (Chapter 7)	Percentage of community homes visited on average once per week	CHW record book
	Level of CHWs' knowledge about prevention and cure of common illnesses	Spot survey Questionnaire
	Percentage of families or individuals able to prevent and self-treat selected illnesses e.g. diarrhoea, scabies	Questionnaire
	Level of satisfaction of community with their CHW	Questionnaire PA methods
Cost effectiveness	This is, broadly: $$\frac{\text{Total cost of project}}{\text{Number people covered by CBHC}}$$ but needs calculating with the aid of an economist	

Notes:

1. *Accurate definitions needed
2. Family folder refers to the survey or resurvey done using the family folder. Full information on each family appears on the outside of the folder (see Chapter 5, page 83). Much of the most useful information for evaluation is best collected during house to house surveys using the folders.
3. Under 'sources of information' several are suggested reflecting the different record systems used by different programmes. Clinic records refers to any records or registers kept in clinics not otherwise specified.
4. For some subjects more than one indicator is usually listed though in practice only one would normally be chosen for any one evaluation.
5. Most information, from whatever source, would be tabulated annually and stored in the master register or computer.
6. For national programmes, official data collecting forms should be used.

For example: We can compare how things are now with how they were when we first started. To do this we will need an accurate baseline survey at the time the project started.

Or we can compare how things are in the project area with how they are in a non-project or 'control' area that we also surveyed originally but in which we have not been working.

Examples of indicators providing soft evidence

1   We want to measure what people think of a development worker from a nearby NGO, or of their own village health worker. We ask a question such as: 'What do you think of your village health worker?' and ask them to select one of the following for each statement: very helpful, helpful, OK, not very helpful, unhelpful. Then the answers can be set out as in

Table 18.2. This way of helping to quantify descriptive evidence is known as coding, and is especially useful in drawing comparisons or showing improvement over a period of time. Adding a few quotes to the table adds further in helping to give an overall idea of the community's assessment of the person in question.

2. We want to measure ways in which women's status has changed as a result of the programme's work. Village workers are asked to select one of the following for each of the statements below: strongly agree, agree, not sure, disagree, strongly disagree.
The statements might be:

- Women are able to participate in decision-making in the family
- Women are allowed to speak to leaders
- Women are able to participate in village affairs

Table 18.2   Differences in reported attitude to a development worker by villages over a two-year period

Attitudes to worker	very useful	useful	OK	not very useful	unhelpful	TOTAL
Baseline survey 2004	2	5	6	8	7	28
Assessment 2006	11	9	9	4	0	33

Adapted from Footsteps 50, Tearfund, p. 9

Then the evidence can be coded in a similar way to the first example.

Other models for the use of indicators can be used. If we are engaged in a national HIV/AIDS programme, we should be aware of the indicators in the box below. If not, this more complex example will not be relevant to us.

WHO/UNAIDS indicators for programmes involved in HIV/AIDS control

The following are used by WHO/UNAIDS in measuring the progress of HIV programmes.

Core indicator sets are used, which are world-wide measurements. These allow widespread comparisons. Examples of indicators include:

- Percentage of respondents who report at least one non-regular sex partner in the past 12 months.
- Percentage who say they used a condom when they last had sex with a non-regular partner.
- Age at first sex.

Locally derived indicators are those that are relevant to a particular programme ideally decided in partnership with the community. Examples of indicators include:

- Number of PLWHAs able to go public.
- Number of people attending voluntary HIV counselling and testing (VCT), percentage of people who return for results.

Long-term impact indicators measure permanent behavioural change, reduction of stigma, and decrease in incidence of HIV/AIDS.

For further ways of gathering and processing information, see Chapters 5 and 6,

Act on the result

Unless action is taken on the findings of M and E the whole process is a waste of time and money. A good evaluation raises hopes that issues will be better understood by all partners. But if everything then continues as before, it can cause disillusionment.

Use results widely

The results of both regular monitoring and less frequent evaluation should be used as widely as possible and the results made known to any who will benefit from seeing them.

- The community should always know about key findings. We will need to present these to leaders, health committees or community meetings in a way each group can understand.

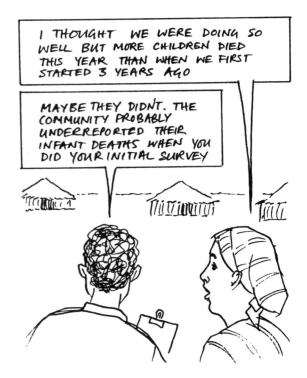

Figure 18.8

- **Health team members** will need to understand the findings and be involved in future planning.
- **The donor agency** will usually receive details, and in the case of evaluations, visiting experts will usually write a report. We should ask to have a copy of this, though agencies may not be willing to share the whole document.
- **The government**, for example, the DMO, TB officer, etc. may want details of any reports, figures or findings directly relevant to their own department or programme.

Respond to recommendations

Regular monitoring gives evidence that helps to fine-tune the programme. We should respond to any unexpected findings and change course if necessary.

An outside evaluation should always lead to recommendations. These should:

- comment on successes and failures;
- recommend courses of action;
- suggest how changes can be carried out;
- propose follow-up to make sure recommendations are acted upon.

The health team, with the community and guided by the evaluation, will then replan the programme or those parts of it that need changing. Usually this will mean rewriting part of the logframe for a new project phase. This will need to include revised objectives, inputs, budgets and plans.

We may find it hard to respond positively if some of the findings are discouraging. We should aim to be:

- organised enough to do something about it;
- brave enough to face up to failure and areas that need changing;
- flexible enough to modify our programme.

Summary

All programmes need regular monitoring and less frequent evaluation to find evidence of how successfully they are achieving their aims and reach-

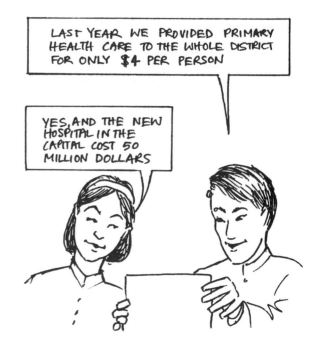

Figure 18.9 Community based health care that is well set up and effectively managed is cost effective.

ing their targets. Monitoring is largely done as a regular annual activity using normal reporting systems set up at the start of the programme. Evaluations usually involve help from outside specialists, and involve a wider look at project activities.

The most important subjects for monitoring and evaluation must be decided and an appropriate indicator set up for each. Sources of information, both numerical and descriptive, need to be decided well in advance. If we are participating in any national programmes such as Stop TB or IMCI we should use their programme indicators. As part of the evaluation, results must be analysed and fed back to the community, donor and government where necessary. Recommendations then lead to joint planning and action by health team and community, which can be incorporated into a new logframe to guide the next project phase.

The community itself should work in partnership with the health team in each stage of the process.

Further reading

1. *Partners in Evaluation*, M.-T. Feuerstein, Macmillan, 1986.
An excellent and well illustrated guide on how to evaluate in partnership with the community. Just as useful as when first written.
Available from: TALC. See Appendix E.

2. *Toolkits: A Practical Guide to Assessment, Monitoring, Review and Evaluation*, L. Gosling and M. Edwards, Save the Children Fund, 1995.
A detailed and useful manual.

3. *A Basic Guide to Evaluation for Development Workers*, F. Rubin, Oxfam, 1995.
Another useful, but shorter, guide.
Available from: IT Publications. See Appendix E.

4. *Participatory Impact Monitoring*, D. Germann, E. Gohl and B. Schwarz, GATE, 1996.
Four very useful booklets.
Available from GATE, PO Box 5180 D-65726, Eschborn, Germany. Website: www5.gtz.de/gate.

5   *Assessing Community Health Programmes; a trainer's guide*, J. Valadez, W. Weiss, C. Leburg and R. Davis, TALC, 2003.
A participant's manual and workbook is also available.
Available from TALC. See Appendix E.

19

Managing Personnel and Finance

In this chapter we shall briefly consider how to manage personnel and finance.

Most chapters of the book include ideas on management for the topics being discussed. In addition, Chapter 4, Initial Tasks, gives ideas on how to obtain and manage project supplies. The index and detailed list of contents will help to locate various areas of management covered in different chapters.

Many health programmes that start well eventually fail through poor management. Management skills are important not only for programme directors but also for all health team and community members who share responsibility.

> In community based health care, management skills are as important as clinical skills. Good management is the key for making programmes efficient and effective.

HOW TO MANAGE PERSONNEL

In this section we shall consider
1. What we need to know
   - Models of leadership
   - Guidelines for leading
   - Ways of encouraging the health team
   - Things that discourage the health team
   - Understand personal and financial pressures on team members
2. What we need to do
   - Write job descriptions
   - Induct new team members
   - Carry out appraisals
   - Resolve conflicts
   - Manage change
   - Delegate to others
   - Enable team and community members to plan effectively

- Manage staff in the day-to-day programme
- Give variety and keep a sense of balance

What we need to know

> A contented, motivated team is the basis for a successful health programme. This will depend in large part on those in charge using appropriate leadership styles and being efficient managers.

Models of leadership

Some people follow the *autocratic* or 'Do what I say approach'. They make the decisions, keep control, give the orders and block discussion. Result: usual disempowerment of team members.

Others follow the open, *consultative* or 'Let's work together approach'. Everyone contributes, authority is delegated, jobs are flexible, self-discipline is encouraged. The leader is 'first among equals'. Result: usual motivation of team members.

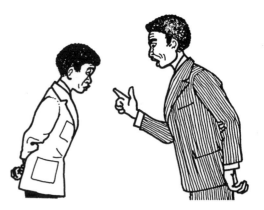

Figure 19.1 The autocratic approach.

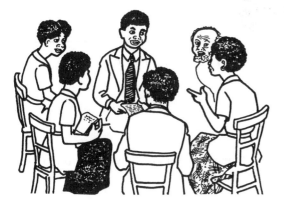

Figure 19.2   The consultative approach.

Most natural leaders are autocratic, and others often become so when put in charge. For this reason leaders will need to learn to become more open and participatory.

One way in which we can undergo change ourselves and help bring it about in others is through the process of transformation described on pages 21–22 and 37–38.

Guidelines for leading

Leaders of all levels should learn to be:

1. **Consultative** – in the day-to-day running of the programme, and decisive when the situation demands it.
2. **Facilitators** – empowering other people to do things themselves. In this way each person learns new skills and grows in self-confidence.
3. **Talent spotters** – learning how to recognise and use the gifts and skills of the health team and community.
4. **Credible** – our team must trust and believe in its leaders. This means leaders must be competent at the skills they use and fair in their ways of handling people.
5. **Patient** – being ready to start at the place where others are, not where we feel they ought to be. In this way people grow more quickly in self-esteem and confidence.

The open model is usually the preferred one in CBHC. However, we need to be aware that:

- Excessive team involvement can lead to perpetual discussion, delayed decisions and slow progress.
- Some team members have little interest in discussion and decision-making and simply want to get on with their job.
- There is a danger that too much consultation means the project moves ahead at the rate of the slowest.
- It is important that leadership is free 'to lead' in order for programmes to be effective.

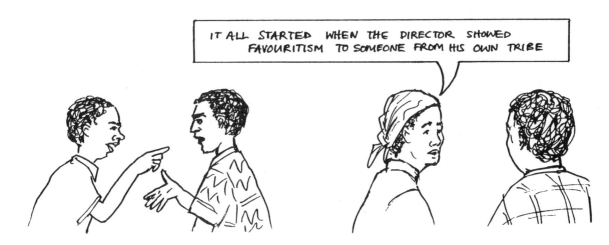

IT ALL STARTED WHEN THE DIRECTOR SHOWED FAVOURITISM TO SOMEONE FROM HIS OWN TRIBE

Figure 19.3

A proverb says: 'People, like plants, grow best by cultivation, not suffocation.'

6. **Unbiased** – we should avoid showing favouritism, being careful to treat everyone with fairness, dignity and respect.

> Even slight favouritism towards one team member can, through jealousy, sow the seeds of tribal and regional infighting, which may seriously damage the project.

7. **Available and supportive** – ready to spend time both with the health team and with individuals. This will include helping with tasks related to work and giving support for personal problems. Sometimes this will be at inconvenient times.

Ways of encouraging the health team

These will include:
1. Sharing objectives. Team and community members will perform best if they are able to share in drawing up aims and setting targets.
2. Commending people for good achievements.
3. Delegating responsibility, with training to support it.

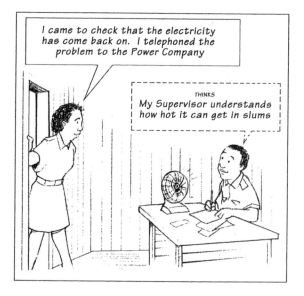

Figure 19.4   Support and understanding help staff bear difficult working conditions.

4. Ensuring salaries are paid on time and that increases and promotion are given when due.
5. Arranging in-service training and regular opportunities for personal and professional development.
6. Handling problems directly and fairly, by finding the root cause of the trouble and trying to solve it.
7. Affirming team members, especially those for whom we have a line management responsibility. This includes such simple things as remembering birthdays and being imaginative during times of crisis and bereavement.

For example: The father of a Congolese team member working in Kenya died during a busy project phase. The manager, knowing that this man was the oldest son and would have many family duties to perform, gave him ten days' compassionate leave, even though the staff member had no contractual right to have this much time off work. As a result, he was able to arrange the funeral and give support to his family. He returned, able to work effectively, and satisfied he had carried out his family duties

Things that discourage the health team

These will include:
1. Poor administration. Leaders who regularly forget, delay, overwork staff or plan inefficiently will annoy and discourage their teams.
2. Lack of personal and professional respect for others.
3. A domineering attitude.
4. Giving too much or too little work.
5. Giving work that is regularly much too easy or much too hard.
6. Cancelling leave or holidays unless there is an important reason.
7. An unwillingness to delegate, or doing so without also giving authority or explaining new management arrangements to the wider team.
8. Lack of training and development opportunities.

It is important to follow good leadership patterns from the beginning. It is easier to keep a team happy than to make a team happy.

Understand personal and financial pressures on team members

In areas where health needs are greatest, we must understand two background factors that will often affect how we manage the programme.

The first is the shortage of health workers, often because of migration to better paid jobs in cities, or transfer to larger programmes: also through illness, death or the need to attend funerals because of locally prevalent illnesses such as HIV/AIDS.

The second is the personal and financial pressure many team members will be under. In many instances they will have multiple home duties, such as caring for the family – often enlarged by orphans because of death through HIV/AIDS or civil conflict. In addition they will often be under serious financial pressure as relatives expect their salary to pay for the needs of other family members, unable or too ill to get work.

We need to understand these issues when it comes to poor attendance, stress and petty corruption amongst our staff, but not always to condone them. We will still need to follow management and disciplinary procedures, but act also from a position of support and understanding when there are genuine pressures.

What we need to do

Write job descriptions

Job descriptions (JDs) list the details and tasks of a job – either for a paid staff member or volunteer.

When a programme first starts it may be unhelpful to define jobs too tightly as there is often a phase when team members are discovering how best they can match their skills with the tasks needing to be done. Later, as different team members take on specific tasks, it is useful to define them. Often this will be formalising what the team members have already been doing.

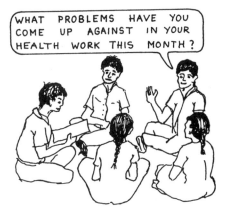

Figure 19.5   Part of the job description for a CHW supervisor.

Established programmes should include Job Descriptions as part of the recruitment process.

All JDs must have a clause that builds in flexibility. Health workers should be ready to do any reasonable task that needs to be carried out.

A well written job description helps each person to know what is expected both of themselves and of others. It gives a sense of security and can increase job satisfaction. It may help to prevent or solve disputes.

A job description includes details of the following:
1. Title and grade.
2. The objectives or main purpose of the job.
3. The tasks and duties to be carried out.
4. The person to whom the staff member is accountable, i.e. their line manager, supervisor or 'boss'.
5. The people for whom the staff member is responsible.

In addition, a contract of employment or a less formal memorandum of understanding can be drawn up. This should include:
- Title and grade
- Length of contract
- Details of appraisal
- Terms and conditions of service.

Sometimes it is helpful to list out the components of a particular task, which can either be included in the JD or listed separately. *For example*: the components of CHW supervision might include:

1. To visit the CHW in her community on a regular basis in order to:
   - give encouragement;
   - check that she is carrying out her duties;
   - teach skills and knowledge;
   - plan future tasks;
   - refill her health kit;
   - complete her records;
   - pay her wages.
2. To assess how well the CHW is functioning and to decide on appropriate guidance for her.
3. To inform the project director or team leader of the CHW's progress.

Induct new team members

During the first one or two weeks after a new team member has joined the project, he/she will need to go through an induction process. This refers to helping a team member to learn as much about the programme as possible. Induction not only helps to raise the confidence of new team members but enables them to be as effective as possible from an early stage.

Induction needs to be planned carefully, and will depend on time available, the experience and seniority of the new team member(s) and other factors specific to the project.

Induction needs to include:

- A clear explanation of all aspects of the programme relevant to the team member's role.
- An opportunity to meet other team members they are likely to work alongside, be answerable to or have management responsibility for.
- An opportunity of joining in a variety of project activities as observer. This enables them to see and enquire about how things are carried out and to understand the style and approaches that the programme uses.
- Being assured that they are free to ask questions whenever unsure of anything that affects their job or undermines their confidence.

Inductions need to be planned in advance so that time is set aside for members of the team who will be involved in doing this, rather than assuming it will 'just happen' in the course of a busy day.

Carry out appraisals

An appraisal is structured time set apart each year for manager (appraiser) and team member (appraisee) to spend together. It does not replace the need for regular meetings nor to sort out significant problems, which are best addressed at the time they arise.

The purposes are as follows:
- To review the past year, looking at what the person has accomplished and comparing this with the objectives set in the previous appraisal.
- To set personal objectives for the coming year.
- To give an opportunity for the appraisee to raise any issues and concerns related to his/her employment.
- To identify areas where there needs to be improvement.
- To identify training needs.
- To recognise and affirm good performance in any area of work.

The advantages of regular appraisals include:
- Opportunities for the manager and team member to strengthen their personal relationship.
- An opportunity for problems and weaknesses to be identified and addressed in a normal work process, before they cause problems.
- An affirmation of the appraisee.

Appraisals need to be regular, confidential, affirming and relational, never disciplinary in character and planned in advance so that both the appraiser and appraisee can think ahead. In this way both gain the most benefit. It is helpful for guidance notes to be issued in advance, and for a form to be filled in by the appraiser at or shortly after the appraisal with a copy given to the appraisee and another kept by the appraiser.

Resolve conflicts

> Preventing disputes is both easier and quicker than solving them.

Guidelines for preventing disputes

To prevent disputes we can follow these guidelines:

1. Manage efficiently and fairly.
2. Meet regularly so that team and community members can plan together, contribute ideas, express feelings and discuss problems.
3. Recruit team members who have friendly and tolerant attitudes. In teams where members of different ethnic or language groups work together we must do everything possible to encourage team members to learn how to respect each other and work together. Those in leadership need to set this example, making sure no favouritism is ever shown.
4. Write clear job descriptions and give clear task instructions.
5. Give spiritual input. There can be a regular time for prayer or meditation, with which all or most team members need to feel comfortable, otherwise it should be optional. We can encourage an appropriate sense of apology and forgiveness if disputes have occurred or there has been perceived unfairness.
6. Assure the team that no one will have special access to the person in charge, nor listen to gossip about other team members.

> Even in the most contented teams conflicts will arise. If they are handled quickly and sensibly they can usually be solved. If they are ignored or mishandled their effects can continue for years.

Guidelines for solving disputes

It is obviously far easier to prevent disputes from arising in the first place through the principles we have already discussed. Also, we should take action early using informal methods that draw on friendship, fairness and common sense so that more serious problems are less likely to occur.

To solve serious disputes between team members or breakdown in relationships we can follow these guidelines:

1. Respond quickly.
2. See each party separately.
3. Listen carefully, making every effort to understand each person's point of view.
4. Ask each party if they are ready for mediation. If they do seem willing, they are encouraged to do this on their own. If they fail or are unwilling we can offer to be a mediator or invite them to name someone else acceptable to both parties.
5. Remain unbiased and slow in giving judgement.

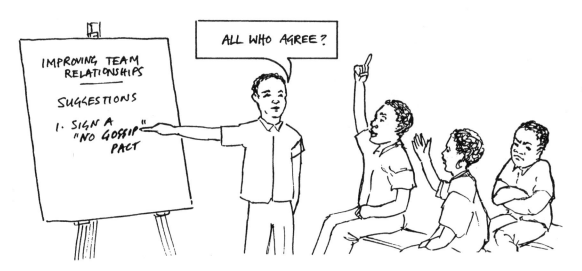

Figure 19.6   Trust between team members is one key to successful programmes.

6. Be ready to act as a scapegoat. One of the causes of the dispute may be our poor management.
7. Record the outcome and what was agreed, and if appropriate ask both parties to sign.
8. Correct any problem that might cause the dispute to happen again.

How to handle more major disputes between team members and managers, or between employees and employers is beyond the scope of this book

Manage change

Any time of change in a programme leads to increased stress. Many people will be frightened by the unknown or worried by loss of control. Some find change harder to cope with than others, especially if they are facing personal problems in other aspects of their life, or have personalities that find change difficult to cope with.

Stressful times include:

1. The appointment of a new director or team leader.
2. Converting a project from a curative, clinical approach to a participatory, community approach.
3. Starting in a new area or beginning a different type of work.
4. Uncertainty about funding, or about the programme's future.
5. A change in management style.
6. Introducing computers or making major IT changes.

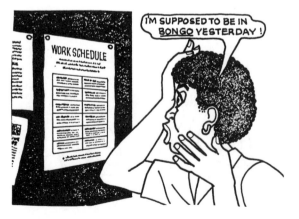

Figure 19.7 Ensure that everyone is fully informed and knows when plans change.

In most effective programmes change will be occurring almost continually, often in one or more of these areas at the same time. Team members will need to understand this and as far as possible be willing for it. Change as an inevitable part of any health programme can be mentioned as part of the induction or recruitment process.

But we need to remember that before any change occurs team members will be asking themselves such questions as:

• How will this affect me?
• Will I have more or less money?
• Will I have more or less status?
• Will I enjoy the job as much?
• Will I be able to do the new job?
• How will I get on with my new colleagues and with my boss?
• If the project closes, where will I find employment?

Because of underlying anxiety, there may be more arguments and complaints than usual, more days lost because of illness, or a general decline of interest in the work.

We can support the team during times of change by:

1. Understanding the stresses they will be feeling and why their standard of work may be falling.
2. Ensuring a good personal relationship with staff.
3. Informing the team as soon as possible and as fully as possible about any developments.
4. Introducing change at the right time.
5. Planning and discussing with the team. We can point out the disadvantage of the present arrangements and explain ways in which they will benefit by the intended changes.
6. Managing change wisely and through carefully planned phases. Each of these can be shared with the team to give them a sense of ownership and control.
7. Very careful and regular communication about what is happening or about to happen and how it will affect their working arrangements.

Delegate to others

Delegation is the art of enabling others to use the gifts and talents they possess, and encouraging them to do as much as, but not more than, they are able.

Learning to delegate is essential for health workers, managers, leaders or anyone who has a line management responsibility for others.

Delegation has two main advantages. It gives the person delegating a task more time to spend on other, more senior or strategic tasks. It gives the person to whom a task has been delegated an opportunity to learn new skills and to grow in self-confidence.

Delegation is the basis of an important principle in community health: 'A job should be done by the person least qualified who can do it well.'

Before delegating we need to ensure that the task is an appropriate one and any person selected to do it is willing and able to carry it out. For all but the smallest tasks we will need to arrange training in advance or at the time the new task is taken on.

Delegation is a skill that has to be learnt. We need to practise it ourselves, then teach others how to carry it out.

In delegating a task to someone else, we need to pass on:

1. Knowledge and expertise on how to do it.
2. Responsibility for the task being delegated with the assurance that the final responsibility lies with us, especially if anything goes wrong.
3. Authority to carry out the task.
   For example: If team members are asked to take control of some aspects of the TB programme, then both they and other members of the team must know they have been empowered to carry this out.

If any of these three is left out, conflict may develop in the team.

Although delegation is an important part of programme management, leaders can become isolated from their team members unless they also regularly take part in team activities, and from time to time join with others in day-to-day or menial tasks.

Enable team and community members to plan effectively

When we plan a new or largescale project activity, we will need to construct a logframe as described on pages 101–6. This section assumes

we will have done an initial needs assessment and defined objectives. It also assumes that we will plan an evaluation of the programme at an agreed period, e.g. after three or five years.

As mentioned previously, for each topic covered in this book the relevant chapter describes the practical ways we can follow to carry out the programmne. The section below reminds us of the four areas where project and community will need to plan together.

Obtaining information

Part of good planning is 'doing our homework' so that we are well informed about all aspects of the activity being considered.

One structure we can use for gathering information is based on the 4 Cs. This needs to be done in full partnership with the community.

* Community need and interest.
* Components or materials needed.
* Construction or how to carry it out.
* Cost expected.

For example: In planning a programme to install smokeless cooking hearths, one mountain programme in Asia used this planning structure as follows:

1. **Community:**
   * Do the people want them?
   * Do the people need them?
   * How do they want them built?
   * Are they ready to do it themselves?
   * Will they need special training?
   * Are they prepared to give their time and skills to this project?
   * Are they ready to pay some of or all the cost themselves?
   * What is the best time of year or season to carry this out?
2. **Components:**
   * What materials are needed?
   * Where can they be obtained?
   * How will they be transported?
   * Where will they be stored?
3. **Construction:**
   * What is the best way of making them?
   * What are the secrets of success that other projects have found?

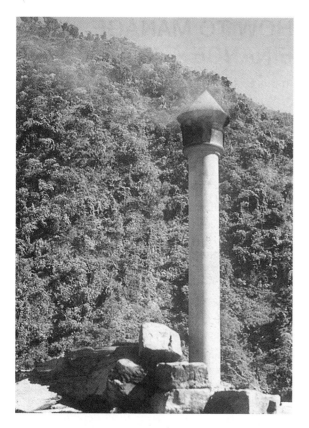

Figure 19.8   Successful management involving community, project and government: the first house to install a smokeless cooking hearth in a north Indian health programme.

  • What are the pitfalls to avoid?
4. **Cost:**
  • What will be the cost of components?
  • What will be the cost of labour?
  • What will be the cost of transport?
  • Will there be other hidden costs?

A similar framework of questions can be worked out for other community health activities.

Setting up a community action group

This will be needed for major programme activities that are sometimes together known as community health development (CHD). They include water and sanitation programmes and other activities that need help from outside agencies and involve community-wide effort or construction.

The CAG will comprise members of the health team, the community (usually representatives of the health committee) and any outside agency involved.

Smaller-scale activities can be based on meetings between health team members and the village health committee. (See pages 27–31 for more details on Village Health Committees and 317–320 on CAGs.)

Carrying out a task analysis

For nearly every task in CBHC we will need to answer the questions in the following list. For CHD activities, each programme stage will need to be broken down and analysed. We will ask:

  • **Who** is going to do it?
  • **When** will it be done?
  • **Where** will it be done?
  • **How** will it be carried out?
  • **What** equipment will be needed?

Communicating with all parties involved

Lack of communication quickly leads to argument and discouragement. We must ensure that everyone is fully informed about any project activity in which they are involved and they are notified as soon as possible if plans change.

Manage staff in the day-to-day programme

Quite apart from planning major project activities, we also need to set up a system for managing the day-to-day programme. This will involve matching the staff available with tasks that need to be done in the field. At an early stage in the programme health committee members can share in day-to-day planning.

A chart can be made that lists out the days of the month, with each day divided into columns either per CH team, per target area or per activity. The chart can have a plastic surface, and coloured, erasable, felt-tip pens can be used to mark different activities and personnel involved in each.

Activities planned are filled in. The names of the team leader and any staff or community members involved are written down. Final details are completed at least one week in advance with instructions about time and place of departure, destination and other important information, such as special equipment needed or important reminders.

This board is displayed in the project headquarters.

Give variety and keep a sense of balance

Balance and variety help to keep a project stable and its members contented. When team members do identical tasks day after day, especially under pressure, it is easy for them to become bored, stressed or demotivated.

Where possible, we need to give variety so that tasks are shared and more than one person is trained and able to do any one task.

For example: Dispensing medicines in a health centre day after day is a job two or more people can be trained to do, while at the same time the main dispenser can be trained to do other tasks, such as helping to register patients. It helps if our team culture ensures multitasking, and encourages the principle that team members are multipurpose.

For example: Project drivers should also be trained to carry out health-related functions so that they don't spend half their days waiting to drive vehicles, but can contribute both to their own satisfaction and to the benefit of the team by being involved in a range of activities.

For individuals and teams, balance might include such things as being involved in:

- Prevention and cure.
- Community and hospital.
- Field and office.
- Serving the rich and serving the poor.
- Health and development.
- Working with men, with women and with children.

Most important of all is work-life balance, when work, family and leisure needs are all considered important. We must ensure that work is not excessive and safeguards are built into the planning, and budget, of the programme (see Further reading 8).

HOW TO MANAGE FINANCE

In this section we will consider:
- Who should handle finance?
- How is the accounting done?
- How are budgets prepared?
- Who needs details of the project accounts?

Who should handle finance?

Anyone involved in handling money will need to be sufficiently well trained so they can comfortably manage the tasks they are asked to do. They must also be thorough, efficient and trustworthy.

> *A project health warning*: many otherwise excellent projects falter, fail, close or cause a scandal because of poor financial management.

Two grades of people are needed:
- **A bookkeeper** to enter cash received and money spent on a daily basis. This can be a relatively junior person, provided they have been shown exactly how to do it. They will need to enter transactions at the time they are made and never delay entry until the following day (or week).
- **An accountant**, who has the following functions:
  - To oversee finances.
  - To prepare accounts at the end of each month, quarter, half-year and year.
  - To prepare a budget (see page 360), in discussion with the programme leaders.
  - To prepare end-of-year accounts for the auditor.

Sometimes the project director will do the accounting, especially when the project first starts. As the project expands an accountant can join the team, possibly working part-time to start with. At each stage of the project, one person needs to take responsibility for financial management, whether this is the Project Director, an accountant or a specially appointed Financial Manager.

Larger size projects may use computers with appropriate accounting software. Small projects

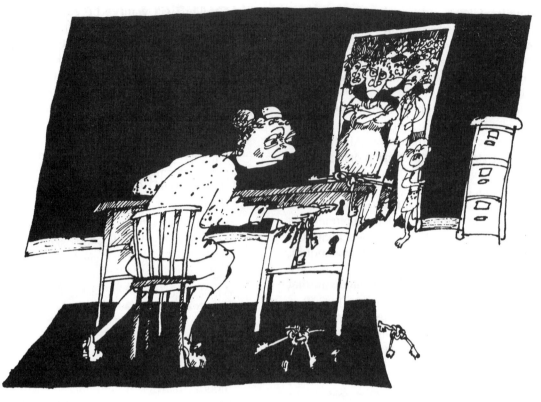

Figure 19.9   A delay in the system, caused by inefficiency.

are advised not to use computers. Only consider computerised accounting if the following can be guaranteed:

- Good quality manual systems that have been well set up and are working efficiently.
- One, preferably two, trained staff members able to manage the system, and do basic trouble shooting.
- Access to expert backup, advice and repair.
- A reliable electricity supply including voltage stabiliser, backup by generator, etc.
- No other more important priorities on which to spend staff time and resources.
- A software package that is easy to use and which can be run side by side with manual systems for at least 12 to 24 months.
- Protection against computer viruses: adequate data backup and security against theft.
- A well planned process for buying, induction and training. This must be built into project planning so as not to cause undue stress to staff or add to their workload in the long term.

- Backup arrangements so that key tasks such as paying bills and salaries can still be carried out even if team members are absent on holiday or on sick leave, or if no computer systems are working.

How is the accounting done?

These are the basic tasks for a smallscale project being set up:

1. **Buy and prepare cash books and files.**
   These will vary depending on the size and style of accounting. Typical books would include:
   - A cashbook or register to enter all money received and paid out, with a column to record current balance.
   - A ledger to list expenditure by category of goods and services bought, and income by source.
   - A petty cashbook or register where minor day-to-day spending is recorded, with

details of each entry also recorded on a Petty Cash Voucher with receipt attached.

- A salary register where details and break-downs of salaries for each project member are recorded and where payments can be signed for.
- Files to keep receipts for items bought, with attached invoices; details of money received with documentation. All should be kept in strict, usually chronological, order or by category.

2. **Open a bank account.**

Unless banks are distant or unreliable we should open accounts and place funds not immediately needed into an account that gathers interest. Remember that cheques, especially from foreign sources, may take weeks to be cleared. Also, in many countries, suppliers will want to be paid in cash or by money order rather than by cheque.

3. **Prepare management accounts.**

These will need to be prepared monthly, quarterly and half-yearly. They include summaries of income received, expenditure by category, amount of money owed by the project (creditors) and owed to the project (debtors). Income and expenditure are compared to the budget for the period under consideration. The purpose of management accounts is for understanding and control. They are essential to help monitor the project finances, ensure the project is on course, and plan for the future.

4. **Prepare cash flow forecasts.**

An example is given in Table 19.1.

Projects very frequently have a 'cash flow crisis' at some point during the year. The best

Table 19.1   Example of cash flow forecast

Women's income generating project
Cash flow forecast for the period 1 January to 30 June 2004

	Jan	Feb	Mar	Apr	May	Jun
	#	#	#	#	#	#
Estimated money coming in:						
Sale of honey	7,500	7,500	7,500	7,500	7,500	7,500
Grant for major equipment					30,000	
Other	600	600	600	600	600	600
Total money coming in [A]	**8,100**	**8,100**	**8,100**	**8,100**	**38,100**	**8,100**
Estimated money to be paid:						
Purchase of equipment					30,000	
Materials		5,350		3,970		
Wages	2,625	2,625	2,625	2,625	2,625	2,625
Rent of premises				13,200		
Vehicle expenses	230	230	230	230	2,190	230
Office expenses	575	575	575	575	575	575
Telephone, electricity	1,517		1,033	1,517		1,033
Total money paid [B]	**4,947**	**8,780**	**4,463**	**22,117**	**35,390**	**4,463**
Opening cash/bank balance	2,340	5,493	4,813	8,450	(5,567)*	(2,857)*
+ Total money coming in [A]	8,100	8,100	8,100	8,100	38,100	8,100
− Total money paid [B]	4,947	8,780	4,463	22,117	35,390	4,463
Closing cash/bank balance	**5,493**	**4,813**	**8,450**	**(5,567)***	**(2,857)***	**780**

* Figures in brackets are negative cash amounts
 # = their currency symbol
Adapted from *Footsteps 57*, Tearfund, December 2003.

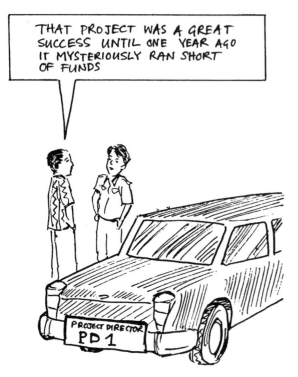

THAT PROJECT WAS A GREAT SUCCESS UNTIL ONE YEAR AGO IT MYSTERIOUSLY RAN SHORT OF FUNDS

PROJECT DIRECTOR
PD 1

Figure 19.10

way to know if funding is sufficient for the coming months is to prepare monthly cash flow forecasts. This involves calculating the amount of money we are likely to spend and to receive each month over the next six months. This helps us to know when income may be especially low or expenditure may be higher than usual, so we can make appropriate plans. Each month we can put in the actual figures for the previous month to replace the forecasted amount for that month, This 'rolling forecast' is an accurate and time-saving way of doing cashflows.

> Management accounts look backwards to the previous few months; cash flow forecasts look forward to the next few months. Together they help us to keep accurate financial control.

5. **Consider setting up an imprest system.**
   Any team member who regularly spends project funds is advanced a fixed sum of money (the imprest) from which purchases are made. When this becomes low, the team member presents his or her receipts for money spent to the director or accountant, who replenishes the imprest up to the original amount.

6. **Prepare annual accounts for the auditor.**
   These will include as a minimum:
   • Details (with documentation) of income, expenditure, money owed to the project (debtors) and money owed by the project to others (creditors). Details of any loans.
   • A profit and loss sheet, and a balance sheet.
   • Donations from overseas, separately listed and accounted for.

Table 19.2 lists out the essential aspects of managing a project and helps us to see how effective our systems are in practice.

How are budgets prepared?

All projects will need to prepare budgets, i.e. listing out the amounts we expect to spend (expenditure) and to receive (income) by different categories. We should do this as accurately as possible for one accounting year, and in outline for two further years.

If we are receiving money from donors, we should prepare budgets the way they advise and according to any conditions they set down. They will often suggest the expenditure headings we should use in order to make it easier for them to coordinate the various projects they support. Sometimes we will need to devise our own headings, especially if our categories of expenditure are different from those of the donor or if we have two or more funding sources that use different headings.

Budgets are usually divided into:

1. **Capital items.**
   This refers to larger sums of money that are received and spent on items lasting a number of years. *For example*: Buildings, vehicles, furniture, computers.

2. **Recurrent items.**
   This refers to income and expenditure for items or services, and includes staff salaries. Some donors have categories they would like us to use for drawing up budgets.
   Typical simplified headings might include:

Table 19.2   Checking your financial management: monitoring good practice

	Always	Mostly	Sometimes	Never
Supporting documents Every financial transaction should be backed up by a 'supporting document', such as a bill, invoice or receipt.				
1. A supporting document is available for every payment.	5	4	1	0
2. A supporting document is available for every item of income.	5	4	1	0
3. Supporting documents are neatly filed, so that it is easy to find any document when it is needed.	5	4	1	0
4. Bank statements are neatly filed.	5	4	1	0
5. Supporting documents and bank statements are kept for the previous seven years.	5	4	1	0
Cashbooks Every transaction should be written down in a cashbook. A cashbook is simply a list of the money that an organisation has spent and received. It can be kept on paper or on a computer.				
6. The date, description and amount of every transaction are recorded in a cashbook.	5	4	1	0
7. All cashbooks are updated at least once per month.	5	4	1	0
8. A separate cashbook is kept for each bank account.	5	4	1	0
Cash records				
9. All cash is kept in a locked cash box or safe.	5	4	1	0
10. Petty cash records are checked every month by a different person from the person who writes them up.	5	4	1	0
11. The balance in the cashbook is checked against the balance on the bank statement every month.	5	4	1	0
12. The balance in the cashbook is checked against the actual amount of cash in the office every month.	5	4	1	0
Budgeting				
13. Budgets are prepared every year.	5	4	1	0
14. Budgets include enough income to pay for all planned expenditure.	5	4	1	0
15. Each month, a cash flow forecast is prepared for the next six month period.	5	4	1	0
Add up the numbers you circled, to give **your score**:				

Adapted from *Footsteps 57,* Tearfund, December 2003.

Expenditure

- Staff salaries
- Services
- Rent and buildings
- Health care supplies including medicines
- Travel and transport
- Training
- Administration
- Maintenance of equipment
- Depreciation (an annual amount to cover the reduced value of capital items bought in the past)
- Contingency (to cover the unexpected).

Income

- By source and amount
- How allocated against expenditure.

We need to make sure that the budget, along with plans for the coming year, is submitted well before the deadline set by any funding agency. See also pages 63–5 and 295–6.

Who needs details of the project accounts?

- The project itself, for its records, and to sort out any questions or problems that may later be raised.

Cashbook A book or spreadsheet that lists all the transactions made into and out of a single account.

Reconciliation The process of comparing and checking information held in two sets of records that describe the same transactions.

Supporting documents The original documents that describe each transaction. They include receipts, invoices and authorising documents.

Transaction Any exchange of goods, services or money in return for other goods, services or money.

Source: Footsteps 11, Tearfund, p. 11.

- Any donor agency supporting the project.
- The government who may inspect them, especially if foreign donations have been received.

Glossary of financial terms

Asset Any item that keeps its value is known as an asset. For NGOs, these are normally stocks of goods, office equipment, vehicles and property.

Bank statement A report produced by a bank, listing all the receipts and payments made into or out of a bank account.

Book-keeping The process of recording the basic details of each transaction.

Budget The best possible estimate of the future cost of activities over a given period of time, and of how those activities will be paid for.

Cash advance A sum of money entrusted to someone to use when precise costs are not known in advance.

Summary

Community health programmes need skilful management of personnel, supplies and finances.

The director and other senior staff must learn how to lead in a fair and consultative style, making sure that their style of leadership encourages and involves the team and community. Systems need to be set up both for planning new or larger-scale activities as well as managing the day-to-day programme. Leaders must learn how to write job descriptions, induct new team members, carry out appraisals, resolve conflicts, delegate and keep a sense of balance in the team.

Careful accounting systems need to be set up and all those involved with finance need careful training, and must be efficient, thorough and trustworthy. Accounts will need to be prepared annually, and, in addition, budgets will need to be prepared well in advance. The preparation of management accounts and cash flow forecasts will become increasingly important as the project grows. Projects that are otherwise successful can fail through poor accounting and financial control.

Further reading and resources

1. *On Being in Charge*, WHO, revised edn, 1992.
    A definitive guide on project management covering all aspects.
    Available from: WHO. See Appendix E.
2. *Medical Administration for Front Line Doctors*, 2nd edn, C. Pearson, FSG Communications, 1995.
    A remarkable book, especially useful for managers of district and base hospitals, but also of relevance to primary health care.
    Available from: TALC. See Appendix E.
3. *Managing for Change: How to Run Community Development Projects*, A. Davies, IT Publications in association with VSO, 1997.
    A valuable book covering aspects of importance to both small and larger projects.
    Available from: IT Publications. See Appendix E.
4. *Basic Accounting for Small Groups*, J. Cammack, Oxfam, 2nd edn, 2003.
    A very useful step-by-step guide to accounting and bookkeeping.
    Available from: Oxfam. See Appendix E.
5. *Management Support for Primary Health Care*, P. Johnstone and J. Ranken, FSG Communications and ODA (DFID), 1994.
    A helpful book covering details of team building, leadership and management of personnel, supplies and finance.
    Available from: TALC. See Appendix E.
6. *Refugee Health*, Médecins sans Frontières, Mavmillan, 1997.
    This covers all aspects of managing health services in refugee camps.
    Available from: TALC. See Appendix E.
7. *Guidance note: Project budgeting and accounting*, J. Cammack, BOND, 2003.
    Valuable information in this booklet.
8. People in Aid is a UK-based organisation that promotes best practice in the management and support of aid personnel. A Code of Best Practice, which helps to promote the well-being of those involved in relief and development programmes for all nationalities, is available from People in Aid, Development House, 56–64 Leonard Street, London EC2A 4JX, UK. Email: info@peopleinaid.org. This is highly recommended.

Websites

BOND is a network of development agencies, which has valuable resources. Website: www.bond.org.uk/pubs.

People in Aid, mentioned above: www.peopleinaid.org.

Mango (Management Accounting for NGOs) provides excellent material, which can be obtained from Mango, 97a St Aldate's, Oxford, OX1 1BT, UK or from www.mango.org.uk.

See Further references and guidelines, page 417.

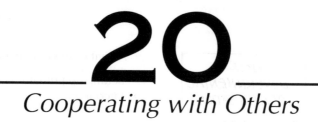

20

Cooperating with Others

In this chapter we shall consider working with the following groups:
1. Government
2. Aid and funding agencies
3. Other voluntary agencies
4. The private sector
5. Doctors and private practitioners
6. Traditional health practitioners
7. Hospitals

Working with government

This section is designed to help organisations that are not officially part of government to work effectively and in a cooperative spirit with government departments.

What is 'government'?

As far as health projects are concerned 'government' includes:

1. **The Health Services or Health Ministry.** These are usually set up on the following levels:
   - Central level: responsible for nationwide health policy and planning.
   - State, provincial or regional level: responsible for adapting and carrying out national health policy according to the needs of the area.
   - District level: responsible through the District Medical Officer (DMO) for organising and carrying out all aspects of health care in the district. The District is seen increasingly as the key component of the health service – large enough to manage health care and small enough to guide and support services at local level. Many countries, e.g. Uganda, also have subdistricts, sometimes called counties, with subdistrict

or deputy medical officers. Often mission hospitals run the services in health subdistricts.
   - Local level: this includes the primary health centre, subcentre, health post or dispensary (the terms used vary from country to country). Health committees and a cadre of community health workers, attached either to government or to NGO, may be linked in.
2. **Other ministries or departments** that have an influence on health such as agriculture, forestry and environment; energy and renewable resources; human resources; education; urban or rural development; water.
   (See also Chapter 8, pages 138–9.)

Who carries out health care more effectively – government or NGO?

Government and Non-Governmental Organisations (NGOs) each have their particular strengths.

Activities often done best by government include:

- Planning health services.
- Funding nationwide health care (though other sources are increasingly necessary).
- Establishing secondary and tertiary health care – district and regional hospitals.
- Being largely responsible for training doctors, nurses and other senior health professionals.
- Co-coordinating nationwide programmes such as Stop TB, Roll Back Malaria, the Integrated Management of Childhood Illness.
- Regulating the activities of other health care providers, both individuals and organisations

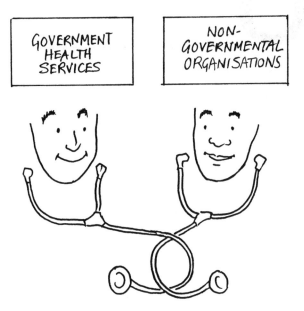

Figure 20.1   An essential partnership to bring health services to the world's poor.

Activities often done best by NGOs include:

- Setting up primary health care.
- Encouraging the participation of the community.
- Training, teaching and motivating health workers and communities.
- Meeting local needs with programmes that are flexible and appropriate.
- Using money, people and resources effectively.
- Working in remote or difficult areas, or with neglected, backward or nomadic groups.
- Integrating primary health care and development activities at local level.
- Establishing urban health care. Working among the urban poor will become an increasing focus for NGOs.

These are tasks that spring from the strengths of the NGO – enthusiasm, flexibility, community involvement and manageable size.

- Replicating or scaling up nationwide methods and ideas often pioneered by NGOs at local or district level.

These are all tasks that require both high expenditure and nationwide planning to be effective.

How can government and NGO work together?

Working relationships between government and NGO usually follow one of these three models:

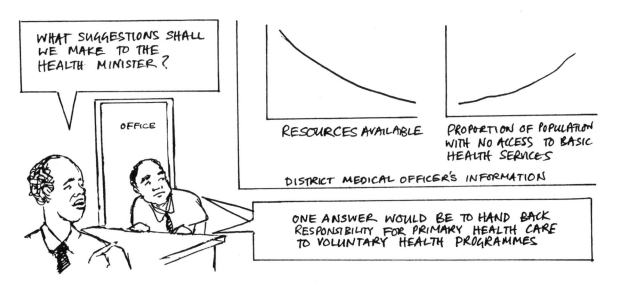

Figure 20.2

1. **NGO and government set up a joint programme.**
   The NGO works closely with the government, and carries out a specific programme or task that government services are not providing.
   For example (1): In parts of Nepal the government concentrates on providing curative services at local level leaving the NGO to train community health workers.
   For example (2): In China, international NGOs are partnering with government health services in many poor or remote communities. Programmes are discussed with each level of the health service. Often the main tasks carried out by the NGO include training village doctors, township or county hospital staff, and helping to improve health care at village level.
   There can be drawbacks in this approach – it may be hard to define who does what and which organisation is responsible for which part of the project. Much time is taken in planning and meeting. The NGO may be restricted and unable to make best use of its enthusiasm and flexibility.

2. **NGO sets up a programme on its own terms.**
   Here the NGO is free to make use of its own resources. However, it must still liaise with and be accountable to government plans, and integrate into national programmes, such as immunisation and TB control. It can respond to the needs of the local people, work in cooperation with them and remain unhindered by bureaucracy.
   If the programme proves to be effective, the government may either help to fund it, learn from it or copy it, using its approach in other areas of the country.
   For example: The Lardin Gabas project in Nigeria made effective use of storytelling for health education. The government adopted its ideas and methods in other areas.

3. **Government delegates or contracts out primary (and sometimes) secondary health care to the NGO for local or district-wide implementation.**
   This is an exciting opportunity for voluntary programmes.
   For example (1): In large areas of the Democratic Republic of Congo many hospital beds are now provided by church-related institutions.
   For example (2): The large-scale ASHA programme working amongst the rural poor of Delhi is responsible under the government for

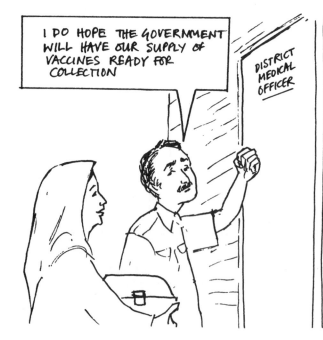

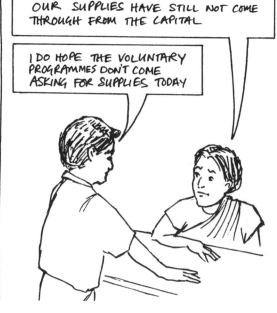

Figure 20.3

providing CHW training, urban health clinics and a variety of other development activities.

For example (3): in Cambodia, health care in several provinces has been contracted out to non-governmental providers. According to some key indicators these have generally proved more cost effective and achieved better results than programmes run by the government.

We are likely to see more health services being provided by civil society organisations in the future.

Practical guidelines for working with government
Build personal relationships

The most strategic person is usually the District Medical Officer, the DMO's equivalent, deputy or any officer with responsibility for liaising with NGOs or with special programmes with which we are involved.

> District medical staff are being transferred continually. We need to keep on friendly working terms with all those we deal with regularly, ranging from the DMO to the junior staff who sign out vaccines or provide supplies.

We can make strategic use of any school, community and family links between health team members and government officials.

Discuss plans for our programme

We should do this with the most senior appropriate government officer. This may be at state, region or district level. If one person is found to be uncooperative, we should try someone else.

When first starting a programme, we may need advice and ideas from the DMO, both about the area in which we should work and the type of project we should carry out.

As the programme develops, we should inform the DMO of any important change of plans or expansion into new areas.

If we have been planning with a government officer other than the DMO we should make sure that the DMO also knows about our plans.

We are likely to be involved in one or more national programmes coordinated by the government, such as Stop TB or Making Pregnancy Safer. In all these situations we will need close and ongoing links with the government and to follow its own adaptations and the recording systems of global control programmes.

It is worth remembering that, in many areas hit by serious poverty, natural disasters or civil conflict, there will be a breakdown in government health care. In each situation we will need to be as well informed as possible, and balance our commitment to the poor with the requests or restraints from government.

Send regular reports, returns and information

We should send in any statistics or reports asked for by the government. This will include immunisation figures for the EPI (page 192) reporting on TB control (page 278), aspects of the Integrated Management of Childhood Illness (IMCI) (Chapter 11) or any other activity that is part of a national health strategy. If our returns are regular, accurate and show good coverage, this will help our standing with the government.

Define areas of responsibility

In joint programmes with government we must ensure that the exact responsibilities of both NGO and government are clearly defined.

> If the government has given us responsibility for part of the programme, we should make sure that it also gives us the authority to carry it out.

Help that may be obtained from the government
Drugs and supplies

The government often provides free or subsidised supplies. These may include TB drugs, antiretroviral therapy for use in HIV/AIDS, family planning

REPORT FORM

Monthly report for ....
(month)

Weighing group (hamlet) ....   Village ....   District ....

Date of weighing ....   Field Worker ....   Number of kaders helping ....

Total hamlet population .... in .... families

1. Total children under 36 months old   ....

2. Total children with weight charts   ....

3. Total newly entered this month   ....

4. Total with increased weight this month   ....

5. Total with no increase in weight   ....

6. Total weighed with last month weight unknown
   (therefore, do not know if weight increased)   ....

7. Total weighed this month   ....

Participation score   = # 2/1
Activity score   = #7/2
Growth score   =#4/(7 − (3 + 6))
Overall score   = # 4/1

Use of supplies this month:
  Weight charts   ....
  Oralyte packets   ....
  Vitamin A high-dose capsules   ....
  Iron folate tablets   ....

Figure 20.4   A report form used in Indonesia for sending monthly statistics to the government.

supplies, Vitamin A, iron and folic acid, midwifery kits and materials for water and sanitation programmes.

EPI vaccines can usually be obtained via the DMO or District Hospital.

We should use government supplies whenever possible, but remember that they may be undependable (we will always need alternative sources), and there may be excessive paperwork (we may need to employ an extra staff member to deal with this).

Financial grants

These may be available, usually for a specific purpose. However, they may be late or never arrive (meaning we should not be dependent on them) and they may have strict conditions (such as defining exactly how the funds should be used).

If possible, we should obtain grants for general purposes, not specific ones, so that the programme can decide on the most appropriate way of using the money, according to the real needs of the community. Some countries are so poor that no funds may be available at all.

Working with aid and funding agencies (see pages 61–6)

Questions asked by projects

From time to time we may wonder:
- Why are the agency's forms so long and complex?

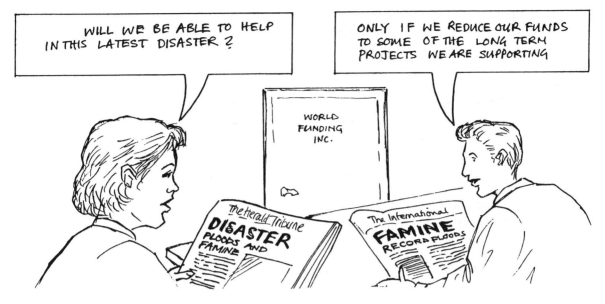

Figure 20.5   Funding agencies themselves can be under great pressure.

- Why does it take so long for funds to reach us?
- Why does the agency send representatives to question us and take photographs? Why instead don't they send experts to give us ideas and information?

It helps to answer these questions if we understand the problems faced by many funding agencies.

Problems faced by agencies

Funding agencies themselves are often under great pressure. We should remember that:

1. **The agency is dependent on its own supporters**, who in turn will expect reassurance that their money is being well spent, and request information including stories and photographs. The more of these that supporters receive, the more money they will give to the agency.
2. **The agency may have insufficient funds**, because so many projects are making requests, often because a major disaster has just occurred, or because famine relief takes priority.
3. **There are problems in communication** because forms may be incomplete or wrongly filled in, and postal delays prevent letters or financial support from arriving. Sometimes unreliable electricity supplies and phone connections make email contact difficult.

Ways in which projects can help

- By sending reports and budgets on time and accurately completed. If projects don't do this they will soon lose the confidence of donors even if they are doing a very good job.
- By keeping costs as low as possible.
- By replying promptly to letters.
- By informing the agency of any major changes of plan.
- By welcoming visitors from the agency.
- By using email and fax.

If two or more agencies are supporting a project, then the area of support and contribution of each should be carefully defined and recorded.

Finally, we should remember that most agencies will want to work in partnership with us. Its members are genuinely interested in what we are doing, and many who visit us will themselves be experts who have previously worked in similar programmes.

Avoid being donor driven

Increasingly, funding is available for clearly defined projects and capital costs, but not usually for running costs. Sometimes, if we participate in vertical programmes such as Stop TB or RBM, some of our running costs will be paid for. But, in practice, the funds our programmes need most are to set up strong community based structures, pay salaries and strengthen local health systems so that a wide variety of needs can be met effectively.

Unless we are aware of these issues and have worked out both needs and goals with the community, we are in danger of being either donor driven or, when it comes to requesting government funding, 'donor battered'. At its worst this can undermine our programme, as we desperately chase funds to carry out the latest programme in the hope that our project will survive and sufficient funding will be included to pay our health workers. This is a dangerous and unsatisfactory situation that all stakeholders, projects, governments and donors need to resist.

For example: A successful programme in south Asia worked out an integrated health programme in three impoverished districts with the local community. They prioritised needs, trained and empowered health workers and made a useful impact in their project area. After some years their main donor changed policy and no longer supported projects in that area. The project had become dependent on a single donor and was only able to continue by bidding for government money for specific programmes, some of which were of doubtful value in the areas where they were working. This project became so donor-battered it had to consider closure.

This should serve as a warning to all of us involved in Community Based Health Care (CBHC) to aim for sustainability and a diverse way of funding our programmes.

Understand partnership and capacity building

Those who provide funds, both foreign governments (bilateral aid), and the best voluntary aid agencies, are increasingly guided by these two principles.

Partnership refers to an agency and its field partner sharing aims and objectives, finding means for mutual benefit and learning from each other. An 'us together' approach replaces a 'we and them' attitude. Partnership needs to be learnt by both sides. It involves regular contact, the building of trust, a direct, open approach and a long-term commitment. Everyone benefits, not least the communities we are serving.

Capacity building (CB) is a form of empowerment: the supporting agency helps to build the field partner's knowledge, capability, and administrative systems. This in turn enables the field partner to become increasingly self-sufficient and non dependent. CB includes training (especially in management skills), providing resources and linking regional partners together for mutual support. It also means empowering the field partner to support other local groups with similar aims.

If we are looking for an outside donor we should ask about their attitude to partnership and capacity building.

Working with other voluntary agencies

We should aim to work as closely as possible with other voluntary programmes present in the target area. These will include development projects who may be tackling the root cause of ill health, through forestry, agriculture, literacy and education.

Although we should always work in cooperation, not competition, we must carefully assess any programme with which we develop special links. We will usually link up with programmes that have followed a community empowerment model.

If the programme seems inappropriate we should be slow to develop formal links.

For example: A new group moves in that has plenty of money but little understanding of development. It gives free handouts and distributes bottles of tonic and vitamins. The people flock to its centre not realising that such a group may have a secret motive, or be 'here today, gone tomorrow'.

If, however, the programme seems appropriate we can:

1. **Cooperate together**. *For example*: By visiting each other's projects, training each other's staff, sharing expensive items of equipment, setting up a combined system for ordering and supplying drugs, sharing leisure activities.

2. **Define project areas**:

> If there is genuine overlap between projects, either in terms of the ground area we are covering or the activities we are carrying out, it will be necessary to define clearly where each project should work and what each project should do.

3. **Join any voluntary health organisation** that encourages local programmes to work together and share activities.

4. **Become a member of a national or international network**, which will enable us to learn, share information and work together. *For*

example: Community Health Global Network is a new global organisation aiming to link together, train and empower community based programmes worldwide (See Appendix E).

Working with the private sector

It is worth considering these three interrelated facts.

1. An increasing amount of wealth is owned by the private sector, both by successful national companies and by multinational corporations.

2. The financial needs of health and development programmes are growing rapidly.

3. The governments of many developing countries are seriously short of money, meaning they struggle to finance health care.

This makes a link between the wealthy private sector and the needy development sector an obvious one to establish. This is one type of

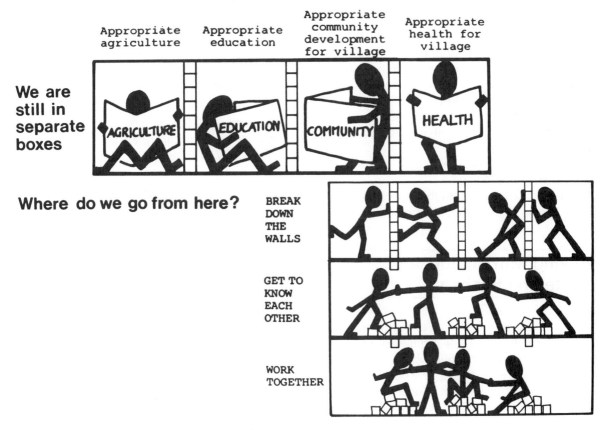

Figure 20.6

Public-Private Partnership. For any link to be successful we need to follow some basic principles:

- Define clearly the needs of the programme in terms of funding, resources, drug supply and other inputs.
- Understand clearly what any company is willing to provide, whether money, supplies or services.
- Work out a way in which both programme and company can benefit from the partnership.
- Ensure that the company does not drive or set the health programme's agenda, either through persuasion, aggressive advertising or illegal incentives.
- Make no links with any company that has unethical policies or products. Obvious examples include tobacco or weapons, unregulated baby milk substitutes or anything that pollutes or damages the environment.
- Set up a careful agreement for a limited period and then review it.

Here are some examples of alliances or PPPs to consider:
- A pharmaceutical company that donates or subsidises an essential drug needed on a wide scale. This could include antimalarials, deworming treatment, TB drugs, antiretroviral drugs for the treatment of HIV/AIDS, or insecticide for impregnating mosquito nets.
- A locally-based company that might sponsor a training programme.
- A bank that might help to set up a cooperative or revolving drug fund.
- Businesses sympathetic to the programme and able to give regular or one-off grants.

Working with doctors and private practitioners

This section refers to trained doctors (those working in government service) and to private practitioners. It does not primarily refer to Traditional Health Practitioners who, despite an overlap, are considered separately below.

Doctors and private practitioners include a wide range of health care providers with varying types of qualification and approach. They are used by an increasing number of patients, including the very poor. In some areas, most patients when they first become ill seek out a private practitioner or Traditional Health Practitioner. (See below and see also pages 8–9.)

There is often no very clear dividing line between public and private sectors as many government doctors also have private practices

Characteristics of doctors

Doctors often tend to show certain characteristics, though there are many exceptions:

1. Much interest in cure, in hospitals, in high-tech equipment, interesting cases, money and status.
2. Little interest in primary or community health – which they often consider to be dull or beneath their status.
3. Some interest in the health programme, either out of social concern, out of fear that successful health prevention will reduce their patient numbers or in hope that serious cases will be referred to them.
4. Many doctors, especially if hospital based, tend to be reactive to situations, e.g. in curing an illness rather than proactive, e.g. in trying to prevent illness.

In other words most doctors, unless converted to a community health approach, are more interested in medical care than in health care (see pages 326–7).

How to work with doctors and private practitioners

We will usually have to follow two different aims that are often in conflict: to protect community members from inappropriate medical care, especially from an approach that leads to dependence; to cooperate with doctors and private practitioners as far as we are able.

We can follow these guidelines:

1. **Build personal relationships.**
2. **Explain who we are and what we are doing**, making clear that our main aim is not primarily to treat patients but to improve the health of the community.

3. **Never publicly criticise** or speak out against other doctors or their practices.

> Even if we strongly disapprove of the way a colleague is treating a patient, we should be slow to criticise either in public or to one of the doctor's patients. If the case is serious we should see the practitioner ourselves.

4. **Provide health education to local doctors and private practitioners.**

   For example: Most private practitioners have little chance for continuing medical education. From the day they qualify, most will receive information largely from the representatives of pharmaceutical companies, biased towards promoting their products. We can, therefore, invite practitioners to our staff training days, run local health courses or seminars, loan health books or journals and allow them access to the project library.

5. **Include practitioners in our health programme.**

The doctor's role in Community Health Programmes (CHPs)

Qualified doctors can have the following roles and senior nurses can have similar roles:

Clinical medical officer

The doctor can see patients referred by other health workers. These may include the very ill or chronically sick, e.g. those with TB or AIDS, cases that are difficult to diagnose or require emergency treatment or surgery.

> In Community Based Health Care doctors should train other members of the health team to care for patients, seeing only those with serious illnesses or referred by other health workers.

Teacher

The doctor's aim should be to pass on relevant skills and knowledge so that other health workers quickly learn to diagnose and treat common and important diseases.

Planner and strategist

Doctors have an important function in identifying health priorities, the best ways of achieving them and helping to draw up plans and strategies. But they should do this alongside the community, who themselves will help to identify problems and solutions. It is easy for programmes to become 'doctor-driven' unless any medic in a leadership role fully understands the CBHC approach.

A liaison role

Doctors are usually best placed to liaise with government officials, medical officers and programme directors of other health care projects. This is especially important when we are involved with national programmes such as EPI or IMCI.

Supervisor

Doctors should supervise the clinical care of patients, including their diagnosis, treatment and rehabilitation.

Compiler of an essential drug list

Because a doctor's training emphasises curing illness and using medicines, any list of essential

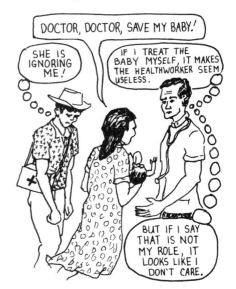

Figure 20.7

drugs a doctor draws up will need to be discussed with others. *For example*: A nurse experienced in CBHC or a medical assistant can advise whether the list is too long; the director or finance officer about whether it is too expensive. (See Chapter 17, page 330 for details.)

Adviser

Doctors can advise on all health-related topics, including clinical care, the use of medicines, immunisation schedules, clean water, latrines, and the setting up of clinics and programmes for mothers and children.

Director

In practice, doctors are often the directors of community health programmes (CHPs), but there are two good reasons why leadership should be either shared or handed over to others:

1. Doctors usually understand CBHC only if they have been strongly exposed to primary health care models or have been 'converted' to CBHC from a hospital based approach. Nurses, on the other hand, often make appropriate CHP leaders, provided that doctors can take on strategic and advisory roles to support them. In practice doctors are often unwilling to work under the leadership of a nurse, especially in areas of the world (e.g. much of Africa and South Asia) where nurses, wrongly, often have much lower social status.
2. Doctors often make poor managers. If doctors direct programmes, they should employ those with management and financial skills as soon as possible, or gain training themselves.

Working with traditional health practitioners (THPs)

What are THPs?

Most patients in the poorest parts of the world, and especially in rural areas, still first seek advice from THPs, often simply known as Traditional Practitioners. Eighty per cent of Africans make use of THPs. In areas with better health services,

increasing numbers of patients first consult scientifically trained (allopathic) health workers. Where health services are declining or becoming too expensive, people are returning to THPs for their main source of health care.

THPs include a huge range of people. Some are following long-established, traditional, medical systems. Examples of these include Ayurvedic, Unani and Siddha practitioners in south Asia, practitioners of traditional Chinese medicine in China and surrounding countries of south-east Asia, and Inyangas (herbalists) in South Africa. What nearly all have in common is a deep understanding and strong connection with the communities they serve, and to which they usually belong. Although many remedies they use are unproven and a few are dangerous, nearly one quarter of all modern medicines used today is derived from traditional medicines. This includes artemesinin, now the most effective treatment for malaria, which has been used for centuries in China and is extracted from the plant *Artemisia annua*.

Most countries have networks of THPs, ranging from those who are ethical, established and registered, to those with little or no training or who use dubious or dangerous practices.

For example: The Republic of South Africa is estimated to have 20 000 THPs and an estimated 80 per cent of the black population uses them. Recently a law has been passed to regulate these THPs, which it is hoped will have two main benefits. First, it gives THPs recognition and second, it seeks to uphold good practice. One part of this law prohibits unregistered THPs from claiming they can relieve or cure HIV/AIDS.

WHO is encouraging the greater regulation, use and integration of THPs into national health services.

In addition to THPs most countries have Traditional Birth Attendants (see pages 238–41), who may sometimes have other healing roles.

The varied knowledge and practices of Traditional Health Practitioners mean that we can never have one universal way of working with them. We must develop a model likely to be effective in our own situation.

Guidelines for working with THPs

1. **Gather information about THPs working in the project area.**
   Do they follow any particular systems? What sorts of treatment do they use? Which members of the community consult them? What types of ailment do they treat? How much do they charge? Are they paid in money or in kind? Do people perceive that their treatments are effective? Are they respected by the local people? Do they use any dangerous or harmful practices? What is their attitude to allopathic medicine?

2. **Devise a model for working with THPs.**
   Once we have answered these questions we can decide how to work with THPs. We should remember that, however we do this, many patients will continue to visit them.
   In practice we will probably work with some types of THP, but may decide that others use approaches or have belief systems that would conflict with the programme. We are probably most likely to select either TBAs, or established practitioners of other traditional systems. For any group of THPs we have three options:

   - To incorporate THPs into our health programme. This will work only if we develop a strong degree of personal trust, if THPs share a broadly similar value system, and if they are prepared to work in close partnership with us.
   - To cooperate with THPs in certain areas of health care. In this model THPs will continue with many of their traditional activities but, through the training we offer, help to promote better health practices in the community.
     For example: In Malawi, THPs within the Queen Elizabeth Hospital catchment area in Blantyre were successfully given briefing sessions on the symptoms of TB, and provided with referral slips so they could refer on patients with chronic cough for sputum testing.
   - To decide against any formal links with THPs.

   Before developing a permanent programme we should run a small scale pilot scheme first.

3. **Set up THP training.**
   Having chosen which THPs to work with and what model to follow, we then need to design training programmes. We have already considered TBA training.
   Our training must be based on trust, a sharing of information, establishing common areas of understanding, correcting harmful beliefs and affirming helpful ones. THPs probably learn best through apprenticeship, and by observation and discussion, rather than formal training. This is especially the case for those who are illiterate or who follow no clearly defined systems.

4. **Ways in which THPs are able to benefit CBHC.**
   Apart from the use of TBAs, many programmes have failed to make the best use of THPs. Where they have been involved in health programmes their contributions have often been valuable. Here are some examples of tasks they can do:

   - Working as CHWs or alongside them.
   - Motivating community members to improve their hygiene and nutrition practices.
   - Becoming advocates for improved sanitation, including the building of latrines.
   - Promoting breastfeeding and the use of ORS.
   - Working alongside TBAs in the care of pregnant women and the newborn.
   - Working as observers in TB DOTS programmes.
   - Cooperating with the project in the prevention and treatment of STIs and AIDS.

5. **Monitor programmes involving THPs.**
   We will need to monitor:

   - The occurrence of any harmful or dangerous practice.
   - The actual or perceived benefit felt by the project, the THP and the community.
   - Ways for wider involvement after a pilot programme.

Working with hospitals

Some community health programmes (CHPs) are attached to a base hospital, others are indepen-

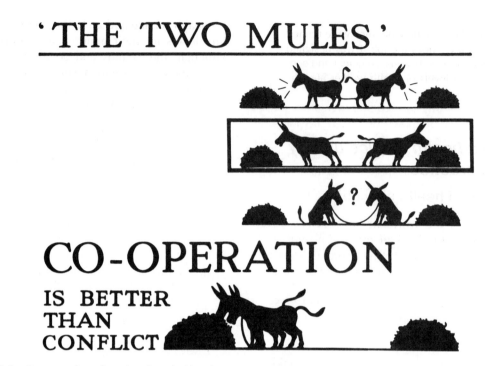

Figure 20.8   Everyone benefits when hospitals and primary health programmes work together.

dent. Whichever arrangement is used, one principle is essential: hospitals and community health programmes (CHPs) must work in partnership.

Hospitals ideally provide a whole range of backup services for the primary health care level.

The way a health service should work

There are usually three levels in a clinical health system. Sometimes a level may be divided into subdivisions and the levels may have different names depending on the country. (See also pages 138–9.)

1. **Primary level.**
   This includes:
   - CHWs working in the community.
   - Health posts, subcentres, primary health centres and their staff to whom CHWs refer patients. Primary health centres usually have a few beds and can carry out uncomplicated deliveries.
2. **Secondary level.**
   This is the district first referral or 'base' hospital, which gives backing to the primary level, and takes referrals from it. It has inpatient beds, can perform routine surgery and carries out a range of investigations.
3. **Tertiary level.**
   This is the large well equipped regional hospital able to do major surgery, complex investigations and offering a range of specialist care. It takes referrals from the secondary level.

When this system works correctly (see Figure 20.9) it is good for patients, health workers and the economy.

It is good for *patients* because they usually receive care at the primary level that is near their home and convenient, so saving them time, money and worry.

It is good for *health workers* because they see patients appropriate to their level of training and receive job satisfaction, neither being swamped by problems that are too easy, nor being frightened by problems that are too difficult.

It is good for the *economy* because highly trained, highly paid doctors or nurses don't spend their time seeing patients with less serious illnesses who could be seen just as well, and at much less cost, by health workers at the level below.

As health workers do the work they were trained for and each level does the job it was designed for, the health service becomes efficient and economical and all levels of health worker become more satisfied.

The way a health service usually works in practice

Breakdown of health services

In many parts of the world health services are severely short of funds. Staff may be absent or demoralised. Equipment may have broken down and drug supplies may have run out. Some levels of the health system may have ceased to function. CBHC has to work within whatever structure is available, drawing support where it can but being self-sufficient when compelled to be.

Non-existent referral systems

Partly because of poor quality health services, many people try to bypass the primary levels of the health service and go to the secondary or tertiary levels for their minor health problems. In particular, the wealthy and powerful like seeing smart doctors in smart hospitals even for their headaches and itchy bottoms.

This has unfortunate results:

1. The rich get overtreated, demanding more expensive drugs and treatments, so setting up an inappropriate pattern, which others start to follow.
2. The poor get undertreated or not treated at all as there is little time left for serious problems referred from the level below. The supply of essential drugs may have run out.
3. Health workers are unfulfilled: doctors spend time seeing patients with minor problems, and so get bored; CHWs and middle level workers are bypassed except by the very poor, and so become discouraged.
4. The referral system breaks down.
5. Costs increase as more hospitals are built.
6. Almost anyone is prepared to see a private practitioner if sufficiently desperate and unable to face the often frightening and unfriendly world of hospitals.

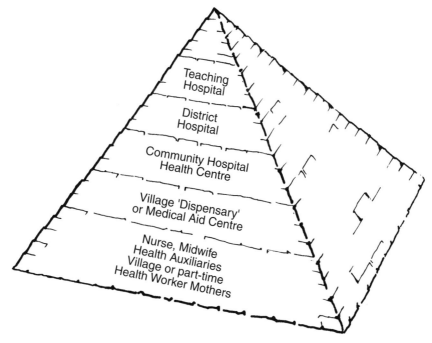

Figure 20.9   The Health Pyramid: Patients should normally enter at the lowest level and only move upwards by referral.

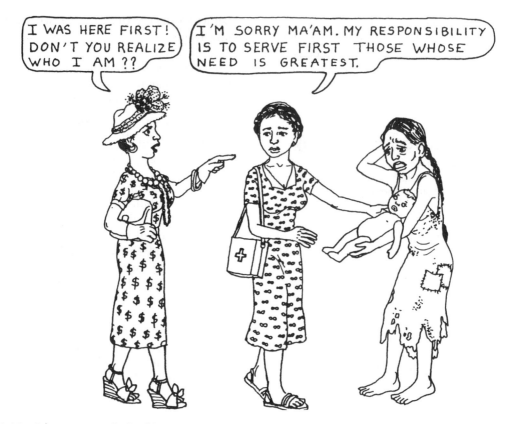

Figure 20.10 A key question for health care in the twenty-first century: 'Will this health worker give in to the demands of the rich or respond to the needs of the poor?'

The correct roles of the base hospital

Acting as a referral centre

Most patients will be referred in from the primary health centre or its equivalent. Seriously ill patients in the community may be referred direct by CHWs bypassing the primary health centre. A few patients will be self-referred. (See page 379.)

Patients requiring referral to hospital will include emergencies; those needing surgery, Caesarean section or assisted delivery; any needing more complex investigations (either as outpatients or inpatients).

In acting as a referral centre the hospital will have three important tasks:

1. **It will receive patients**, trying where possible to admit any patient referred, especially if from a long distance.

2. **It will care for patients** in the ward, where staff will need to be taught to show kindness and special care for the poorest, the most uninformed and the most sick. Often in practice staff respect the rich and push the poor aside.

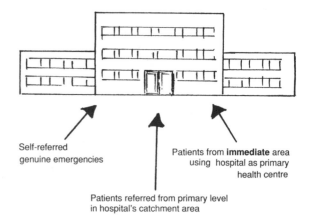

Figure 20.11 The correct use of a referral hospital.

3. **It will discharge patients** back to the community, first contacting the primary health centre team to arrange a suitable time, and means of transport. A doctor or nurse will write a discharge summary.

> The time immediately after discharge is often difficult for patients. They may not know who should be looking after them, when they should be seen again or what treatment they should be taking. To avoid these problems, base hospitals and the CHP team must communicate and follow agreed procedures.

Whenever patients are admitted to a ward or seen as outpatients, they should be offered 'primary health activities' such as health education, immunisation, family planning or other appropriate services. Any procedures given should be written on the patient's self-retained record card.

Acting as a teaching centre

In some programmes, teaching of the health team, including the CHWs, is done in the hospital – in others it is done mainly in the community with occasional visits to the hospital.

Backing up with supplies and equipment

The hospital may be the simplest place to obtain medicines, vaccines and equipment. It may arrange to sterilise instruments and needles. It may have more expensive items that community health programmes can borrow or use, such as teaching aids, projectors or vehicles.

Backing up with management

The hospital may do the CHP's accounting, prepare statistics or help produce the annual report. It may have salary structures and management systems that can be adapted. It may have a fax machine and computer with email facilities and access to the internet.

Backing up by giving the same health message

Hospitals should be using simple drugs and an Essential Drugs List. They should be giving the same basic health teaching.

> Patients will usually pay more attention to what the hospital says than to what the primary health team says. It is important therefore that both give the same message and that the hospital supports the teaching of the primary health workers.

Hospitals are also in a good position to fight those who promote illicit liquor and drugs, smoking and artificial baby foods.

Base hospitals should sign up to the WHO's Baby-friendly and Mother-friendly hospital initiatives and set up systems for implementing and monitoring these. Breastfeeding should be promoted and no artificial baby milk be advertised, unless this is part of an integrated programme to help prevent the mother-to-child transmission of HIV/AIDS.

Backing up by discouraging self-referrals

The role of the hospital is to treat serious cases referred from the primary level, not to act as a primary health centre for anyone who walks in. The hospital should discourage patients from attending unless they have a referral letter, are a genuine emergency or come from the hospital 'core area' (see below and Figure 20.11).

One way of doing this is to charge non-emergency self-referred patients double rates or agree to see them only if they have first seen a member of the community health team and brought a letter with them.

Providing a 'core' primary health programme

People who live in communities very near the hospital, especially the poor, can use the hospital as their primary health centre.

The hospital can set up a programme or section of the hospital, with appropriate staff, for those in the core area. They can carry out community health activities just as would be done by a regular CHP. CHWs can be selected and trained, immunisations and mother and child care set up. Those needing to be seen in a clinic can be referred direct to the main hospital by the CHW.

How hospitals and community health projects relate to each other

Models

There are several different models of how hospital and CHP can relate. Here are some common ones:

A. Community health programme under hospital management

This is the traditional plan. The hospital has been set up in the past and now for various reasons decides to start a community health programme. This may be because the funding agency has asked for it or because of genuine interest among health workers or because of a request from the community.

B. Community health programme separate from hospital

1. No fixed hospital for referral.
   Here the CHP is truly on its own and dependent on its own resources, planning and expertise. Patients needing referral will be sent to different practitioners, clinics or hospitals, with whom arrangements are made. Many urban projects follow this model.
2. Fixed hospital(s) for referral.
   The programme remains detached but builds up special contacts with one or two hospitals that act as referral centres. This pattern has much to commend it and if well set up enables a project to be self-dependent, while still retaining use of a base hospital for referral.

C. Community health programme served and supported by base hospital

This radical pattern, though rarely followed, is probably the best. The hospital is actually part of

the community health programme and has been set up with the chief aim of providing referral and support services. Staff move freely between hospital and community; patients feel welcomed in the hospital and are treated with understanding. An excellent example of this approach is provided by the Comprehensive Rural Health Programme in Jamkhed, west India (see Further reading below). In practice some rural hospitals both in the past and in the present have started with this vision but it has gradually been lost as the demand for curative services becomes so overwhelming.

Problems in practice

The following problems tend to be worse when CHPs are managed by hospitals. They tend to be least when a CHP sets up its own hospital as a referral base.

1. Poor cooperation – misunderstandings or even rivalry between the hospital and CHP may be very longstanding.
2. Poor care for the poor patient – hospital staff prefer looking after the rich who can pay rather than the slum-dweller or poor villager who 'can't pay and can't understand'.
3. Priority to the hospital – the hospital is seen as the most important service, the community health project as an extra. When shortages of money or staff develop, the CHP suffers.
   The hospital may have started a CHP because this was the only way it could attract extra funding.

Practical solutions

The secret of a successful partnership is the development of a friendly working relationship between the primary level and the secondary level, between the CHP and the base hospital. We should set this as a definite aim of our programme.

There are several keys to good CHP–hospital relations and one leads from the other:

1. Mutual understanding of each other's role. CHP members need to spend time working in the hospital, understanding how it works and

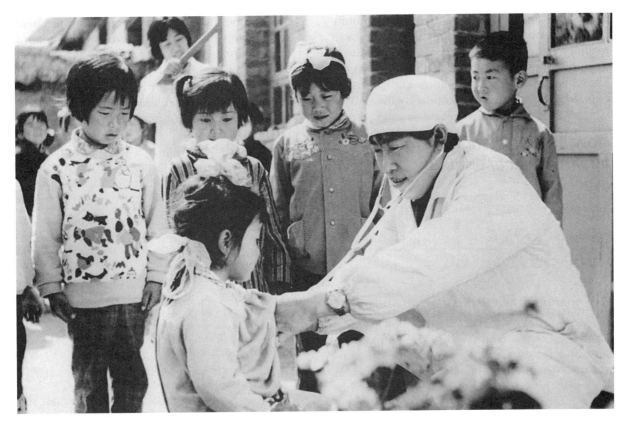

Figure 20.12   Close links between hospital doctors and primary health services in China benefit all members of the community.

getting to know its staff. Hospital staff need to spend time in the community, understanding the way of life of its members and sharing in their problems and solutions.

2. Mutual respect.

   As each branch of the health team understands the other, so mutual respect grows, which in turn leads on to:

3. Mutual cooperation.

   Where everyone benefits, and through which the poor receive appropriate treatment.

This partnership between primary and secondary levels will not just happen if we hope for the best. Staff continually change and everyone is busy. One or two people with the respect of both hospital and CHP must encourage and manage this process.

Summary

Community health programmes work best when they cooperate, rather than compete, with other branches of the health service.

They need to learn to cooperate with government in a well defined partnership, each recognising the strengths and roles of the other.

They must cooperate with donor agencies, providing the necessary information without undue delay. They should work with other voluntary health or development programmes in the project area, provided that goals are similar.

They should be open for alliances with the private sector, provided there are strict safeguards. Community health programmes will use and relate to doctors in a variety of ways. They should consider carefully how to work in cooperation with any private practitioners or traditional health practitioners in the project area.

Finally, CHPs should integrate with other levels of the health service, including referral hospitals, so that each tier carries out the jobs for which it was designed. This causes increased job satisfaction to health workers, provides more effective services for patients and greatly reduces costs.

Underlying all cooperation is the building of friendship and trust between the health programme and colleagues in government, neighbouring programmes and hospitals.

Further reading

1. *District Health Care*, 2nd edn, R. Amonoo-Lartson, G. Ibrahim, H. Lovell and J. Rankin, Macmillan, 1996.
   A clear description of how District Health Services function.
   Available from: TALC. See Appendix E.

2. New WHO Guidelines to promote proper use of alternative medicines, 2004.
   The definitive guide on this subject.
   Available from WHO. See Appendix E.

3. *Medicinal Plants in The Republic of Korea*, WHO, 1998.
   Documents the 150 plants used in traditional Chinese medicine. This book helps understanding in how to respect and work with complementary forms of health care.
   Available from: WHO. See Appendix E.

4. *Jamkhed: A Comprehensive Rural Health Programme*, M. and R. Arole, Macmillan, 1994.
   An account of this inspirational programme as relevant now as when first written.

5. *Building the Capacity of Local Groups*, I. Carter, Tearfund, 2001.
   Full of down-to-earth practical advice on this important subject.
   Available from TALC. See Appendix E.
   Also see reading lists in other chapters that have an overlap with this, e.g. Chapters 4 (Funding) and 17 (Using Medicines Correctly).

See Further references and guidelines, page 417.

21

How to Make a Programme Sustainable

In this chapter we shall consider:

1. What we mean by sustainability
2. Some important background
3. Ways to reduce programme costs
4. Ways to increase programme resources
5. User fees and co-financing
6. Revolving drug funds
7. Health insurance schemes
8. Other methods of cost recovery

Central to all we discuss in this chapter is our priority to make sure that those who are the poorest and most vulnerable in the community are the main focus of our programme. We must take care that, even though we do everything possible to make our programme sustainable, we never turn away those who are in the greatest need (see reality check in Table 21.1 below).

What we mean by sustainability

As all of us in CBHC soon come to know, sustainability is one of the 'buzz words' we continually hear and talk about. Usually we think of sustainability in financial terms. We consider ways in which our project can be less dependent on outside supporters.

It is helpful to try to define more clearly what sustainability actually means. Here is one definition.

Sustainable projects are those whose internal and external methods of raising finance are likely to ensure their long-term survival.

This does not mean these projects are entirely self-sufficient, i.e. depending on their own resources alone. Rather it means they are self-reliant, i.e. are able to assume responsibility for their own futures. This will usually be through a varied mix of cost recovery from users, income generation and selective support from outside.

Understanding the difference between self-sufficiency and self-reliance is important. Few if any projects will manage to be entirely self-sufficient (free from any dependence on outside funding) especially in the poorest areas where

Table 21.1 *Any misfortune to a slum household may precipitate utter destitution*

To individuals	To communities
Serious or fatal accidents, on the road, in the house or at work Fire Flood Electrocution or electrical burns Tuberculosis AIDS Loss of job Imprisonment Drug addiction Demands from creditors	Demolition Fire Flood Civil disorder Severe weather

Source: *Urban Health and Development*, Macmillan, TALC and Tearfund 2001.

CBHC is of the greatest value. But all projects must work towards self-reliance, always making sure that the poorest community members and subgroups have priority.

However, we should not think of sustainability purely in financial terms, though most of the time we will be concentrating on financial aspects. From a holistic viewpoint there are other ways in which a project must be sustainable.

The first way is in terms of the environment. A project must not exploit, undermine or devalue the local environment and ecology. It must take care to maintain the quality of the land and to preserve the local flora and fauna. This is all the more important in areas such as tropical forests and mountain areas where environments are fragile and any ecological damage is hard to reverse. *For example*: Soil erosion in hill areas caused by deforestation or overgrazing in turn leads to floods and widespread devastation as is seen annually in Bangladesh. *Another example* comes from east Africa: On the Kenyan coast the Muhindi project aims to provide cooking fuel from cheap sustainable resources so as to reduce charcoal burning from indigenous trees. At the same time trees are being replanted by community members to reverse the destruction of past years.

The second way is in terms of the culture and ethical values of the population. A correct approach to CBHC must ensure that we tackle the root causes of poverty. We can do this in a variety of ways, such as promoting justice and equality in access to services for women and children, and working towards behavioural change, such as reducing the amount of family income spent on alcohol and cigarettes. But we must be careful to interfere as little as possible with the culture, ethnic distinctiveness and customs of the community.

The third way is in terms of the personal welfare of staff and community members employed by the project or working closely with them. We should ensure employment practices that protect people from overwork, exploitation, dangerous practices or prolonged separation from family members. We need to set up an ethical personnel policy.

The fourth way is in terms of the local community feeling connected with the programme, and

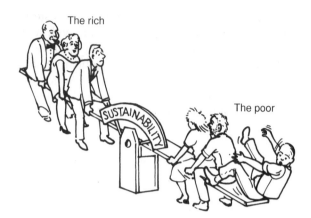

Figure 21.1   The greatest danger of sustainability: those needing care the most don't receive it.

demonstrating, through its continued use and interest, a long-term commitment. This will largely come about through the community's being involved in as wide a range of activities as early as possible including its involvement in helping to shape the programme. This will help people to feel the programme belongs to them and has not been planted from outside. 'Community ownership' may be the single most important factor in terms of long-term sustainability

Some important background

Before looking at practical ways to help our programmes become sustainable, it is useful to understand some background to health and development in the recent past.

Since the 1978 Alma-Ata Declaration, (see page 3) primary health care was originally given greater priority by many governments and the number of health programmes set up by NGOs increased dramatically. In the 1970s there was a general belief that poverty could be tackled successfully and that donors would be able to help achieve this by supporting both government programmes and the growing number of NGOs. But by the mid-1980s severe economic hardship had already started to hit many countries, for a variety of reasons, including debt repayment to western donors and falling commodity prices. Governments in developing countries started to cut back on spending for health and social welfare.

These problems coincided with the western world electing right-wing governments with less sympathy for the plight of the poor. In the 1980s, the World Bank and International Monetary Fund introduced a series of measures called Structural Adjustment Programmes. It was thought that, if countries could strengthen their economies, then the poor would automatically be helped. Unfortunately a side effect of these policies was that countries spent less on basic services and subsidies. Rather than reducing poverty, they actually increased it, often widening the gap between the rich and the poor at the same time.

During the late 1980s and the early 1990s, many of these policies continued and the concepts of sustainability and cost recovery (i.e. patients paying towards the cost of their health services) became key slogans. In 1987 the Bamako Initiative was launched, which tried to combine the ideas of cost recovery with the genuine needs of the poor. This series of reforms originating out of a meeting in Bamako, the capital of Mali, introduced the idea of community financing to help pay for essential drug costs, often through the setting up of revolving drug funds. It was hoped that, as users paid for their medicines, sufficient funds would become available not only to pay for drugs but also to help improve health services in general.

Evidence since that time shows that several things have been occurring:

- Many cost recovery schemes, and in particular the charging of user fees, seriously reduce the number of poor people who use health services.
- It is difficult to raise a large percentage of costs through user fees; the general guidance to governments of just 15 per cent is quite an ambitious target.
- If fees are introduced into a previously free service, users really must see an improvement in the service they receive, otherwise they will feel resentful and stop using the service. We can help to overcome this by meeting with the community and helping people to understand the need for change.
- If the community realises that by charging fees it will receive more reliable medicines, people may use the health services more, but the poorest may be unable to afford what we provide – the very people we most want to serve.

All these factors have added to the difficulty of programmes trying to combine sustainability with a just and open-handed approach to the poor.

However, the fact remains that if programmes can prove to be sustainable they will survive, if they can't they will fold up. In order to attract start-up funding we will need to persuade donors that we have practical ideas about how we can make sure our programmes will last into the future. This in turn will force us to use a variety of methods to keep our costs as low as possible and to search out ways of increasing project income.

Ways to reduce programme costs

Sustainability consists of a mix and match of two different components: reducing costs and raising resources. This section looks at the first of these.

Programmes are more likely to survive if they keep their costs to a minimum and if they are run as efficiently as possible. Cost-cutting can save the equivalent of large annual donations. Here are some suggestions:

1. **Increase efficiency.**
   - Ensuring good time management and the best use of staff time and skills.
     Because salaries are usually the largest single cost, anything that increases productivity will improve sustainability. But we must ensure that efficiency is never at the expense of staff health and welfare, nor of the environment.
   - Cutting costs in all project areas.
     We need to carry out an audit of all project activities to see if costs are being kept as low as possible. This will include fuel and transport costs, and buying supplies at the lowest rates we can find, provided quality does not suffer. We need to reduce wastage in all areas of the project.
   - Recruiting staff with high motivation, appropriate training, and the willingness to take on tasks outside their main job description.

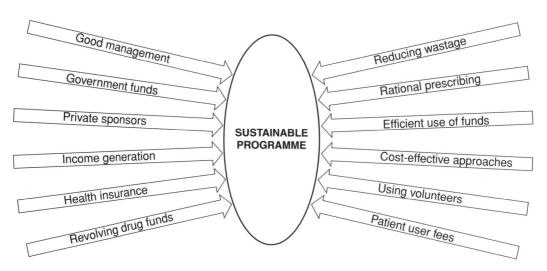

Figure 21.2   Twelve ways to help a project become sustainable.

- Considering limited-term contracts coupled with career development plans and ongoing training. This enables staff to see their time with the project as part of their career, not a job for life. Training empowers them to do the job better and improves motivation.
- Ensuring that staff are affirmed and motivated: that disputes are minimised and, if they occur, they are handled swiftly and appropriately (pages 352–4).

2. **Use an Essential Drugs List** (see pages 330–1). Huge amounts of money are wasted by overprescribing. We can reduce this by:

- Using only medicines on the EDL.
- Obtaining supplies from the least expensive good quality producer of generic drugs.
- Training all staff members who prescribe drugs to use the minimum necessary for effective care.
- Training all staff to use Disease Protocols or Standing Orders to treat common ailments, and banning expensive alternatives or unnecessary additions.
- Obtaining any free supplies to which we may be entitled. Depending on country and district these might include: TB drugs, anti-retrovirals for PLWHA, immunisations, Vitamin A, iron and folic acid supplements, any drugs donated free for mass distribution

for locally prevalent diseases, such as praziquantel for schistosomiasis, ivermectin for onchocerciasis (river blindness), azithromycin for trachoma. Sometimes, however, these sources suddenly cease to be available and this can leave us with a dilemma. We should not become overly dependent on any of them.

- Ensuring drugs are not wasted through poor storage and theft. Buy drugs with as long an expiry date as possible and use old stocks first.

One example: Kenya has set up an innovative programme to encourage essential drug use. Community pharmacies stocking 9–12 essential drugs have been opened and run by CHWs. Charges cover drug costs, and give a small profit for the CHWs. They also sell impregnated mosquito nets at subsidised prices.

3. **Concentrate on low cost approaches.** Curative care and the use of medicines is only one part of CBHC. A great deal can be done to raise health awareness and work towards behavioural change at very low cost. Here are some examples:

- Training community health workers.
- Raising health awareness in the community through meetings, focus groups, drama and puppet shows.

- Starting female literacy classes, ideally in the context of women's groups (see pages 31–34).
- Keeping transport costs as low as possible by using public transport or bicycle rather than motorbike or project vehicle.

4. **Do 'Planned Preventive Maintenance' (PPM).** This refers to planning ahead so we look after equipment before it permanently breaks down. It will involve us in auditing the needs we have, obtaining the funds and expertise needed for repair and maintenance, and setting aside time to make sure that repairs take place. Vehicles, office and clinical equipment will be priorities. PPM avoids crisis breakdowns, which can be more expensive to deal with, waste staff time and cause a lot of discouragement.

For example: the NGO Transaid works in some African countries to build the capacity of programmes to maintain vehicles and motorbikes in good working order. See Resources, below.

Related to PPM is planning ahead for capital expenditure. We calculate when major items of equipment will need replacing and budget for this accordingly so that we are not suddenly left without transport and other essential systems on which our programme depends.

5. **Use volunteers.**
Many communities have members who are willing to volunteer, provided they have the time, are adequately trained and have a strong religious or humanitarian motivation.

The skilful use of volunteers can reduce project salary costs. However, it is important not to exploit or overuse volunteers, and to be

---

Dear Friends,

The main reason for the death of people in our villages is lack of money to pay for healthcare. In 1995 health unions (Mutuelles de Santé) were begun in Nikki, bringing together farmers and health staff. The health unions help people to face together the problem of illness by improving the health of members and helping people to plan for possible illness in the future. They raise funds from entrance fees and annual subscriptions collected from the member families.

The health unions are small groups - there may be several groups or just one in each village. There are also district unions and a regional association, which co-ordinate all the health unions. In the last year over 10,000 members registered in health unions. Members receive a membership card which gives their family the right to one year's free healthcare for childbirth, treatment of small wounds, snake bites, malaria, diarrhoea, vomiting and surgery. Minor illnesses and the cost of doctors' consultations are not included in the free treatment
                    yours sincerely

Figure 21.3   Part of a letter written in 1999 from the Republic of Benin. *Source, Footsteps*, Tearfund.

sensitive to their feelings. Volunteers, unless strongly affirmed and valued by other team members, can become demotivated, especially if their families do not approve of what they are doing. The project should pay their transport costs, other out-of-pocket expenses and, where appropriate, a small honorarium. CHWs are a good example of the use of volunteers (see page 129) but the concept can be extended to other project workers, both junior and senior. Volunteers need to be well managed just like other team members, and it is helpful to draw up an informal contract or memorandum of understanding with them. They need to be welcomed as full members of the team.

Ways to increase programme resources

Cost recovery refers to a system where the users of the health facility, i.e. patients, pay for some of or all the costs of the service, in particular for the cost of medicines. They can do this through paying user fees at the time of their visit to the clinic, or through an insurance system via a fixed regular premium.

Of course, it is not only the cost of drugs that needs to be paid for. However, community members are more willing to pay for curative care than for other aspects of CBHC where benefits are longer term and seem less obvious. Cost recovery (if successful) can pay for drugs with a certain amount left over. This can be used for what is known as cross subsidy; that is, paying for other parts of the programme such as the training and payment of CHWs. However, the community must understand the way in which any money it has paid is being used.

For most health systems to function, the users themselves need to contribute. Unless this happens there is insufficient money to run clinics, pay health staff and provide essential drugs. Supplies fail, the number of patients attending declines, and community members either receive no care at all, return to traditional healers or attend private practitioners. The main health facility may cease to function altogether.

Much experience has been gained worldwide on how best to encourage communities to pay towards their health care. First we will list guidelines taken from a variety of successful projects. Then we will describe some practical methods for estimating and collecting fees. First the guidelines:

• **Involve the community at all stages**
  This is the key to success. If a plan is dumped on a community it will fail. If it arises from a community that comes to understand the issues involved, it will have ownership of the scheme and is more likely to give it its support. In our explanation to the community, we must help people to understand that, if the project

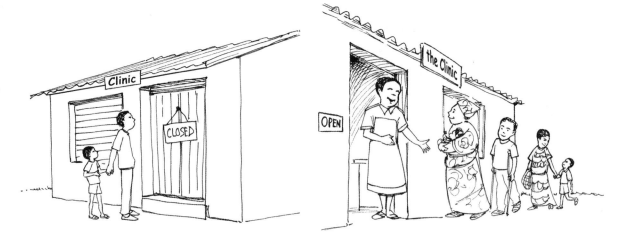

Figure 21.4 Provided prices are not excessive, many patients will continue to use clinics if they are friendly, convenient and accessible.

runs out of money and can't pay for medicines and salaries, it will have to close and then they will be worse off than before.

- **Make use of payment schemes already familiar to the community**
  For example: in parts of Tanzania, traditional healers have sliding scales of the amount they charge, based on ability to pay. Other communities have traditions of contributing to community activities such as funerals or festivities. These systems can be used as models to help explain and guide the fixing of fair user fees or insurance premiums.
- **Make sure the community has confidence in the health facility**
  Health workers must be friendly and competent. Essential drugs must be always available. Nothing so undermines a health service as a frustrated health worker turning away the mother of a seriously ill child because antimalarials have run out.
- **Investigate other schemes being used nearby**
  We should find out about cost recovery systems used in other parts of the country or health district. We can join them, use them or adapt them as appropriate to our situation.
- **Consider the use of cross subsidy to help pay drug costs**
  For example: in Ghana one project made a 'profit' from Vitamin B complex, which people really wanted, (despite little clinical need and taking care that the health programme did not actively promote it). This helped to pay for snake-venom, normally expensive, but which could now be charged at a subsidised rate, in particular for the farming breadwinner during sowing and harvesting.
- **Manage the scheme at the most local level possible**
  Schemes work best when user fees and insurance schemes are managed at the most peripheral level, such as the health post or the primary health centre, provided people have sufficient skills to manage it. This demonstrates to the community that the fees paid are used to improve its own health facility, not siphoned off for use elsewhere. A health committee should run the scheme (see page 271).
  This committee will need careful training, outside support and encouragement.

- **Make sure that finances are honestly managed**
  Large sums of money may be generated, which can be both daunting and tempting for staff to handle. There will need to be systems and audits to guard against mistakes and theft.

In addition to these general guidelines we will need to draw up careful, practical methods for the collection of fees. It is helpful to consider these under three headings:

1. **Decide on how much money needs to be recovered.**
   To help us fix fees and premiums we will need to calculate two things.

   - How much on average will patients be able to afford?
     This figure will need to take into account the sliding scales and exemptions. A good starting point is to look through any previous clinic records (or those of similar projects) to calculate the total of money taken per patient. Then decide whether people might afford to pay more per head, providing fair levels and exemptions are set up.
   - How much does the project have to charge in order for the clinic to be viable?
     We need to decide whether we are aiming to recover the partial cost of drugs, the full cost of drugs, or the full cost plus extra for cross subsidy (to contribute towards staff salaries, transport costs, etc.). Obviously we cannot charge a fee or premium that is more than the community on average can afford, but we still need to know the ideal amount we are aiming to recover. Then we can calculate the balance that will need to be raised from other sources.

2. **Set up a policy on fee levels and exemptions.**
   As we know, fee collection often triggers bargaining or argument. We can reduce this by drawing up a simple, fair system, agreed by the community and easy to operate. It is not appropriate for the health worker, CHW or health committee member to be mainly responsible for assessing a person's ability to pay, though they can help if disputes arise.
   A policy will need to have clear statements on categories, exemptions (whether for all drugs and procedures or some only), what happens

if fees or premiums are not paid, and the level of authority of health centre staff.

For example: In one programme in Bangladesh a system of four categories has been established, which has worked well in the community being served. Group 1 is the poorest and Group 4 the wealthiest and each is charged a different rate. We can use this as a model and adapt it for our situation.

Group 1. Families with no male earner or with a disabled male earner. Lowest user or membership fee.

Group 2. Families that cannot afford two meals per day throughout the year.

Group 3. Families that can afford two meals per day all year but do not have a surplus.

Group 4. Families that have an agricultural or financial surplus.

A family survey is one way we can assess the rate of exemption (see page 88).

3. **Put the policy into practice.**
   We will need to decide questions such as:

   * Who actually collects the fees or premiums?
   * How will money be handled, stored or banked?
   * How will the fee or premium category and exemption be identified?
   * What forms will be needed?
   * Who will arbitrate if a dispute arises?

User fees and co-financing

User fees are the charges patients incur at the time they attend a health facility. Charges are usually made for drugs, and can also be raised for services provided or procedures carried out.

Co-financing refers to the partnership between project and community, where costs are raised between them by mutual agreement.

User fees have become a standard and simple way of recovering at least some of the cost of providing health care. However, experience has shown that user fees tend to dissuade certain people from attending. These include those needing antenatal care, those with certain infectious illnesses, (in particular sexually transmitted illness) and, as we have seen, the very poor. In some communities the proportion of women attending also falls.

An example of a successful health centre that charges user fees is Mabuku in the Democratic Republic of Congo. Here a number of factors together helped this to work well:

* A competent and respected head nurse, able to balance immediate needs with long-term development.
* A community with high confidence in its health workers, both clinic and community based.
* An active health committee, which meets regularly and represents a wide range of the local population.
* An understanding that people who can't pay their bills in cash can contribute in produce or livestock, which is either sold or contributes to staff salaries.
* Using an outside grant to build maternity waiting rooms where high-risk or distant mothers can wait near to the health centre for delivery.

The Mabuku Health Centre is an example of co-financing where the community had a strong input in setting up the scheme, both in decision-making and management.

There are two common ways in which user fees can be charged at clinic level:

1. **Per clinic attendance as a charge taken on registration.** (See also pages 159–61.)
   One main *advantage* is simplicity: a single charge is taken on one occasion. There can be different rates, e.g. for adults and children, and by category of wealth. A further advantage is that people know in advance what they have to pay so they can plan accordingly. This also reduces disputes. Exemptions can be made; e.g. for the very poor, antenatal patients, or those coming for immunisations only.
   The main *disadvantage* is that patients want their 'money's worth' of drugs for the charge they have paid. They may expect or demand unnecessary injections or medicines, or feel cheated if they don't receive them. This can be overcome by partial reimbursement if no medicines are necessary, and training staff to explain why medicines may not be needed.

2. **Per medicine dispensed or procedure carried out.**

   The *advantage* of this is that patients are charged according to the actual medicine or procedure they need.

   A *disadvantage* is that collecting the fees and accounting can be more complex and time-taking.

Revolving drug funds (RDFs)

RDFs, also known as Drug Revolving Funds (DRFs), are an effective way of setting up a long-term method of paying for medicine costs. Drugs are sold to patients, via clinic or CHW, and the money paid is used to buy more drugs. A grant or loan enables the project to buy sufficient essential drugs at the start to last, say, for a period of six months. Schemes, if carefully managed, may be able to revolve the original money in buying replacement drugs so that little or no outside funding is needed for further drug purchase.

The *advantages* of RDFs are several. It is an attractive option for donors, and a good way to demonstrate self-sufficiency to the community. The *disadvantages* are that the administration can be difficult, especially at local level, when large sums of money may be involved. RDFs have a high failure rate unless they are very carefully planned.

The secrets of success are largely those already mentioned in the guidelines for successful cost recovery. RDFs work best when there is simplicity

in the paperwork, and careful training (both initial and ongoing) for all those administering the scheme. If there are too many exemptions the fund runs out of money. Unless there are careful checks and balances, monies received and banked can get lost, confused or stolen, which causes the community to lose confidence in the scheme, and in the clinic.

Setting up RDFs involves considerable time and expense. Ongoing monitoring and training are essential for success.

Health insurance schemes

Health insurance is also known as a prepayment scheme. Community members pay a regular amount into a fund, and only those who have paid this premium or membership fee are eligible for benefits. In practice an insurance scheme only works effectively if a majority, e.g. 75 per cent, of a community belongs to it. In some countries or districts there are national not-for-profit insurance schemes that can be joined.

Guidelines for success are largely those already mentioned. These will help the scheme to get off to a good start, but even so community members may be reluctant to pay when they are not feeling ill.

There are various ways of increasing uptake. *For example*: Members who have not yet paid can be charged a penalty when they attend the clinic, or more appropriately, they can pay their annual premium, plus the price of the immediate

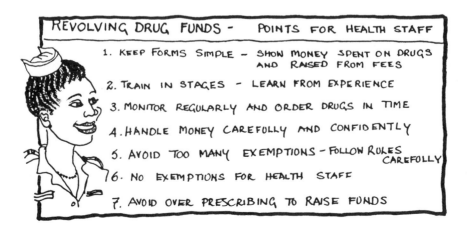

REVOLVING DRUG FUNDS -   POINTS FOR HEALTH STAFF

1. KEEP FORMS SIMPLE - SHOW MONEY SPENT ON DRUGS AND RAISED FROM FEES

2. TRAIN IN STAGES - LEARN FROM EXPERIENCE

3. MONITOR REGULARLY AND ORDER DRUGS IN TIME

4. HANDLE MONEY CAREFULLY AND CONFIDENTLY

5. AVOID TOO MANY EXEMPTIONS - FOLLOW RULES CAREFULLY

6. NO EXEMPTIONS FOR HEALTH STAFF

7. AVOID OVER PRESCRIBING TO RAISE FUNDS

Figure 21.5

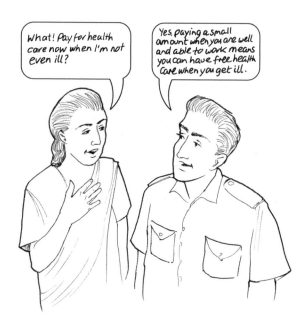

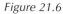
Figure 21.6

medical care together, thus becoming members at the same time as receiving treatment. Hard-to-persuade community members can be encouraged to join the scheme as a fair way of guaranteeing health care for their children. There can be special family rates.

Rates of insurance can be set at various levels. *For example*: A low premium would pay for care, (including medicines) from the community health worker. A small extra premium would cover additional care from the nearest health post or clinic. For a larger premium the primary health centre or referral hospital could be included. However, this will work only where there is excellent local administration and good integration between different levels of the health service. A 'bypass' fee can be levied if people go straight to the PHC or hospital without first seeing the CHW or attending the health post.

One example: an effective nationwide programme known as Dana Sehat has been set up in Indonesia. Each scheme is adapted to the particular needs of the community. In many cases funds are raised partly through annual insurance premiums, fundraising events, or the sale of commodities or handicrafts. This enables sufficient funds to cover all medicine costs, and also to extend loans to community members for specific projects such

as latrine construction. These schemes work best when women are actively involved.

The main *advantages* of health insurance schemes are that most people pay into the fund when they are well and at a time of year when their resources are greatest, e.g. harvest. When illness occurs they have no worry about paying.

There are several *disadvantages*:

- It may be hard to persuade fit people to pay when they have no felt need.
- If people pay a premium they may be tempted to overuse the health facility and expect medicines for trivial illnesses. One way round this problem is to charge a small co-payment at the time of attending the clinic.
- Members may pay their premium when they first start feeling ill. We can get round this problem by not allowing people to use insurance-paid health care within two weeks of buying their insurance
- Sometimes health workers overprescribe, knowing that the insurance scheme will pay for the medicines.
- In areas with high rates of HIV, it is very difficult to make insurance schemes work because of high demands being made on the system
- As with RDFs, there can be quite high failure rates but schemes that have been carefully thought through, have the ownership of the people and are efficiently and honestly managed can be very successful.

Finally we must guard against the development of a two-tier system: those who are insured and those who are not. There must be strong encouragement to enlist as many community members as possible. At the same time those genuinely unable to afford to join must be protected and never be denied access to health care.

Other methods of cost recovery

1. **Income generation**
   An increasing number of projects are now raising income to help them remain sustainable. Here are some examples currently used by primary health programmes. For many of

these, capital grants are necessary to set up the income generating activities:

- Making and selling handicrafts.
- Setting up plantations, and selling fruit and vegetables.
- Running bakeries.
- Hiring out vehicles (with strict guidelines and never undermining the needs of the project).
- Running a petrol/diesel station (which also gives opportunities for HIV education for long-distance truck and bus drivers).
- Obtaining capital funds to set up a tourist lodge, and then using the income.

In addition to year-round income generation, some projects arrange special fund-raising events.

For example: One company in Delhi with personal links to a slum development programme arranged an evening banquet for top industrialists in the city. Large numbers attended, paid a high price for tickets and in addition to having an enjoyable evening, learnt firsthand about the project through meeting both the project director and slum community volunteers. Considerable funds were raised and much good will and understanding generated. The press was invited in order to further increase the impact.

2. **Micro-finance**

In many countries schemes are being set up to provide loans for community groups to help them develop their own local businesses and income generating activities. These micro-finance schemes are usually managed by projects with special expertise in this area or by banks and other institutions with trained field workers able to provide the loans and help communities use them successfully. The Grameen bank in Bangladesh is a well known example (see Further reading 3).

Sometimes we can work alongside such groups so that income raised can be used to help fund essential health care needs for the family. Any such project needs to be carefully set up with built-in safeguards and clear agreement between the micro-finance institution, the health project and the community.

There have been some programmes, notably in Ghana and the Philippines, where micro-

finance officers themselves have received basic health training so they can include health education in their visits to customers.

3. **Partnerships with funding agencies**

As described at the beginning of this chapter, programmes are unlikely to become fully self-financing for several years. In addition to raising money through cost recovery schemes, most projects also need to establish partnerships with one or more donor agencies. Such agencies often help to pay start-up costs, grants for new initiatives and capital expenditure.

But we will also need to discover any particular priority a funding agency may have (these can vary over a one-, three- and five-year period); also how the agency judges success. Having this information can help us to target funding agencies more successfully. (See also pages 61–65, 295–6.)

Partnerships with funding agencies should usually go beyond simple financing. They should involve a two-way learning process, with visits, training and technical help from the funding agency or through local consultants or other partners of the agency working in the country or region.

4. **Strategic alliances with the private sector**

Local industry, pharmaceutical companies and philanthropists may be interested in supporting some project activities. *For example*: Several drug companies are distributing free medicines for special illnesses (e.g. albendazole for intestinal worms). We will need to monitor any commercial links for ethical standards. We should also remember that drug companies will sometimes create demand so they can achieve higher sales, so we should only enter into agreements when we need essential medicines over a period of time.

Many links with the private sector come about through networking via project leaders, board members or trustees.

For example: In Zambia, a number of non-profit trading and production companies have been set up to provide basic health equipment and supplies, both through health shops and through supplying NGOs direct.

There may be a major employer nearby who will have an interest in the improved health of

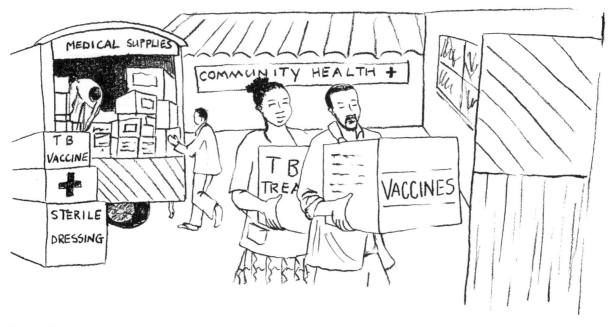

Figure 21.7   Tap into government supplies where possible.

its workforce and may be able to help sub-sidise the services we provide.

5. **Tapping into government funding**

    As already stated elsewhere in this book, we should link up with national programmes and develop relationships with government at dis-trict level. Funds may often be available for specific programmes, such as TB control, impregnated bed-nets, and vaccines through the Expanded Programme on Immunisation. Whether funds are available will often depend on multilateral and bilateral aid being sup-plied to national governments or programmes.

6. **Contracting out**

    Governments are increasingly contracting out services to NGOs. *For example*: in Cambodia health care for whole districts has been con-tracted out to voluntary or private providers. As our own programmes grow in size and effectiveness we should be open for any such opportunities that come our way.

Summary

With health needs outstripping the amount of outside funding available, all health programmes need to work towards becoming sustainable. Only those who succeed in this are likely to survive into the future.

All projects need to ensure that they remain financially viable through a variety of measures. Important methods are cost cutting and increased efficiency in programme management. Most pro-jects will also need to recover costs either by charging user fees, through insurance schemes or from a variety of other means for generating income, of which several examples are described.

Projects should also develop alliances with one or more partner agencies, with the private sector and with government. Both the methods of cost recovery and any alliance formed need to be monitored to ensure that the poor are never denied health care, and that ethical values are maintained.

Further reading

1. *Financing Health Care*, H. Goodman and C. Waddington, Oxfam, 1993.
    This is an excellent practical manual with a wealth of useful information, still very relevant.
    Available from: Oxfam. See Appendix E.

2. *Sustaining Primary Health Care*, A. Lafond, Save the Children Fund, 1995.
    This is more a useful policy document than a practical manual.
    Available from: Save the Children Fund. See Appendix E.
3. The Grameen Foundation www.grameen foundation.org is a worldwide network devoted to microcredit and income generation for poor communities. This is worth accessing and studying.

4. Transaid works in some countries to train in transport and driving skills; www.transaid.org.

Certain journals and newsheets frequently have articles on sustainability. These include *The Health Exchange*, and *Footsteps*. See Appendix D.

The Panos Institute specialises in information on sustainable development. See Appendix E.

See Further references and guidelines, page 417.

PART V
Appendices

Appendix A: Suppliers of Equipment

General supplies, equipment, vehicles

1. **International Dispensary Association (IDA)**: PO Box 37098, 1003 AB Amsterdam, The Netherlands.
   Email: info@ida.nl. Website: www.ida.nl/en-US.
   Suppliers of a large range of medical supplies, including medicines, suitable for developing countries. Also sterilisers, water filters, generators, equipment for cold chain, and various publications.
2. **Durbin plc**, Durbin House, 180 Northolt Rd, South Harrow, Middlesex HA2 OLT, UK.
   Website: www.durbin.co.uk.
   Major suppliers of medicines and pharmaceutical supplies to many parts of the world, including generics.
3. **Mission Supplies Ltd**, Airport House, Kingsmill Lane, South Nutfield, Surrey, RH1 5JY, UK. Email: enquiries@missionsupplies.co.uk
   Website: www.missionsupplies.co.uk.
   Supply a variety of appliances, office equipment, computers, audiovisual aids, vehicles.
4. **Unimatco**: Bulstrode, Oxford Road, Gerrards Cross, Bucks, SL9 7SZ, UK.
   Email: sales@unimatco.co.uk. Website: www.unimatco.co.uk.
   Provides an extensive range of equipment supplies, vehicles, invertors, solar fridges and lighting.

Community health supplies

1. Teaching Aids at Low Cost (TALC): PO Box 49, St Albans, Herts, AL1 4AX, UK. Tel: +44 (0) 1727 853869; Fax: +44 (0) 1727 846852.
   Email: info@talcuk.org. Website: www.talcuk.org.
   TALC is a major community health resource centre in the UK. Supplies a complete range of books on community health, plus child weighing scales, height measurers, arm measurers, growth charts, sets of teaching slides, CD Roms, etc. TALC is a distributor of this book.
2. **Tropical Health Technology**, PO Box 50, Fakenham, Norfolk NR21 8XB, UK.
   Email: thtbooks@tht.ndirect.co.uk. Website: www.tht.ndirect.co.uk.
   Supplies laboratory equipment and books, bench aids and microscopes, AIDS/HIV test kits, etc. Also publishes appropriate laboratory manuals.
3. **PATH**, 1455 NW Leary Way, Seattle, WA 98107, USA. Email: info@path.org. Website: www.path.org.
   PATH is a large-scale not-for-profit organisation carrying out many initiatives to further global health and provides an extensive range of books and supplies of relevance to community health.

Steam sterilisers

1. **Prestige Medical**, PO Box 154, Off Clarendon Road, Blackburn, Lancashire BB1 9UG, UK.
   Email: info@prestigemedical.co.uk. Website: www.prestigemedical.co.uk.
   Produces a wide range of sterilisers, autoclaves, pressure cookers and spare parts. A commercial company: compare prices.
   Sterilisers can also be obtained from most general suppliers listed on this page.

Further information on supplies and resources

Practical Action, formerly Intermediate Technology (ITDG), Schumacher Centre for Technology and Development, Bourton Hall, Bourton-on-Dunsmore, Rugby, Warwickshire, CV23 9QZ, UK. Tel: +44 (0) 1926 634400; Fax: +44 (0) 1926 634401.
Email: enquiries@practicalaction.org.uk.
Website: www.practicalaction.org.uk.
ITDG is a world leader on applied technology and a source of information on many areas of interest in community based health and development.
See also Appendix E under Intermediate Technology.

Appendix B: Supplies Needed by a Small Health Centre

Each project will need to draw up a list specific to its needs. Here are items that are likely to be needed by most clinics. Specifications for sizes, types and numbers of medical items are available from IDA, see Appendix A.

Medical equipment

Ambubag
Ampoule file
Aural forceps
Blood pressure machine
Clinical thermometers
Crutches adult/child
Dental forceps/gum retractor/syringes/needles
Dressing tray
Ear syringe
Eye bath
Eye testing lenses and charts
First aid equipment
Foetal stethoscope
Forceps, various
Gallipots
Haemoglobinometer
Hair clippers
Height measurer
Jugs
Kidney bowls
Medicine measurers/pill counters
Microscope
Nasal hook for foreign bodies
Nasal speculum
Needle holders
Ophthalmoscope/spare batteries, bulbs
Otoscope/spare batteries, bulbs/speculums
Patella hammer
Plaster knife/shears
Portable suction
Probe
Scalpels

Scissors
Sigmoidoscope/proctoscope
Splinter forceps
Splints
Stethoscope
Tape measure
Tourniquets
Trolley
Tuning forks
Vacuum extractor
Vaginal speculums
Weighing scales adult/child

Renewable medical supplies

Adhesive tape
AIDS testing kit
Aprons
Bandages, various including crepe/triangular
Bottles, etc. for dispensing
Butterfly needles
Child feeding tubes
Cotton wool
Delivery kits
Dressings, various
Elastic (crepe) bandages
Episiotomy set
Family planning supplies including IUDs
Gauze bandages
Gauze compresses
Gloves (rubber), large, small/maternity and non-latex
Intravenous giving sets and cannulas/butterfly sets
Insect repellent containing DEET
Labels for dispensing
Laboratory supplies
Lancets for malaria tests
Lubricant, e.g. KY jelly
Malaria rapid diagnostic tests
Mediswabs

Micropore (non-allergenic) tape
Midwives' kit
Mosquito nets, impregnated
Nailbrush
Needles gauges 26, 22,18
Paraffin gauze dressings
PVC sheeting
Safety box (sharps containers)
Safety pins
Soap and soapdishes
Spoons, plastic
Steristrips for small wound closure
Sugar/salt/spoon for demonstrating ORS
Suturing materials
Swabs and swab sticks
Syringes 2 ml, 5 ml, 10 ml
Tongue depressors
Tweezers
Umbilical cord clamp/tie
Urinary catheters, varying sizes/spigot
Urinary dipsticks
Urine drainage bag
Vaccine vial monitors
Water buckets and dippers

General equipment

Autoclave/steriliser/pressure cooker with drums/
autoclave tape, labels, wrapping cloths
Batteries
Blankets, pillows, etc.
Brooms, dustpans, etc.
Candles
Chairs/benches
Cold boxes
Computer, software and accessories
Examination couches
Fuel
Generator/cable

Kettle
Keys/locks
Lamps/lanterns
Matches
Money box
Projector for films/slides
Refrigerator
Storage cupboards
Stove
Tables
Teaching aids, e.g. flashcards, drama props,
videos
Tool and repair kit
Torch
Typewriter, word processor/PC
Video/DVD player
Water filter with replacement 'candles'
Whiteboard/chalkboard and coloured crayons

Records, registers, etc.

Books (medical)
Calculator
Cash books, ledger, etc.
CHW notebooks/diaries
Clinic Essential Drug list
Family folders
Patient numbers (cardboard)
Folders and files
Petty cash container
Record cards (including self-retained), tally
sheets, report forms, etc.
Referral letters
Registers (strong)
Rubber stamps/ink pads
Standing Orders/Treatment Protocols
Stationery including paper, pens, drawing pins,
paper clips, etc.
Stock cards/order forms

Appendix C: An Essential Drugs List

This is a suggested list of commonly used medicines at the community health centre level. Each project will need to draw up its own list after consulting the following sources: the latest WHO Model List of Essential Drugs, any National Essential Drugs List, any nationally or locally used Essential Drugs List for Primary Health Care, and the advice of a medical advisor who is guided by rational drug policies.

Drug lists may differ considerably from one area or one programme to another. Factors influencing choice include local patterns of disease, drug availability and expense, population covered and level of training of health personnel. Equivalent drugs can be used depending on what is available and current price levels.

Many smaller projects with no regular doctor in attendance at the clinic, or those with good hospital backup, would be able to use a shorter list (suggestions are marked*).

A list suitable for use by CHWs is included in Chapter 7.

Drugs listed here are based on the WHO *13th Model List of Essential Drugs* (2003). The order and classification have been slightly simplified.

Anaesthetics
Ketamine injection 50 mg/ml, 10 ml (general anaesthetic)
Lidocaine injection 1% or 2% (local anaesthetic)

Analgesics and anti-inflammatories (pain-killers)
* Acetylsalicylic acid tablet 300 mg (aspirin)
Ibuprofen tablet 200 mg
Morphine injection 10mg/1ml (drug subject to international control)
* Paracetamol tablet 500 mg and 100 mg or paediatric syrup 125 mg/5 ml

Antiallergics
* Adrenalin injection 1 mg/ml (Epinephrine)
* Chlorphenamine tablet 4 mg (Chlorpheniramine)
* Chlorphenamine injection 10 mg in 1 ml
Dexamethasone injection 4 mg in 1 ml
Prednisolone tablet 5 mg

Antidotes
* Ipecacuanha syrup 0.14% strength (as non-specific emetic after poisoning)

Anti-amoebics, antigiardials
Diloxanide tablet 500 mg (for amoebic cysts)
* Metronidazole tablet 200 mg or 400 mg

Anti-anaemia drugs
* Ferrous salt tablet, equivalent to 60 mg iron
* Folic acid tablet 1 mg
Ferrous salt (60 mg equiv Fe) + folic acid 0.40 mg (this combined preparation often used in pregnancy)
* Iron dextran injection equivalent to 50 mg iron/ml in 2 ml ampoule

Antibacterials
* Amoxycillin tablet or capsule 250 mg
Chloramphenicol injection 1 g/vial
* Ciprofloxacin tablet 250 mg
Doxycycline capsule or tablet 100 mg
* Erythromycin capsule or tablet 250 mg
Phenoxymethylpenicillin tablet 250 mg
* Procaine benzylpenicillin injection 1 g (1 million IU)
* Sulfamethoxazole 400 mg + trimethoprim 80 mg tablet (co-trimoxazole)
(Many smaller health centres may choose not to keep all these antibiotics)

Anticonvulsants
* Diazepam injection 5 mg in 2 ml
* Phenobarbital tablet 30 mg, 50 mg or 60 mg (phenobarbitone)

Antifungals
Fluconazole 50 mg
* Griseofulvin tablet 125 mg or 250 mg

*   Nystatin tablet 500 000 IU and pessary 100 000 IU

Anthelminthics (for worms)

Diethylcarbamazine tablet (DEC) 50 mg (for filaria)

Ivermectin tablet 6 mg (for onchocerciasis, etc.)

*   Mebendazole tablet 100 or 500 mg (alternative to mebendazole 500 mg is albendazole 400 mg)

Niclosamide tablet 500 mg

Praziquantel tablet 600 mg (for schistosomiasis)

Antileprotics

Clofazimine capsule 50 mg or 100 mg

Dapsone tablet 50 mg or 100 mg

Rifampicin tablet or capsule 150 mg or 300 mg (also in antituberculous list)

Antimalarials

It is essential to use drugs to prevent and treat malaria recommended by your national programme. See latest WHO List of Essential drugs, and details in Chapter 11. They include: artemether 20 mg and lumefantrine 120 mg (co-artemether, one form of Artemisinin Combined Therapy)

*   Chloroquine tablet 150 mg base, or syrup

Doxycycline 100 mg capsule

*   Quinine tablet 300 mg
*   Quinine injection 300 mg/ml, 2 ml
*   Sulfadoxine 500 mg + pyrimethamine 25 mg tablet ('Fansidar')

Antiretrovirals

The drugs used for treating HIV/AIDS must follow national guidelines and are deliberately omitted from this list.

Antiseptics

*   Chlorhexidine 5% solution

Antituberculous drugs

It is essential to use drugs to treat tuberculosis that are recommended by your national TB programme. They are likely to include:

Ethambutol tablet 200 mg or 400 mg

Isoniazid tablet 100 mg or 300 mg (INH)

Pyrazinamide tablet 400 mg

Rifampicin tablet or capsule 150 mg or 300 mg

Streptomycin injection 1 g (various combined preparations also available and recommended)

Cardiovascular drugs

*   Atenolol tablet 50 mg

Digoxin tablet 0.25 mg

*   Furosemide tablet 40 mg (Frusemide)

Hydrochlorothiazide tablet 25 mg or 50 mg

Dermatological drugs (for applying to skin)

*   Benzoic acid + salicylic acid ointment or cream 6% + 3% (Whitfield's ointment)
*   Benzyl benzoate lotion 25%, bottle 1 litre
*   Calamine lotion
*   Gentian violet aqueous solution 0.5%

Hydrocortisone cream or ointment 1%

*   Neomycin and bacitracin ointment 5 mg + 500 IU
*   Permethrin cream 5% or lotion 1%

Gastro-intestinal drugs

*   Aluminium hydroxide tablet 500 mg
*   Atropine tablet 1 mg or equivalent

Cimetidine tablet 200 mg

*   Metoclopramide tablet 10 mg
*   Oral rehydration salts, powder 27.9 g/l

Senna tablet 7.5 mg or equivalent

Gynaecological/Obstetric/Contraceptive preparations

*   Condoms

Copper-containing intrauterine device

*   Ethinyloestradiol + levonorgestrel tablets (30 μg + 150 μg or 30 μg + 250 μg) ethinyloestradiol + norethisterone (35 μg + 1 mg) (contraceptive pills)
*   Ergometrine tablet 0.2 mg and injection 0.2 mg in 1 ml

Immunisations/serum

Anti-venom snake sera where relevant

*   BCG vaccine
*   Hib vaccine
*   Diphtheria–pertussis–tetanus (DPT) vaccine
*   Hepatitis B vaccine
*   Measles vaccine or MMR
*   Poliomyelitis vaccine
*   Tetanus vaccine

Tetanus–diphtheria vaccine (Td)

(Others as indicated locally e.g., meningitis, pneumococcal, rabies, typhoid, yellow fever vaccines.)

Intravenous solutions
Compound solution of sodium lactate injectable solution
Glucose injectable solution 5%

Ophthalmic drugs (for eyes)
Atropine eye drops 0.1%, 0.5% or 1%
* Gentamicin eye drops 0.3%
Pilocarpine eye drops 2% or 4%
Tetracaine eye drops 0.5%
Tetracycline eye ointment 1%

Psychotherapeutic drugs (for mental disturbance)
Amitriptyline tablet 25 mg
* Chlorpromazine tablet 100 mg and injection 25 mg/ml in 2 ml
Diazepam tablet 5 mg

Respiratory drugs
Adrenalin as under **antiallergics**
Salbutamol tablet 2 mg or 4 mg or aerosol inhaler
* Theophylline tablet 100 mg or 200 mg

Vitamin and mineral preparations
* Iodised oil 1 ml (480 mg) in ampoule (oral or injectable)
* Vitamin A capsule 200 000 IU or oily solution 100 000 IU (retinol)
* Vitamin C 50 mg (ascorbic acid)
(Other vitamins and minerals will depend on local deficiencies.)

Water for injection
* 2, 5, 10 ml ampoules

Appendix D: Useful Journals and Newsletters

Addresses in most cases are given in **Appendix E**, which lists resource agencies.

General community health topics

Footsteps

A free international newsletter on practical aspects of health and development, each issue read by approximately one million readers. Published four times per year in English, French, Spanish, Portuguese and other languages. .
Available from: Tearfund, Resources Department, PO Box 200, Bridgnorth, Shropshire WV16 4WQ.
Fax: +44 (0) 1746 764594. Email: roots@tearfund.org.uk. Website: www.tearfund.org/tilz from which back copies can be downloaded.

Specific community health topics

Developing Mental Health: an international journal for mental health care
A key resource for community mental health care, a subject of growing importance. Published by ICTHES World Care, PO Box 408, Bankhead Avenue, Edinburgh EH11 4HE, UK. Email: m.mcgavin@icthesworldcare.com.
Icthes also publishes other relevant information for doctors and senior health care workers on ears and hearing, dermatology, and repair and reconstruction.

The Health Exchange

Topic based, challenging and informative issues of this magazine are available from RedR-IHE, 1 Great George Street, London SW1P 3AA. Email: info@redr.org. Website: www.redr.org.

Women's Health Exchange

A free newsletter providing information on women's health.
Available from: the Hesperian Foundation, 1919 Addison Street #304, Berkeley, CA 94704, USA.
Email: hesperian@hesperian.org

Journals with community health emphasis mainly written for doctors or administrators

Tropical Doctor

A useful journal for doctors and nurses working in community health programmes and rural hospitals.
Available from: The Royal Society of Medicine Press Ltd, PO Box 9002, London W1A 0ZA, UK. Tel: +44 (0) 207 290 2928. Fax: +44 (0) 207 290 2929. Email: rsmjournals@rsm.ac.uk. Quarterly: English

Bulletin of the World Health Organization
Published monthly and containing many articles of interest and relevance. Available from: WHO, see Appendix E.

Appendix E: Addresses of Resource and Information Centres

African Medical Research Foundation (AMREF); HQ Langata Road, PO Box 00506, 27961 Nairobi, Kenya. Email: info@amrefhq.org. Email of Kenyan Office: info@amrefke.org. Website: www.amref.org. (Offices in various other countries.) Publishes books, journals and other literature. Runs training courses and seminars. Acts as a comprehensive advisory centre on primary health care.

Centre for International Child Health (CICH), Institute of Child Health, 30 Guilford Street, London WC1N 1EH, UK. Email: cich@ich.ucl.ac.uk . The information centre at CICH has this email: source@ich.ucl.ac.uk and website: www.ich.ucl.ac.uk. CICH runs a large variety of courses relevant to CBHC. It also has an extensive library and SOURCE has a large information centre on all aspects of child health and community based health care. It has close links with TALC.

Child-to-Child, Institute of Education, 20 Bedford Way, London WC1H OAL, UK. Tel: +44 (0) 207 612 6648 Fax: +44 (0) 207 612 6645 Website: www.child-to-child.org Child-to-Child publishes a whole range of resource books, readers and activity sheets to enable children to teach other children and family members, or for schemes who include children as partners in health and development. Many of these materials are also available from TALC.

Community Health Global Network Website: www.communityhealthglobal.net. This is a new networking and training organisation that aims to link, share information and strengthen community based health programmes.

Healthlink Worldwide, Cityside, 40 Adler Street, London E1 1EE, UK. Tel: +44 (0) 207 539 1570 Fax: +44 (0) 207 539 1580. Email: info@healthlink.org.uk.

Website: www.healthlink.org.uk. Previously known as AHRTAG. This is a major resource and information centre.

Hesperian Foundation, address in Appendix D. Outstanding books, health information and newsletters. Original publishers of *Where There is No Doctor*; www.hesperian.org.

Intermediate Technology. Further details in Appendix A. Website for publications: www.itdgpublishing.org.uk. Email: itpubs@itpubs.org.uk. ITDG Publishing publishes many books and also has a comprehensive book catalogue covering all aspects of health, development and technology. This organisation has been renamed Practical Action.

International Centre for Eye Health, London School of Hygiene and Tropical Medicine, Keppel Street, London WC1E 7HT, Email: icehorg@iceh.org.uk. Website: www.lshtm.ac.uk/iceh. Advises and publishes information on all aspects of eye care, including prevention of blindness.

International Planned Parenthood Federation (IPPF), Regents College, Regents Park, London NW1 4NS, UK. Tel: +44 (0) 207 487 7900. Fax: +44 (0) 207 487 7950. Email: info@ippf.org. Website: www.ippf.org. Advises and publishes information on all aspects of family planning and child spacing.

Macmillan, For all publications write to: Macmillan Direct, Houndmills, Basingstoke, RG21 6XS, UK. Tel: +44 (0) 1256 302687 Fax: +44 (0) 1256 364733 Email: mdl@macmillan.co.uk. Or order from your local Macmillan office. For general enquiries, email Africa@macmillan.co.uk. This company, the publisher of this book, also publishes a wide range of books on all aspects of health care and education appropriate for health programmes worldwide.

MAP International, HQ at PO Box 215000, Brunswick, Georgia 31521-5000, USA. Tel: +1 912 265 6010 Fax: +1 912 265 6170 Email: map@map.org. Website: www.map.org. A resource and information consultancy on community health development with offices throughout the world. MAP also supplies essential drugs and medical equipment for primary health care programmes and runs training courses.

OXFAM Publishing, Oxfam's main address is: Oxfam House, 274 Banbury Road, Oxford, OX2 7DZ, UK. Website: publications.oxfam.org.uk/Oxfam. Their book distributors are BEBC, PO Box 1496, Parkstone, Dorset BH12 3YD, UK. Email for orders: oxfam@bebc.co.uk. Oxfam also has regional offices in many countries. It advises about community health, development and funding and publishes a variety of useful books and manuals, including valuable country profiles.

Pan-American Health Organization, 525 23rd Street, NW, Washington DC, 20037, USA. A major health resource centre for the Americas. Website: www.paho.org.

The Panos Institute, 9 White Lion Street, London N1 9PD, UK. Email: info@panos.org.uk. Website: www.panos.org.uk. This institute specialises in information and communications for sustainable development.

Save the Children UK, 1 St John's Lane, London EC1M 4AR, UK. Website: www.savethechildren.org.uk/scuk/jsp/resources. This large international organisation dedicated to bringing lasting benefits to children is committed to the principles of CBHC. It helps to set up long-term health and development programmes worldwide. Publishes a wide range of books on all aspects of children, including conflict, emergencies, development and food security.

Swiss Centre for Development Co-operation in Technology and Management (SKAT) (Includes both SKAT Consulting and SKAT Foundation)

Vadianstrasse 42, CH-9000 St Gallen, Switzerland. Email: info@skat.ch. Website: www.skat.ch. Produces lists of publications in various languages on development, appropriate technology, water and sanitation. Also a quarterly newsletter.

Teaching Aids at Low Cost (TALC), PO Box 49, St Albans, Herts, AL1 4AX, UK. Tel: +44 (0) 1727 853869. Fax: +44 (0) 1727 846852. Email: info@talcuk.org. Website: www.talcuk.org. For further details see Appendix A. It is helpful to be on TALC's free mailing list.

SOURCE at the Centre for International Child Health, London (See Above under CICH.)

Tropical Health Technology, THT has its prime focus in laboratory services and associated information and technology. See Appendix A.

UNICEF (United Nations Children's Fund) UNICEF House, 3 UN Plaza, New York 10017, USA. Website: www.unicef.org/publications. Advises governments and agencies on programmes for children. Provides a large range of resource materials, journals and books. Their regional offices will provide advice on all aspects of child health care, and they also publish regional journals. The State of the World's Children is a major report published yearly.

Voluntary Health Association of India, B 40 Qutub Institutional Area, South of IIT, New Delhi, 110 016, India. Email: vhai@vsnl.com and vhai@sify.com. Website: www.vhai.org. VHAI publishes journals, e.g. *Health for the Millions* and health educational materials in regional languages. Runs training programmes, acts as resource and advisory centre on all forms of community based health care. Has associated branches in each state of India. Its website is worth accessing by all programmes working in South Asia and beyond. VHAI also publishes an Indian and a Hindi version of this book (2nd edition).

Water, Engineering and Development Centre (WEDC), Loughborough University, Loughborough, Leics LE11 3TU, UK. Email: wedc@lboro.ac.uk. Website: wedc.lboro.ac.uk. A resource centre and consultancy on all aspects of water supplies and sanitation.

World Health Organization (WHO), Marketing and Dissemination, CH-1211 Geneva 27, Switzerland

Website: www.who.int/publications which gives details of how to order and information about all WHO publications. Also on their website is a vast range of health information, which, with careful searching, will give valuable information about many aspects of community based health care. Most chapters in this book have links to particular areas on their website for more information on their specific programmes.

WHO is the definitive United Nations Agency that advises governments worldwide on all aspects of health care. WHO publishes a huge number of books, journals, reports and other publications, and has specialists available to advise on almost any health related subject. Details of their regional offices can be obtained from their website.

Appendix F: Family Folder and Data Recording Form

The use of the Family Folder is described on pages 85–9, in the section on carrying out a survey.

The folder shown here was developed for use in SHARE Project, and with modifications has been used in a number of programmes in North India. The folder should be made of thick card. The upper side is shown on page 410, the underside or inside on page 411.

Details on the family folder are those recorded on the day of the survey and they should not be altered, except to complete any births, deaths and migrations in the section labelled Vital Events Since Survey.

Insert Cards for any at risk family members can be kept in the folder, thus keeping an updated record for any significant health problems affecting the family. These can be completed at the time of the survey and updated when family members attend the clinic. How this is done is described on pages 83, 158–9.

The Family Folder and Insert Cards are best kept in the clinic or health post and should be available for the health worker to make use of whenever a member of that family attends. This gives an opportunity of enquiring about health concerns in any other member of the family.

Each project will need to adapt this card with appropriate headings, design and health priorities.

a) NAME OF HEAD OF FAMILY _____   OCCUPATION _____   FOLDER NO. _____

VILLAGE/TOWN/COLONY _____   DISTRICT _____   REGION _____   STATE/PROVINCE _____   DATE OF SURVEY _____

b) Felt Problems – see inside folder

No	FAMILY PROFILE c)				DISEASES d)				IMMUNISATION e)						FAMILY PLANNING f)					ADDICTION g)		EDUCATION h)		REMARKS
	NAME	AGE + D.O.B. IF UNDER 5	SEX	RELATION TO HEAD	RELATION TO EACH OTHER	TB	LEPROSY	OTHER	NUTR. under 5	BCG	DPT	POLIO	MEASLES	TET TOX	TUB	VAS	O/C PILL	COIL	IF PREGNANT	ELIG FOR FP	ALCOHOL	TOBACCO	ADULT LIT	SCH. ATT.	
01																									
02																									
03																									
04																									
05																									
06																									
07																									
08																									
09																									
10																									
11																									
12																									
13																									
14																									

VITAL EVENTS SINCE SURVEY

BIRTHS				DEATHS					MIGRATION					
NAME	SEX	FATHER'S NAME	DATE OF BIRTH	NAME	AGE	CAUSE	DATE OF DEATH	NAME	AGE	SEX	DATE OF MIG.	RELATION TO HEAD	In / out	REASON

Figure F.1   Upper side of a family folder.

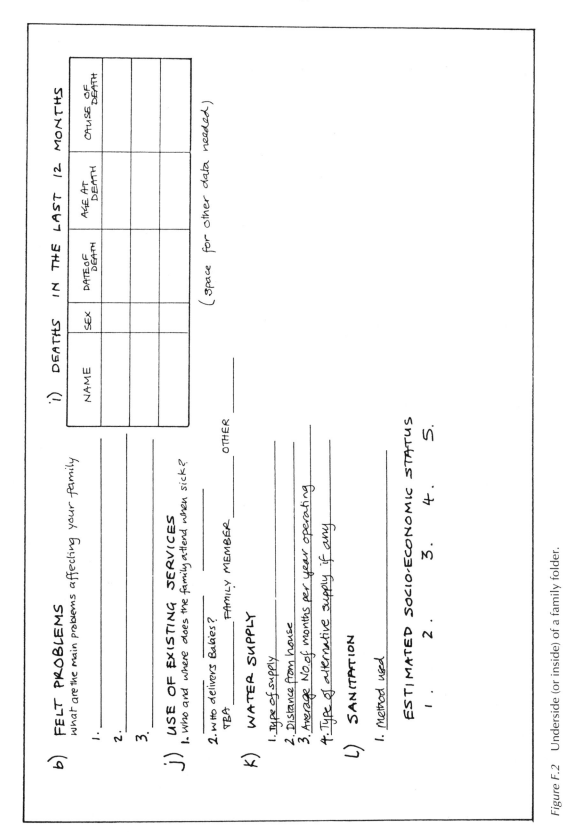

Figure F.2 Underside (or inside) of a family folder.

Further References and Guidelines

Updated research articles and details of good practice can be found on the website of Community Health Global Network, www.communityhealthglobal.net.

Please note the references below are in addition to the Further reading sections at the end of each chapter and give sources of information of original research and other papers and publications from which good practice and case histories are drawn.

A variety of papers was used for material in the first and second editions of this book, which are not recorded below.

Chapter 1

Chen, L. et al. 'Human resources for health: overcoming the crisis', *Lancet*, 2004, 364:1984–2004.

Chowdhury, M. 'Community participation in health care', letter, *Bulletin of the World Health Organization*, 2004, 82(11):881.

Victora, C. G. et al. 'Achieving universal coverage with health interventions', *Lancet*, 2004, 364:1541–8.

Mudur, G. 'India launches national rural health mission', *BMJ*, 2005, 330:920.

WHO, 'World Health Assembly raises global public health to new level', Press Release WHA/4, 2004, Geneva, World Health Organization.

WHO, 'Number of work-related accidents and illnesses continues to increase', Joint Media Release, WHO/ILO18, Geneva, World Health Organization.

WHO, World Development Report and Annex: 'Health in the Millennium Development Goals', A56/11, 2003, Geneva, World Health Organization.

Chapter 2

DFID, 'Children want a say, not a vote', *Developments*, first quarter, 2003, London, Department for International Development.

Chapter 3

Brown, H. 'UN urges broadcasters to air AIDS programmes', *Lancet*, 2004:363:295.

Carter, I. 'Mobilising the community', *Footsteps* 2003:53–5, London, Tearfund.

Gousseine, A. 'Theatre for disease prevention', *Footsteps* 2001:46:13–14, London, Tearfund.

'Music, dancing – and a national policy – are challenging violence in Brazil', *Bulletin of the World Health Organization*, 2002:80(10): 841–2.

Uwamariya, Irene J. and Narcisse, K. 'Country life; rural drama in Rwanda', *Developments*, fourth quarter, 2003,10–11, London, Department for International Development.

Chapter 4

See Further reading list at end of chapter.

Chapter 5

Aid Workers Exchange, Reach out and practice participation, internal communication, London, 2003.

Min, L. Participatory rural appraisal. Community Health Education Interest Group, internal communication, Singapore, 2005.

Tearfund, 'Risk mapping', *Footsteps* 2003, 56:8–9, London, Tearfund.

USPG, Health project review forms: internal publications, London, United Society for the Propagation of the Gospel, 2005.

Chapter 6

Included in Further reading at end of chapter.

Chapter 7

Adamson, S. et al. 'Practice points in utilizing local volunteers in community health projects', *Tropical Doctor*, 2004, 34:182–3.

Beltramello, C. and Zagaria, N. 'Where there is no health worker: saving children's lives in southern Sudan', *Health Exchange*, 2002, 22:19–22.

Birbeck, G. L. and Kalichi, E. M. 'Primary healthcare workers' perceptions about barriers to health services in Zambia', *Tropical Doctor*, 2004, 34:84–86.

International Centre for Eye Health, 'What's new in trachoma control?' *Community Eye Health*, 2004, 17:49–68.

Kumar, A. et al. 'Community perception and readiness for anti-helminth programmes in rural Nepal', *Tropical Doctor*, 2004, 34:87–89.

Kumar, S. 'Palliative care can be delivered through neighbourhood networks, *BMJ*, 2004, 329:1184.

Chapter 8

Included in Further reading at end of chapter.

Chapter 9

Collins, S. 'Community-based therapeutic care: a new paradigm for selective feeding in nutritional crises', Network Paper No. 48, 2004, London, Humanitarian Practice Network.

Filteau, S. 'Reducing childhood mortality in poor countries: infant feeding strategies to prevent post-natal HIV transmission', *Transactions of the Royal Society of Tropical Medicine and Hygiene*, 2003, 97:25–29.

Finch, L. 'Fighting for food aid – the struggle to assist groups affected by HIV/AIDS', *Lancet*, 2004, 364:1650–1.

Shrimpton, R. et al. 'Zinc deficiency: what are the most appropriate health interventions?', *BMJ*, 2005, 330:347–9.

Sur, D. et al. 'Periodic deworming with albendazole and its impact on growth status and diarrhoeal incidence among children in an urban slum of India', *Transactions of the Royal Society of Tropical Medicine and Hygiene*, 2005, 99:261–7.

Tomkins, A. 'Helping those with small voices', *Footsteps*, 2004, 61:10–12, London, Tearfund.

WHO, 'Anti-retroviral drugs for treating pregnant women and preventing HIV infection in infants', 2004, Geneva, World Health Organization.

WHO. 'Cambodia protects 75% of children against parasites, becoming first country', Press release, WHO/46, 2004, Geneva, World Health Organization.

WHO, 'Global Strategy for infant and young child feeding', 2004, Geneva World Health Organization.

WHO, 'Increased benefits found from wide use of anti-parasite drugs', Press Release, Geneva, 2004, World Health Organization.

Young, H. et al. 'Public nutrition in complex emergencies', *Lancet*, 2004, 365:1899–1907.

Chapter 10

Ding, D. et al. 'Cost effectiveness of routine immunization to control Japanese Encephalitis in Shanghai, China', *Bulletin of the World Health Organization*, 2003, 81:334ff.

Drain, P. et al. 'Introducing auto-disable syringes to the national immunization programme in Madagascar', *Bulletin of the World Health Organization*, 2003, 81:553–8.

Drain, P., Nelson, C. and Lloyd, J. 'Single-dose versus multi-dose vaccine vials for immunization programmes in developing countries', *Bulletin of the World Health Organization*, 2003, 81:726–730.

Hutin, Y. et al. and members of the Injection Safety Best Practices Development Group, 'Best injection practices for intradermal, subcutaneous and intramuscular needle injections', *Bulletin of the World Health Organization*, 2003, 31:491–500.

Kabir, Z. 'Non-specific effects of measles vaccination on overall child mortality in an area of rural India with high vaccination coverage: a population-based case control study', *Bulletin of the World Health Organization*, 2003, 81:244ff.

Lancet editorial, 'Globalization of Hib vaccination – how far are we?' *Lancet*, 2005, 365:5–6.

McGuigan, K. and Kehoe, S. 'Cooking the waste', *Lancet* editorial, 2003, 362:1251.

Moss, W., Clements. C. and Halsey, N. 'Immunization of children at risk of infection with human immunodeficiency virus', *Bulletin of the World Health Organization*, 2003, 81:61ff.

Murray, C. et al. 'Validity of reported vaccination coverage in 45 countries', *Lancet*, 2004, 362:1022–7.

Nelson, C. et al. 'Hepatitis B vaccine freezing in the Indonesian cold chain: evidence and solutions', *Bulletin of the World Health Organization*, 2004, 82:99–104.

Papani, M. and Strebel, P. 'Measles surveillance: the importance of finding the tip of the iceberg', *Lancet* editorial, 2005, 365:100–101.

WHO, 'Hepatitis B vaccines: WHO position paper', *Weekly Epidemiological Record*, 2004, 28:255–263, World Health Organization.

WHO, 'Measles deaths worldwide drop by nearly 40% over 5 years', Press Release WHO/UNICEF/11 and Fact Sheet WHO/286, 2005, Geneva, World Health Organization.

WHO, 'Vaccinating African children against pneumococcal disease saves lives', Press release WHO/3, 2005, Geneva, World Health Organization.

WHO, 'Websites providing information on vaccine safety recognized for good information practices', Press Release WHO/9, 2005, Geneva, World Health Organization.

Chapter 11

General

Al Fadil, S. et al. 'Integrated management of childhood illnesses strategy: compliance with referral and follow-up recommendations in Gezira state Sudan', *Bulletin of the World Health Organization*, 2003, 81:708–716.

Alves, J. and Correia, J. 'Ability of mothers to assess the presence of fever in their children without using a thermometer', *Tropical Doctor*, 2002 32:145–6.

Becher, H. et al. 'Risk factors of infant and child mortality in rural Burkina Faso', *Bulletin of the World Health Organization*, 2004, 82:265–272.

Gouws, E. et al. 'Improving antimicrobial use among health workers in first-level facilities: results from the multi-country evaluation of the Integrated Management of Childhood Illness strategy', *Bulletin of the World Health Organization*, 2004, 82:509–513.

Gwatkin, D. 'Integrating the management of childhood illness', *Lancet* editorial, 2004, 364;1557–8.

Lancet editorial, 'The world's forgotten children', *Lancet*, 2003, 361:1.

WHO, 'A new model for child survival in Africa', Press Release, WHO/UNICEF/91, 2004, Geneva, World Health Organization.

Diarrhoea

Curtis, V. et al. 'Evidence of behaviour change following a hygiene promotion programme in Burkina Faso', *Bulletin of the World Health Organization*, 2001, 79:518–27.

Kumar, R., Bodakhe, S. and Tailang, M. 'Patterns of use of rehydration therapy in Srinagar, Garhwal, Uttaranchal India', *Tropical Doctor*, 2003, 33:143–5.

Robberstad, B. et al. 'Cost-effectiveness of zinc as adjunct therapy for acute childhood diarrhoea in developing countries', *Bulletin of the World Health Organization*, 2004, 82:523–531.

WHO, 'Five simple measures could significantly reduce the global incidence of food borne disease', Press Release WHO/72, 2004, Geneva, World Health Organization.

WHO, 'New formula for oral rehydration salts will save millions of lives', Press Release WHO/35, 2002, Geneva, World Health Organization.

Pneumonia

Addo-yobo, E. 'Oral amoxicillin versus injectable penicillin for severe pneumonia in children aged 3 to 59 months: a randomized multi-centre equivalence study', *Lancet*, 2004, 364:1141–48.

Hadi, A. 'Management of acute respiratory infections by community health volunteers: experience of Bangladesh Rural Advancement Committee (BRAC)', *Bulletin of the World Health Organization*, 2003, 81:183–9.

Pakistan multi-centre Amoxicillin short course Therapy Pneumonia Study Group, 'Clinical efficacy of 3 days versus 5 days oral amoxicillin for treatment of childhood pneumonia: a multicentre double-blind trial', *Lancet*, 2002, 360:835–41.

Malaria

Acceng, J., Byarugaba, J. and Tumwine, J. 'Rectal artemether versus intravenous quinine for the treatment of cerebral malaria in children in Uganda', *BMJ*, 2005, 330:334–6.

Adam, I. et al. 'Artemether in the treatment of falciparum malaria during pregnancy in Eastern Sudan', *Transactions of the Royal Society of Tropical Medicine and Hygiene*, 2004, 98:509–513.

Amexo, M. et al. 'Malaria misdiagnosis effects on the poor and vulnerable', *Lancet*, 2004, 364:1896–8.

Deressa, W., Ali, A. and Enqusellassie, F. 'Self-treatment of malaria in rural communiies, Butajira, Southern Ethiopia', *Bulletin of the World Health Organization*, 2003, 81:261–7.

Diablo, D. et al. 'Child mortality in a West African population protected with insecticide-treated curtains for a period of up to 6 years', *Bulletin of the World Health Organization*, 2004, 82:85–91.

Hanson, K. et al. 'Cost-effectiveness of social marketing of insecticide-treated nets for malaria control in the United Republic of Tanzania', *Bulletin of the World Health Organization*, 2003, 81:269ff.

Hung le Q. et al. 'Control of malaria: a successful experience from Vietnam', *Bulletin of the World Health Organization*, 2002, 80:860ff.

Kroeger, A. et al. 'Combined field and laboratory evaluation of a long-term impregnated bednet, Permanet', *Transactions of the Royal Society of Tropical Medicine and Hygiene* 2004, 98:152–5.

Mueller, M. et al. 'Randomized controlled trial of a traditional preparation of Artemisia annua in the treatment of malaria', *Transactions of the Royal Society of Tropical Medicine and Hygiene*, 2004, 98:318–321.

Mwangi, T. et al. 'The effects of untreated bednets on malaria infection and morbidity on the Kenyan coast', *Transactions of the Royal Society of Tropical Medicine and Hygiene*, 2003, 97:369–72.

Reyburn, H. et al. 'Overdiagnosis of malaria in patients with severe febrile illness in Tanzania: a prospective study', *BMJ*, 2004, 329:1212–5.

Wendo, C. 'Uganda leads the way on Africa Malaria day', *Lancet*, 2002, 359:1494.

Rosen, J. and Breman, J. 'Malaria intermittent preventive treatment in infants, chemoprophylaxis and childhood vaccinations; rapid review', *Lancet*, 2004, 363:1386–8.

Shulman, C. and Dorman, E. 'Reducing childhood mortality in poor countries: importance and prevention of malaria in pregnancy', *Transactions of the Royal Society of Tropical Medicine and Hygiene*, 2003, 97:30–35.

Whitty, C., Ansah, E. and Reyburn, H. 'Treating severe malaria with rectal artemether may be as good as intravenous quinine', *BMJ* editorial, 2005, 330:317–8.

Chapter 12

Banajeh, S. 'Investing in traditional birth attendants may help reduce mortality in poor countries', *BMJ*, 2005, 330:478.

Bellagio Child Survival Study Group, 'Child survival 11: How many child deaths can we prevent this year?' *Lancet*, 2003, 362:65–71.

Brugha, R. and Pritze-Aliassime, S. 'Promoting safe motherhood through the private sector in middle and low income counties', *Bulletin of the World Health Organization*, 2003, 81:616–623.

Bulterys, M. et al. 'Role of traditional birth attendants in preventing perinatal transmission of HIV', *BMJ*, 2002, 324:222–5.

Costello, A., Osrin, D. and Manandhar, D. 'Reducing maternal and neonatal mortality in the poorest communities', *BMJ*, 2004, 329:1166–8.

Darmstadt, G., Lawn, J. and Costello, A. 'Advancing the state of the world's newborns', *Bulletin of the World Health Organization*, 2003, 81:224–6.

En Hamed, M., van Rheenen, P. and Brabin, B. 'The early effects of delayed cord clamping in term infants born to Libyan mothers', *Tropical Doctor*, 2004, 34:218–222.

Martinies, J. et al. 'Neonatal survival 4: a call for action', *Lancet*, 2005, 365:1189–97.

Mswia, R. et al. 'Community-based monitoring of safe motherhood in the United Republic of Tanzania', *Bulletin of the World Health Organization*, 2003 81:67–94.

Murakami, I. et al. 'Training of skilled birth attendants in Bangladesh', *Lancet*, 2003, 362:1940.

Osrin, D. et al. 'Cross-sectional, community-based study of care of newborn infants in Nepal', *BMJ*, 2002, 325:1063–6.

Osrin, D. et al. 'Implementing a community-based participatory intervention to improve essential newborn care in rural Nepal', *Transactions of the Royal Society of Tropical Medicine and Hygiene*, 2003, 97:18–21.

Potts, M. and Campbell, M. 'Three meetings and fewer funerals: misoprostol in post-partum haemorrhage', *Lancet*, 2004, 364:1110–11.

Safe Motherhood, 'Skilled attendants: the way forward', *Safe Motherhood*, 2002, Issue 29:1–5, Geneva, World Health Organization.

Shrimpton, R. 'Reducing childhood mortality in poor countries: preventing low birthweight and reduction of child mortality', *Transactions of the Royal Society of Tropical Medicine and Hygiene*, 2003, 97:39–42.

Shulman, C. and Dorman, E. 'Reducing childhood mortality in poor countries: importance and prevention of malaria in pregnancy', *Transactions of the Royal Society of Tropical Medicine and Hygiene*, 2003, 97:30–35.

Tsu, V. 'New and underused technologies to reduce maternal mortality', *Lancet*, 2004, 363:75–6.

WHO, 'Assessment of neonatal tetanus elimination in Rwanda', *Weekly Epidemiological Record*, 2004, 79:409–416, Geneva, World Health Organization.

WHO, 'Making Pregnancy Safer', Fact Sheet No. 276, 2004, Geneva, World Health Organization.

Wilder-Smith, A. 'Current status of "essential obstetric care" activities internationally: a literature review', *Tropical Doctor*, 2003, 33:135–8.

Chapter 13

Adler, M. 'Reproductive and sexual health of older women in developing countries', *BMJ*, 2003, 327:64–5.

Brown, H. 'Feature: marvellous microbicides', *Lancet*, 2004, 263:1042–3.

Freedman, L. et al. 'Transforming health systems to improve the lives of women and children', *Lancet*, 2005, 365:997–1000.

Grown, C., Gupta, G. and Pande, R. 'Taking action to improve women's health through gender equality and women's empowerment', *Lancet*, 2005, 365:541–3.

Mabey, D., Ndowa, F. and Maher, D. 'Control of sexually transmitted infections', *Tropical Doctor*, 2002, 32:49–53.

Philpott, A. 'Putting protection in female hands', *Health Exchange*, 2004, Feb: 15–18.

Shattock, R. and Solomon, S. 'Microbicides: aids to safer sex', *Lancet*, 2004, 263:1002–3.

Sleap, S. 'Sexual and reproductive health – activating an emergency response', *Health Exchange*, 2004, Feb:22–25.

Smith, G., Pell, J. and Dobbie, R. 'Inter-pregnancy interval and risk of preterm birth and neonatal death: retrospective cohort study', *BMJ*, 2003, 327:313–6.

Von Hertzen, H. et al. 'Low dose mifepristone and two regimens of levonorgestrel for emergency contraception: a WHO multicentre randomized trial', *Lancet*, 2002, 360:1803–10.

WHO, 'Nonoxynol-9 ineffective in preventing HIV infection', Press release WHO/55, 2002, Geneva, World Health Organization.

Chapter 14

Chen, X. et al. 'The DOTS strategy in China: results and lessons after 10 years', *Bulletin of the World Health Organization*, 2002, 80:430–36.

China Tuberculosis Control Collaboration, 'The effect of tuberculosis control in China', *Lancet*, 2004, 364:417–22.

Chintu, C. and Mwaba, P. 'Is there a role for chest radiography in identification of asymptomatic tuberculosis in HIV-infected people?' *Lancet*, 2003, 362:1516.

Elzinga, G., Raviglione, M. and Maher, D. 'Scale up: meeting targets in global tuberculosis control', *Lancet*, 2004, 363:814–19.

Frieden, T. et al. 'Tuberculosis: a seminar', *Lancet*, 2003, 362:887–99.

WHO, 'Drug resistant tuberculosis is ten times higher in Eastern Europe and Central Asia', Press release WHO/17, 2004, Geneva, World Health Organization.

Gajalakshmi, V. et al. 'Smoking and mortality from tuberculosis and other diseases in India: retrospective study of 43,000 adult male deaths and 35,000 controls', *Lancet*, 2003, 362:507–15.

Harper, M. et al. 'Identifying the determinants of tuberculosis control in resource-poor countries: insights from a qualitative study in the Gambia', *Transactions of the Royal Society of Tropical Medicine and Hygiene*, 2003, 97:506–510.

Islam, Md et al. 'Cost-effectiveness of community health workers in tuberculosis control in Bangladesh', *Bulletin of the World Health Organization*, 2002, 80:445–450.

Lonnroth, K. et al. 'Public-private mix for DOTS implementation: what makes it work?', *Bulletin of the World Health Organization*, 2004, 82:580–86.

Maher, D. et al. 'Treatment of tuberculosis: concordance is a key step', *BMJ*, 2003, 327:821–2.

Mwaungulu, F. et al. 'Cotrimoxazole prophylaxis reduces mortality in human immunodeficiency virus-positive tuberculosis patients in Karonga District Malawi', *Bulletin of the World Health Organization*, 2004, 82: 354–63.

Mwinga, A. 'Challenges and hope for the diagnosis of tuberculosis in infants and young children', *Lancet* editorial, 2005, 365:97–8.

Newell, J. 'The implications for TB control of the growth in numbers of private practitioners in developing countries', *Bulletin of the World Health Organization*, 2002, 80:836–7.

Pungrassami, P. and Chongsuvivatwong, V. 'Are health personnel the best choice for directly observed treatment in southern Thailand? A comparison of treatment outcomes among different types of observers', *Transactions of the Royal Society of Tropical Medicine and Hygiene*, 2002, 26:695–9.

Sterling, T., Lehmann, H. and Frieden, T. 'Impact of DOTS compared with DOTS-plus on multidrug resistant tuberculosis and tuberculosis deaths: decision analysis', *BMJ*, 2003, 326:574–7.

Chapter 15

A small selection:

Brugha, R. 'Antiretroviral treatment in developing countries: the peril of neglecting private providers', *BMJ*, 2003, 326:1382–4.

Chintu, C. et al. 'Cotrimoxazole as prophylaxis against opportunistic infections in HIV-infected Zambian children (CHAP): a double-blind randomized placebo-controlled trial', *Lancet*, 2004, 364:1865–71.

Gupta, J. et al. 'Scaling up treatment for HIV/AIDS: lessons learned from multidrug resistant tuberculosis', *Lancet*, 2004, 363:320–4.

Hogan, D. and Salomon, J. 'Prevention and treatment of human immunodeficiency virus/acquired immunodeficiency syndrome in resource-limited settings', *Bulletin of the World Health Organization*, 2005, 83:135–43.

Painter, T. et al. 'Women's reasons for not participating in follow-up visits before starting short course antiretroviral prophylaxis for prevention of mother to child transmission of HIV: qualitative interview study', *BMJ*, 2004, 329:543–6.

Shelton, J. et al. 'Partner reduction is crucial for balanced ABC approach to HIV prevention', *BMJ*, 2004, 328:891–4.

WHO, 'Recommendations of the interim policy on collaborative TB/HIV activities', *Weekly Epidemiological Record*, 2004, Jan. No.1/2:6–11.

Chapter 16

Bartram, J. et al. 'Millennium project: focusing on improved water and sanitation for health', *Lancet*, 2005, 365:810–12.

Curtis, V. and Cairncross, S. 'Water, sanitation and hygiene at Kyoto: hand washing and sanitation need to be marketed as if they were consumer products', *BMJ*, 2003, 327:3–4.

Emerson, P. et al. 'Role of flies and provision of latrines in trachoma control: cluster-randomized controlled trial', *Lancet*, 2004, 363:1093–8.

Khan, A. 'Chasing water uphill', *Developments*, 2003, fourth quarter: 30–31, London Department for International Development.

MacDonald, R. 'Providing the world with clean water', *BMJ*, 2003, 327:1416–7.

Meddings, D. et al. 'Cost effectiveness of a latrine revision programme in Kabul, Afghanistan', *Bulletin of the World Health Organization*, 2004, 82:281–9.

Nanan, D. et al. 'Evaluation of a water, sanitation and hygiene education intervention on diarrhoea in northern Pakistan', *Bulletin of the World Health Organization*, 2003, 81:160–65.

Rego, R., Moraes, L. and Dourado, I. 'Diarrhoea and garbage disposal in Salvador, Brazil', *Transactions of the Royal Society of Tropical Medicine and Hygiene*, 2005, 99:48–54.

Van Geen, A. et al. 'Community wells to mitigate the arsenic crisis in Bangladesh', *Bulletin of the World Health Organization*, 2003, 81:632–8.

WHO, Almost 2 billion more people need access to basic sanitation by 2015', Press release WHO/23, 2005, Geneva, World Health Organization.

WHO, 'Arsenic: mass poisoning on an unprecedented scale', Feature No. 206, 2002, Geneva, World Health Organization.

WHO, 'The atlas of children's environmental health and the environment', 2004, Geneva, World Health Organization.

WHO, 'WHO issues revised drinking water guidelines to help prevent water-related outbreaks and diseases', Press release WHO/67, 2004, Geneva, World Health Organization.

Chapter 17

Huntin. Y., Haauri, A. and Armstrong, G. 'Use of injections in health care settings worldwide: literature review and regional estimates', *BMJ*, 2003, 327:1075–8.

Peters, E. et al. 'Traditional healers' practices and the spread of HIV/AIDS in south eastern Nigeria', *Tropical Doctor*, 2004, 34:79–82.

Rishi, R. et al. 'Prescription audit: experience in Garhwal, Uttaranchal India', *Tropical Doctor*, 2003 33:76–9.

Ruxin, J. et al. 'Millennium Project: emerging consensus in HIV/AIDS, malaria, tuberculosis and access to essential medicines', *Lancet*, 2005, 365: 618–21.

Vandebroek, I. et al. 'Use of medicinal plants and pharmaceuticals by indigenous communities in the Bolivian Andes and Amazon', *Bulletin of the World Health Organization*, 2004, 82:243–250.

Wammanda, R., Ejembi, C. and Lorliam, T. 'Drug treatment costs: projected impact of using the integrated management of childhood illness', *Tropical Doctor*, 2003, 33:86–8.

WHO, 'Antimicrobial resistance', *Fact Sheet No. 194*, 2002, Geneva, World Health Organization.

WHO, 'Injection Safety', *Fact Sheet No. 231*, 2002, Geneva, World Health Organization.

WHO, 'Promoting rational use of medicines saves lives and money WHO experts say', Press release No. 9, 2004, Geneva, World Health Organization.

WHO, 'Substandard and counterfeit medicines', *Fact Sheet No. 275*, 2003, Geneva, World Health Organization.

Chapter 18
Included in further reading at end of chapter.

Chapter 19
WHO, 'How underpaid staff survive', Press release No. 7, 2002, Geneva, World Health Organization.

Bell, R., Ithindi, T. and Low, A. 'Improving equity in the provision of primary health care: lessons from decentralized planning and management in Namibia', *Bulletin of the World Health Organization*, 2002, 80:675–81.

Radford. R. and Laurance, L. 'How to mediate in a dispute', London, *People Management*, 2003, 25 Sept., 54–55.

Chapter 20
Palmer, N. et al. 'A new face for private practioners in developing countries: what implications for public health?', *Bulletin of the World Health Organization*, 2002, 80:292–7.

British Medical Journal, 'South Africa to regulate healers', *BMJ*, 2004, 329:758.

Mills, A. et al. 'What can be done about the private health sector in low-income countries?', *Bulletin of the World Health Organization*, 2002, 80:325–330.

Harris, A, et al. 'Traditional healers and their practices in Malawi', *Tropical Doctor*, 2002, 32:32–3.

Chapter 21
Burnham, G. et al. 'Discontinuation of cost sharing in Uganda', *Bulletin of the World Health Organization*, 2004, 82:187–95.

Gillespie, G. 'Buying health in Honduras', *Lancet* editorial, 2003, 364:1996–7.

Hope, R. 'Paying in potatoes; community based health insurance for the rural and informal sector', *Lancet*, 2003, 362:827–9.

Morris, S. 'Monetary incentives in primary healthcare: effects on use and coverage of preventive health care interventions in rural Honduras', *Lancet*, 2004, 364:2030–7.

Mugisha, F. et al. 'The two faces of enhancing utilization of health-care services: determinants of patient initiation and retention in rural Burkina Faso', *Bulletin of the World Health Organization*, 2004, 82:572–9.

Palmer, N. et al. 'Health financing to promote access in low income settings – how much do we know?', *Lancet*, 2004, 364:1365–70.

Preker, A. et al. 'Effectiveness of community health financing in meeting the cost of illness', *Bulletin of the World Health Organization*, 2002, 80:143–50.

Ridde, V. 'Fees-for service, cost recovery and equity in a district of Burkina Faso operating the Bamako initiative', *Bulletin of the World Health Organization*, 2003, 81:532–8.

Index

List of Commonly Used Abbreviations

ACT	Artemisinin combined therapy
AD	Auto-disable devices
AIDS	Acquired immune deficiency syndrome
ARF	At-risk factor
ARI	Acute respiratory infection
ART	Antiretroviral therapy – sometimes known as HAART
ARVs	Antiretrovirals
CAG	Community action group
CB	Capacity building
CBHC	Community based health care
CHD	Community Health Development
CHGN	Community Health Global Network
CHP	Community health programme
CHW	Community health worker
CTC	Community-based therapeutic care
DMO	District medical officer
DOT	Directly Observed Treatment
DOTS	Directly Observed Treatment – Short course
EDL	Essential drugs list
EPI	Expanded Programme on Immunization
FP	Family planning
FPP	Family planning provider
GAVI	Global Alliance for Vaccines and Immunisation
HFA	Health For All
HIV	Human immunodeficiency virus
HRC	Home-based record card
HW	Health worker
IMCI	Integrated Management of Childhood Illness
IUD	Intra-uterine device
KAP	Knowledge, attitude and practice
LLITN	Long-lasting insecticide-treated net
MDG	Millennium Development Goal
MDR-TB	Multi-drug resistant TB
M & E	Monitoring and evaluation
MPW	Multipurpose health worker
MRSA	Methicillin-resistant Staphylococcus aureus
MUAC	Mid-upper arm circumference
NGO	Non-governmental organisation
NID	National immunisation day
NTP	National tuberculosis programme
ORS	Oral rehydration salts/solution
ORT	Oral rehydration therapy
PA	Participatory appraisal
PLWHA	People living with HIV/AIDS
PHC	Primary health care
PPM	Planned preventive maintenance
PPP	Public-private partnership
RBM	Roll Back Malaria
RDF	Revolving drug fund
RUTF	Ready-to-use therapeutic food
STI	Sexually transmitted infection
TALC	Teaching Aids at Low Cost
TBA	Traditional birth attendant
TB	Tuberculosis
THP	Traditional health practitioner
TOT	Training of trainers
UNDP	United Nations Development Programme
UNICEF	United Nations Children's Fund
VCT	Voluntary (HIV) counselling and testing
VHC	Village health committee
VIP	Ventilated improved pit latrine
VVM	Vaccine vial monitor
WHO	World Health Organization